Biochemical Methods
in
Medical Genetics

Publication Number 1008

AMERICAN LECTURE SERIES®

A Monograph in

The BANNERSTONE DIVISION *of*
AMERICAN LECTURES IN LABORATORY MEDICINE

Edited by

Gilbert Dalldorf, M.D.

Oxford, Maryland

Biochemical Methods

——in——

Medical Genetics

By

SALLY KELLY, Ph.D., M.D.

Research Physician (Genetics)
Birth Defects Institute
New York State Department of Health
Albany, New York

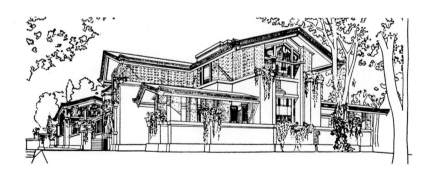

CHARLES C THOMAS • **PUBLISHER**
Springfield • *Illinois* • *U.S.A.*

Published and Distributed Throughout the World by

CHARLES C THOMAS ● PUBLISHER

Bannerstone House

301-327 East Lawrence Avenue, Springfield, Illinois, U.S.A.

© *1977, by* CHARLES C THOMAS ● PUBLISHER

ISBN 0-398-03630-6

Library of Congress Catalog Card Number: 76-54363

With THOMAS BOOKS *careful attention is given to all details of
manufacturing and design. It is the Publisher's desire to present books that
are satisfactory as to their physical qualities and artistic possibilities and
appropriate for their particular use.* THOMAS BOOKS *will be true to those
laws of quality that assure a good name and good will.*

Printed in the United States of America
R-1

Library of Congress Cataloging in Publication Data

Kelly, Sally.
  Biochemical methods in medical genetics.

  (American lecture series ; publication no. 1008)
  Includes index.
  1. Metabolism, Inborn errors of--Diagnosis.
2. Diagnosis, Laboratory. 3. Medical genetics--
Technique. I. Title. [DNLM: 1. Metabolism, Inborn errors--Diagnosis--Laboratory manuals. 2. Mass
screening. 3. Genetics, Biochemical--Laboratory
manuals. WD205 K29b]
  RC627.8.K44   616'.042'028   76-54363
  ISBN 0-398-03630-6

FOREWORD

Medicine is finding many new opportunities in the expanding field of heritable diseases where the combined attention of biochemists and physicians has yielded revolutionary advances. Doctor Kelly, who was highly competent in biochemistry before undertaking her medical studies, ideally expresses the advantages of this broad approach.

Her book includes those assays she has found useful in her direction of the biochemical laboratory of the Birth Defects Institute, New York State Department of Health. The value and reliability of the methods have been established by Doctor Kelly both in the study of patients and in the laboratory.

The compilation is also a step toward the standardization of laboratory techniques, a desirable sequel to the development of a diagnostic methodology. In this respect the work perpetuates the character of Wadsworth's *Standard Methods,* for many years the model in the public health laboratory field.

The book is highly recommended for its completeness and its trustworthiness.

Gilbert Dalldorf, M.D.

---

*Wadsworth, Augustus B.: *Standard Methods of the Division of Laboratories and Research of the New York State Department of Health,* 3rd ed. Baltimore, Williams & Wilkins Company, 1947.

PREFACE

THE modern observer of heritable diseases faces unfamiliar territory, as the fresh breeze of genetics clears horizons and brightens the dark corners of medicine. Like other taxonomists, he gains confidence by thumbing his manual, relating the unknown to familiar species. May this slim handbook be such a tool!

The manual contains the procedures we use in providing physicians with laboratory data needed for the diagnosis, treatment, and control of heritable metabolic disease. Included are the diseases or groups of diseases in which the biochemical abnormalities are either pathognomonic or clearly associated; excluded are those in which the biochemical lesions are poorly defined, nonspecifically expressed or inaccessible. The procedures have been selected empirically, organized according to the metabolic pathway or structural protein affected, and the emphasis placed on assays which provide the biochemical facts necessary for the recognition of disease.

I hope that presentation of the details will encourage laboratory technicians to add to their armamentarium of diagnostic tests, that the brief clinical facts will alert medical workers to the laboratory's diagnostic potential, and that the compilation will serve as a sourcebook of methods for investigators who study other facets of biochemical medical genetics.

Many have helped me: Dr. Victor Tompkins, who introduced medical genetics into the concerns of the New York State Department of Health, invited me to contribute and directed me to the field; Dr. Ian Porter continued the leadership and gave me time to undertake the task; the editor encouraged its fruition by many years of friendly support. I also thank my laboratory staff for initiative and competence in providing the details, especially Lucille Desjardins, Edward Leikhim, Lewis Schedlbauer,

Rani Bakhru-Kishore, Alice Dagle, and James Seeger; Constance Christo for patiently typing the manuscript through many revisions; Dr. Marilyn Cowger for critically reading the manuscript; and Philomena Sculco for the drawings.

S.K.

CONTENTS

ix

Biochemical Methods
in
Medical Genetics

Chapter 1

BASIC CONCEPTS OF BIOCHEMICAL MEDICAL GENETICS

WHAT ARE INHERITED METABOLIC DISEASES?

THE inborn errors and other heritable metabolic diseases excite both clinicians and biochemists. Indeed, their combined efforts developed the field to its present fertility. The two approaches help us to understand and control these diseases; the energies and skills of both disciplines bear jointly on the problems and find solutions together.

The clinician and biochemist cooperate intimately in managing these diseases. The clinician sees the disease — the biochemist identifies the underlying cause and means of control. Together they uncover the facade of overt disease in the patient and find a larger skeleton of biochemical disease hidden in the family.

GENES AND METABOLIC DISEASE

Most heritable metabolic diseases appear only in one generation of a family. They are caused by mutant genes which express themselves as disease only when present in pairs. Thus, the patient usually has two mutant genes, one from each parent. Geneticists refer to this kind of disease as "recessively inherited." If the patient inherits a pair of mutant genes, he is homozygous for the gene and usually has clinical signs; if he inherits the gene from one parent only, he is heterozygous for, or a carrier of, the mutant gene. He has a corresponding normal gene for the trait and, consequently, rarely has the clinical signs. Both patient and carrier, however, have biochemical disease expressed in varying degrees.

Diseases which appear as the expression of single mutant genes, i.e. in heterozygotes, are considered dominantly inherited, are not associated with specific metabolic defects, and thus are not referred to here, unless the clinical signs are similar to those of certain recessively inherited metabolic diseases.

Single mutant genes for recessively inherited diseases, not present as a pair, will cause disease under some circumstances, as, for example, those carried on the "female" or X-chromosome. Boys receive an X chromosome from their mothers; if it contains a mutant gene, the mutation is not balanced by a normal gene, because a boy's other sex chromosome is a Y chromosome received from his father, rather than another X chromosome. Only boys have the disease, and they receive the mutation only from their mothers. Such recessively-inherited diseases are considered X-linked.

The actions of mutant genes are at the core of inherited metabolic disease. The mutation triggers a chain of metabolic mistakes which lead to biochemical and, finally, clinical abnormalities.

The metabolic pathway through which the cells change nutrients into energy is often the target of mutant genes. The molecular changes proceed by steps, each step catalyzed by a specific enzyme, the production or regulation of which is governed by a gene. If the enzyme is absent, the step is blocked, and the metabolic pathway is interrupted. Immediate and precursor substrates accumulate, expected products do not form, abnormal derivatives appear, and alternative and less efficient pathways emerge. The primary result is deranged metabolism. Cells in the homozygous patient usually lack the enzyme entirely, so that the metabolic block is complete. The cells of carriers, however, form enough normal enzyme under normal gene direction to maintain the metabolic flow at relatively normal rates.

If, on the other hand, the mutation's target is cell structure, structural proteins, like hemoglobin, will be affected. The homozygous patient has none of the normal protein, e.g. hemoglobin A, but survives with a substitute and often less functional form. The heterozygote, however, forms both the substitute protein and enough normal protein for normal function.

How do genes regulate the production of structural and enzymic proteins? Molecular biologists theorize that genes direct the manufacture of both forms of cytoplasmic protein. Mutation interferes with this role by directing, instead, the manufacture of changed and nonfunctional molecules. The direct effect of the mutation is a change in the primary structure of the protein which forms structural protein, e.g. hemoglobin, or enzyme protein, i.e. a change in the kind or sequence of amino acids which form the protein's "backbone" of polypeptide chains. Ordinarily, the manufacture of polypeptide chains in the cytoplasmic organelles is directed by normal genes. This theory of gene action is based on the Watson-Crick model of deoxyribonucleic acid (DNA), the major molecular component of nuclear chromatin, whereby a triplet of base pairs in the double-stranded helix functions as the gene, codes for an amino acid in the cytoplasm, and transfers the information by a messenger molecule of ribonucleic acid (RNA). The mechanism is clearly applicable to the manufacture of proteins like hemoglobin, whose structure is known, and is probably applicable to the enzymic proteins, whose primary structures are still mostly unknown.

NATURE OF "MARKERS"

The clinical expression of a mutant gene for a recessively inherited disease usually appears only in the homozygote. The biochemical expression, however, may also appear in other members of the family — the carriers — and is thus a truer indication of the mutant gene's distribution in a family than is disease.

The biochemist searches for clues to the gene among the metabolic products of the patient's or carrier's cells, tissues, and body fluids. If biochemical abnormalities appear consistently in association with clinical signs, we accept them as a "marker" of the disease and, since the disease is caused by a mutation, a marker of the mutant gene.

The way or ways a mutant gene manifests itself to us is considered its phenotype. Thus, there are both clinical and biochemical phenotypes of the mutant genes for heritable metabolic diseases. Homozygous persons usually express both phenotypes. The heterozygous person usually expresses only the biochemical phenotype in a mild form. Conversely, the degree of expression is useful in predicting genotypes. When the expression is complete or severe, one predicts a homozygous genotype; if mild, one predicts the heterozygous state. If absent, the family member may be homozygous for the normal gene.

"Markers" reflect the metabolic systems affected by the mutant gene. Fat storage is involved in Tay-Sachs disease, for example, carbohydrate degradation in galactosemia, and energy transfer in the red cell enzyme deficiency diseases. The particular process and step affected are characteristic of the individual gene and disease. The crux of the biochemist's problem is to identify the metabolic pathway involved and the step affected.

The biochemist chooses a laboratory test or battery of tests to expose the particular marker. He employs specific chemical or histochemical procedures for the suspected metabolite, measures enzyme function, or deciphers structure.

These tests implicate the metabolic system involved and may even identify the exact site of the biochemical error.

One also chooses the biological sample carefully, as gene-induced changes (and markers) are often found only at specific anatomic sites. Fortunately, many sites are accessible and pose no sampling problem. The body fluids and formed elements of the blood, for example, are obtained easily and contain a great many markers. Other sites are equally accessible, such as nail scrapings and hair bulbs, but contain only few or single markers. Fibroblasts, muscle, liver, and amniotic cells, on the other hand, are less accessible and samples must be obtained surgically. In certain tissues, furthermore, the markers are so weak that cells must be cultured before analysis, or, if lymphocytes, artificially stimulated to divide.

The structural proteins, the hemoglobins and myoglobins, for example, are reliable indicators of mutation because their formation and deviation from normal can be traced back to a single change in the DNA molecule. Indeed, the synthesis of the various polypeptide chains of the hemoglobins was the model for the current molecular theory of gene action! Furthermore, other phenotypic expressions of the mutant gene — a particular syndrome or constellation of clinical signs; clear-cut pedigree pattern including usually dominant inheritance of the marker itself; qualitative, "all-or-none" evidence for the cellular protein involved, based on demonstration of protein mass or its absence — are consistently associated with abnormal structural protein.

Abnormality in enzyme protein, on the other hand, is a somewhat less reliable marker of mutation. The primary structures are for the most part unknown; therefore, changes are not directly traceable to mutational events. That the mutation results in a structural change in the immediate gene product is part of current molecular genetic theory. The uncertainty lies in where the errors are in the polypeptide chains. The association of enzymic protein markers with syndromes, pedigree patterns, etc., however, is consistent, like that of the structural protein markers. The test data, on the other hand, are valuable chiefly for their quantitative, rather than qualitative, feature. The quantitative data often consist of measures of enzyme activity. The enzyme proteins, furthermore, are more subject to variation and are found in a greater variety of anatomic sites than the structural proteins. Thus they are more variable markers of mutations.

The products of deranged metabolism which appear in response to the metabolic block form another group of markers — unused substrate, intermediary metabolites, storage products, and abnormal derivatives. They accompany the enzyme protein marker and, like the enzymes, are found in both cells and body fluids. Although their appearance is secondary to that of the enzyme protein markers and thus are less closely related to the mutation itself, they are useful when the defect is unknown, is detectable only in less accessible tissue or is more difficult to demonstrate.

These markers are subject to greater variability than the structural or enzymic proteins: Their molecular structures are byproducts of the metabolic block rather than abnormalities deriving from a gene-directed amino acid substitution. They are nonspecific in that, as the product of deranged metabolism, they may arise by one of several metabolic routes, none of which is necessarily the result of a mutation. Since several synthetic and regulatory steps, furthermore, may intervene between the mutation and the appearance of the marker, nongenic influences may interfere with the mutant gene's expression.

Other dissimilarities to the structural or enzymic protein markers are their association with variable clinical signs and other nongenic diseases. The biochemical pedigrees of families traced by this kind of marker are often incomplete, as the marker usually appears only in the homozygous patient. The data, furthermore, are primarily quantitative and can be interpreted variably. Galactosuria, for example, occurs in several diseases and conditions to varying degrees, and from several causes; it is a less certain marker of the mutant gene for galactosemia than is absence of the specific transferase protein.

HOW "MARKERS" ARE DETECTED

The biochemist searches for markers among the products of cells, the formation of which is governed, directly or indirectly, by gene action. He recognizes the molecular changes mutant genes cause in structural protein by comparing the properties of the mutant protein with those of normal structural protein. The marker may have electrophoretic mobility, for example, or solubility or refraction properties which differ from those of the normal protein if the mutation results in the substitution of an amino acid with a change in net electric charge.

He recognizes the effects of mutant genes on enzymic protein through changes in kinetic rather than physical-chemical properties of enzymes. The marker is usually less or no activity. Factors which affect activity — substrate specificity and sensitivity, and pH optima or heat stability — are also useful markers, especially when searching for variant *forms* of disease. The discovery of isozymes or multiple forms of enzymes by electrophoresis reveals that enzyme protein, like structural protein, may be structurally heterogeneous. We infer, further, that the synthesis of enzyme protein, like that of structural protein, involves gene-directed changes in molecular structure.

The biochemist detects markers comprised of substrates, intermediates, and storage products by a variety of chemical or physical procedures, chosen either to demonstrate their presence or absence or to measure quantity by chromatography, colorimetry, turbidity, solubility, microbiological assay, or histochemistry.

APPLICATION OF "MARKERS"

Diagnosis

Biochemical "markers" are the physician's means of confirming clinical impressions. Markers are especially informative when the clinical and laboratory findings are variable or nonspecific, as in infants, in whom the clinical signs may be of short duration or not fully expressed, e.g. failure to thrive, hypotonia, etc., or when, in older children and adults, the clinical signs mimic those of diseases without biochemical markers, e.g. homocystinuria versus Marfan syndrome.

Markers have special diagnostic value in the patient whose pedigree is short, whose family history is inappropriate, or whose clinical signs are the disease's initial appearance in a family. Markers are hardly necessary for the diagnosis, on the other hand, if the pedigree is long and typical and the clinical signs unique, as in Duchenne-type muscular dystrophy.

Physicians can make minute distinctions between the disease in one patient and a similar one in another patient by searching for slight differences in the biochemical marker, i.e. revealing variant forms of a disease. The isozyme pattern of galactose-1-phosphate transferase activity, for example, distinguishes between the classical and Duarte variant form of galactosemia; in this particular genetic defect, the distinction is prognostic, one form being progressive and the other relatively benign. Patients with hemolytic anemias from deficiencies of glucose-6-phosphate dehydrogenase may have one of several kinds of mutation, discernible by kinetic studies of the enzyme. The fate of markers in complementation is yet another means of recognizing variants. The curing or noncuring of the metabolic defect in fibroblasts, especially those from patients with storage diseases, by hybridizing with fibroblasts from patients with different or similar defects, respectively, indicates the similarity to previously-diagnosed forms of the disease.

Treatment

The effects of treatment can be judged by changes in the biochemical markers. The success or failure of treatment may be reflected in the amount of marker remaining. The indirect markers of mutation, i.e. the substrate, storage product, and derivative markers like phenylalanine, glycogen, and the imidazoles, respectively, are best suited to the purpose. Since their appearance in cells and body fluids is variable and modifiable, the non-genic factors of diet and medication affect them. Structural proteins, on the other hand, play a small role and are relatively constant. Nor are the enzymic markers useful, other than in following the treatment of patients receiving allografts and enzyme replacement, as their levels also remain fairly constant.

Carrier Identification

Structural protein, which is certain evidence of the mutant gene's presence, is the chosen marker for detecting heterozygous or carrier states. Enzymic protein is more often a convenient marker, and its variable degree of expression makes it a useful clue to heterozygous phenotypes. The storage product markers, on the other hand, are seldom found in carriers, or appear only when forced by loading doses, fasts, culture techniques, or other manipulations.

Screening

Biochemical markers are frequently used in screening large populations for inherited metabolic disease. In this application, the marker may identify the patient before he comes to medical attention, and a tentative diagnosis may be made on the basis of a simple laboratory test. The marker is often an efficient means of case finding.

Markers selected for use in screening are often sensitive and practical, rather than specific. The substrate marker found in the serum, hyperphenylalaninemia, for example, is widely used in screening newborns for phenylketonuria (PKU), although deficiency of the liver enzyme, phenylalanine hydoxylase, is more specific. The structural and enzymic proteins are preferable markers, if appropriate, since they are less variable. In any event, the choice should be modified by adhering to the marker's physiologic timetable: Substrate, metabolite, and storage product markers, especially, may be age-related. Some require induction, others may be masked temporarily by extrinsic factors, and some are delayed manifestations of the mutation.

Application of markers in screening newborns has great value because the patient is usually identified while in a preclinical state — early enough to prevent irreversible damage by treatment.

Preclinical Disease

The structural, enzymic, and storage product markers help to identify the patient with preclinical disease, i.e. patients whose biochemical phenotype appears before the clinical phenotype. In addition (to finding him through a screening program), the marker usually locates this kind of patient among the younger siblings in an affected family. The chosen marker should be reliable, since the prognosis is dependent on the test result. Conversely, family members who are free of the marker can then be reassured with confidence.

Prenatal Diagnosis

Markers are used to predict fetal genotypes in families at high risk for certain heritable metabolic diseases. The attendant information usually applies to decisions concerning the pregnancy's future. In most instances when genotypes are predicted by ascertaining biochemical phenotypes *in utero*, the abortus or newborn phenotype reinforces the prediction. Infants whose *in utero* phenotypes suggest homozygosity for galactosemia and methylmalonic aciduria, furthermore, can be helped by treatment during the mother's pregnancy. Conversely, ascertainment of a normal prenatal phenotype is reassuring in families whose offspring are at high risk.

The prenatal samples, comprised of amniotic fluid and cells withdrawn from the uterine cavity (amniocentesis), are examined for markers by the same methods as postnatal samples. The variables that affect the appearance of markers in postnatal specimens apply to prenatal samples: The marker may or may not be present in the fetal cells, require manipulation for its demonstration, follow physiologic timetables, or appear late in the disease. The same restriction on the validity of markers in tissues from postnatal life applies to those from fetal life, i.e. their presence or absence in controls should be demonstrated before their contrary appearance in the patient's (fetus's) specimens is accepted as evidence of the mutation.

The structural proteins are not necessarily satisfactory markers of mutant genes in prenatal life: Some change from fetal to adult forms during gestation; others comprise integral parts of the fetal structures. The enzymic protein, metabolite, and storage product markers, however, are usually present in anatomic sites which can be sampled without harming the fetus. Enzyme protein, for example, forms in sufficient amount for marker tests during culture of fibroblast and/or epithelioid elements, and a few enzymes are present in amniotic fluid immediately after the tap. Marker data from the fluid, however, are less reliable than from cultured cells. Regardless of source, the fluctuating activity of enzymes during gestation requires that appropriate control data accompany attempts to interpret them as markers. The substrate, derivative, and storage product markers, in some instances, appear in accord with their status in postnatal specimens. Metachromasia, for example, a cytologic marker in mucopolysaccharide store diseases, is demonstrable in amnion cells, but mucopolysaccharide excess in amniotic fluid may not be.

SUMMARY

The once-immutable problems associated with inherited disease may now be approached through the use of biochemical markers. The markers in cells and body fluids play an important role in the diagnosis, treatment, prevention, and control of heritable metabolic disease. Marker studies also reveal the distribution of mutant genes in a family or population group. The data are helpful in genetic counseling and prenatal detection of disease in affected families. Ideally, the clinical signs can be prevented or ameliorated by early detection of the genetic marker, a goal underlying the rationale of newborn screening programs. Many variants of genetic disease, furthermore, have been revealed by the discovery of minute, precise, biochemical differences in individual patients with essentially similar clinical signs.

Success in searching for markers depends on recognizing the proper timing and anatomic site for their appearance in the course of the disease. The techniques of demonstration are relatively new, for the most part, and must be learned, practiced to develop competence, and adequately controlled. The satisfaction of knowing that a patient and his family are alive or healthier through the application of knowledge gained from a reliable laboratory test is a rich reward.

THE AMINOACIDOPATHIES

THE primary aminoacidopathies are a group of diverse diseases caused by mutant genes controlling the synthesis or function of enzymes which regulate protein and amino acid metabolism. The clinical signs are referable to the particular metabolic pathway involved; since they frequently overlap those of other kinds of defects, the diagnosis usually rests on the laboratory demonstration of a particular amino acid abnormality.

The basic metabolic lesion is usually a defect in enzymic protein, which sets off a chain of biochemical events leading to overt disease. Two common defects arising from mutation in enzymic protein are reduction in amount produced or failure of molecular fit, either of which reduces the cells' supply of functional enzyme. Normal cycles of protein and amino acid metabolism, consequently, are interrupted at the site regulated by the affected enzyme. Unused substrate accumulates in blood (aminoacidemia) and overflows into urine (aminoaciduria); the amino acids patterns, in most instances, are distinctive. They and/or demonstration of the enzyme defect itself are markers. (see Table I).

Enzyme defects have not been identified in some aminoacidopathies. In these instances, the marker consists of the amino acid pattern only.

The biochemical defects of the more common aminoacidopathies are described more fully in the sections referring to the specific disease.

Amino acid abnormalities are generally identified in the laboratory by examining the body fluids for one or more amino acids. One narrows the choice initially by performing a single test for several possible amino acid abnormalities, e.g. by chromatography or electrophoresis. Positive findings are confirmed with a definitive assay, e.g. by specific chemical or microbiologic methods for the probable amino acid involved.

When clinical findings are distinctive, or one particular

14

Table I

DISTINCTIVE SERUM AND URINARY AMINO ACID PATTERNS OF THE AMINOACIDOPATHIES

Pattern of Amino Acids in Excess

Disease	Blood	Urine	Clinical Signs	Mentality
Argininosuccinaciduria	—	Argininosuccinic acid	Seizures, ataxia, friable hair	Retarded
Citrullinemia	Citrulline	Citrulline	Seizures	Retarded
Cystathioninuria	—	Cystathionine	Anomalies, psychosis	Retarded
Cystinuria	—	Cystine, lysine, arginine, ornithine	Stones	Normal
Cystinosis	Cystine	Cystine, others	Rickets, stones	Retarded
Hartnup disease	Several	Aminoaciduria, especially neutrals	Intermittent attacks of ataxia, rash, psychosis	Normal or retarded
Histidinemia	Histidine	Histidine	Speech defects	Normal or retarded
Homocystinuria	Methionine	Homocystine	Dislocated lens, seizures, fine sparse hair	Normal or retarded
Hydroxyprolinemia	Hydroxyproline	Hydroxyproline	Small size, hyperactive	Normal or retarded

Disease	Blood	Urine	Clinical Signs	Mentality
Hyperglycinemia	Glycine and others	Glycine	Protein-induced vomiting, lethargy, coma in the neonate	Retarded
Hyperlysinemia	Lysine	Lysine, ornithine, γ-aminobutyric	Seizures, hypermobility	Retarded
Hyperprolinemia	Proline	Proline, hydroxyproline, glycine	Renal disease, anomalies	Normal or retarded
Hypophosphatasia	—	Phosphoethanolamine	Stillbirth, rickets, fractures	Normal
Maple syrup urine disease	Valine, leucine, isoleucine	Keto derivatives	Urine odor, seizures	Retarded
Phenylketonuria	Phenylalanine	Phenylketones	Slow development	Retarded
Tyrosinemia	Tyrosine	Tyrosine, phenylalanine derivatives	Failure to thrive, hepatomegaly	Retarded

aminoacidopathy is being sought, as in newborn screening programs, the specific chemical or microbiological assay for the amino acid in question is performed directly, without preliminary chromatography or electrophoresis.

SCREENING BY ONE-DIMENSIONAL PAPER CHROMATOGRAPHY

Principle

One can discern several amino acid abnormalities and examine several samples simultaneously by chromatographing the body fluids in one dimension on paper. One learns the normal pattern easily and recognizes the abnormality readily (Figure 1).

The amino acids applied to absorbent paper separate when washed with organic solvents, according to their individual solubilities. A convenient solvent system for separating over a dozen amino acids contains butanol, acetic acid, and water. Ninhydrin and isatin stain the amino and imino acids blue, purple, or red. The position and color identifies the amino acid when compared with control chromatographs. The basic amino acids are less soluble in the system, travel slowly during development, and appear near the application point of the sample (origin); neutral, acidic, and aromatic (ring-structured) amino acids remain in solution longer and appear nearer the top of the paper (solvent front). Concentrations are estimated by matching the spot densities with those of standard amino acid solutions chromatographed simultaneously. Excretion rates per day and concentrations per unit volume are calculated from excretion volumes and creatinine concentrations, respectively. Amino acids with unique structures or similar solubilities can be distinguished by overstaining the ninhydrin-stained spots with specific dyes (see Table II).

Procedure

1. Saturate a PKU filter paper card, i.e. fill the circle on both sides with whole blood (venepuncture or finger-prick) from a clean, disinfected, dry surface, without contaminating spots

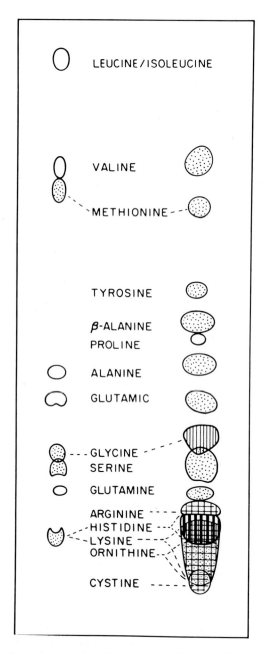

Figure 1. One-dimensional paper chromatographic separation of amino acids in serum (left) and urine (right), likely to be excessive in the aminoacidopathies. Amino acids requiring overstaining (citrulline, hydroxyproline) are not shown. Sheet developed overnight in butanol:acetic acid:water, 12:3:5, and stained with ninhydrin-isatin.

Table II

DIFFERENTIAL STAINS FOR THE IDENTIFICATION OF AMINO ACIDS IN
BLOOD, SERUM OR URINE SEPARATED BY ONE-DIMENSIONAL PAPER
CHROMATOGRAPHY IN BUTANOL-ACETIC ACID-WATER SOLVENT AND
STAINED WITH NINHYDRIN-ISATIN

Stained Amino Acid Spot	*Amino Acid Identified*	*Stain*
Cystine-Cystathionine	Cystine	Pauly (neg)
	Cystine	Nitroprusside
Histidine-Lysine	Histidine	Pauly
Arginine	Arginine	Sakaguchi
Glutamine-Homocystine	Homocystine	Nitroprusside
Citrulline-Serine	Citrulline	Ehrlich
Hydroxyproline	Hydroxyproline	Ehrlich
Glutamic-Threonine-Homocitrulline	Homocitrulline	Ehrlich
Tryptophane-β Aminoisobutryic	Tryptophane	Ehrlich

with saliva or perspiration. Air-dry for at least an hour. Precipitate hemoglobin and minimize diffusion by autoclaving blood spots for three minutes with 15 lbs pressure at 250°F. Cards saturated with serum or plasma samples need not be autoclaved.

2. Prepare catch urine samples and twenty-four-hour collections as follows: Estimate concentration of creatinine in 1 ml aliquot (p. 25). Lyophilize 2 ml aliquot until dry (approximately one hour). Store at -20°C. Reconstitute on the day of test with demineralized water (2 ml or less), so that 10 μl of sample contain 15 μg of creatinine, using formula below:

$$ml = \frac{\textit{creatinine concentration (mg/100 ml)} \times 2}{150}$$

3. Wearing clean, disposable plastic gloves, identify samples in

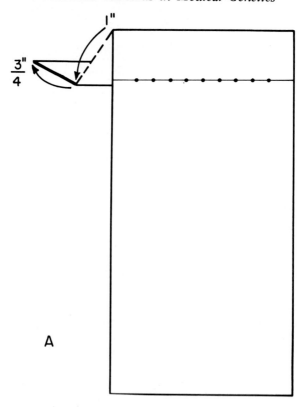

Figure 2. Preparation of sheet and tank for one-dimensional paper chromatography. (A) Folding and marking sheet for application of samples.

pencil at respective origins on chromatography sheet.
4. Punch 1/4-inch discs of the dried blood samples from PKU cards, matching holes at the origin end of the chromatography sheet. Insert discs into the labelled origin holes with forceps, wearing plastic gloves. When all holes are filled, press discs into position by holding a plastic ruler against them and rubbing briskly with the forceps' handle.
5. Pipette 10 μl reconstituted urine samples at the notch marks on chromatography sheet. Air-dry.
6. Pipette 10 μl standard amino acid solutions in graded concentrations on a separate sheet. Air-dry.
7. In hood, equilibrate atmosphere in tank with 50 ml portions

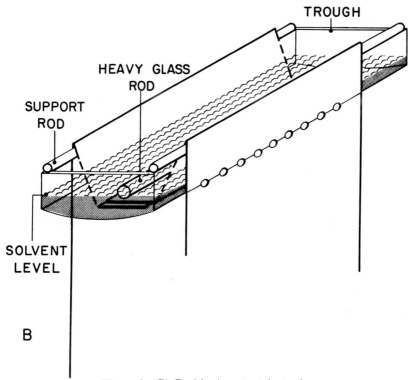

TROUGH

HEAVY GLASS
ROD

SUPPORT
ROD

SOLVENT
LEVEL

B

Figure 2. (B) Positioning sheet in tank.

of solvent in two 250 ml beakers on floor of tank for at least thirty minutes before use. Leave beakers in position throughout development.

8. Hang sheet carefully in chromatography tank (Slip glass rod under second fold and fasten with Teflon®-coated clips at both ends. Dip folded ends into trough.) (see Figure 2.)

9. Saturate folded ends with 90 to 100 ml of solvent. Anchor under surface with glass rod.

10. Seal lid with silicone grease and develop at room temperature (68 to 72°F) fifteen to sixteen hours or until the solvent front approaches end of sheet.

11. Dry on portable rack in hood sixty minutes and five minutes

in vented, spark-proof oven at 70°C.

12. Stain by passing chromatography sheets twice through ninhydrin-isatin stain in glass baking dish. Dry five minutes in hood and fifteen minutes in vented, spark-proof oven at 70°C.

13. Cut upper portions into longitudinal strips, leaving origin ends intact.

14. Match spots with those on strips containing standard amino acids. Identify by position and color. Estimate concentrations by matching spots with those on strips containing standard amino acids in graded concentrations. Record as mg per 100 ml.

15. Confirm presence of histidine by circling probable histidine spots with pencil and dipping lower portions of sheets into petri plate containing freshly made Pauly test reagent. Observe immediately for brick-red spot. If spot is disproportionately less intense than the ninhydrin-stained spot, an amino acid other than histidine is also present, e.g. lysine, ornithine, cystathionine, or cystine. These should be distinguished, if possible, by alternative methods. Estimate concentrations of histidine by matching Pauly reagent-stained spots with similarly stained spots on strips containing histidine and other standard amino acids in graded concentrations. Record in mg per 100 ml.

16. Confirm presence (or absence) of citrulline and hydroxyproline, by circling appropriate spots with pencil and dipping middle portions of sheets into petri plate containing freshly diluted Ehrlich's solution. Air-dry. Hydroxyproline appears pink in ten minutes, citrulline, in three hours. Homocitrulline appears orange in three hours. Estimate concentrations by matching appropriate Ehrlich reagent-stained spots with similarly stained spots on strips containing hydroxyproline, citrulline, and other standard amino acids in graded concentrations. Record in mg per 100 ml.

Calculations

1. Estimate the concentrations in blood, serum, or plasma sam-

ples directly from the standard amino acid strips and record as mg per 100 ml.

2. Estimate the concentrations of amino acids in catch samples of urine in mg/g Cr:

   Since the lyophilized sample was reconstituted to a volume containing 150 mg creatinine per 100 ml of sample,

$$\text{mg AA/g Cr} = \frac{\text{mg\% AA}}{150 \text{ mg\% Cr}} \times \frac{1000 \text{ mg}}{1 \text{ g}}$$

   or

   since $\dfrac{1000}{150} = 6.67$,

$$\text{mg AA/g Cr} = \text{mg\% AA} \times 6.67$$

3. Estimate the excretion rates of amino acids in mg/day: Since the lyophilized 2 ml sample was reconstituted to a volume (V_2) containing 150 mg creatinine per 100 ml of sample,

$$\text{mg}^{AA}/24 \text{ hrs} = \text{mg\% AA} \times \frac{V_2}{2} \times \frac{24 \text{ hr volume (ml)}}{100 \text{ ml}}$$

$$= \text{mg\% AA} \times V_2 \times 0.005 \times 24 \text{ hr volume (ml)}$$

Interpretation

Unusual amino acids and abnormal concentrations are readily discernible on the chromatograms. Concentrations in urine and excretion rates vary with age and other nongenetic factors; test values, therefore, should be compared with normal values acquired by similar methods, preferably the testing laboratory's own. (See Color Illustration 3.)

Reagents

1. *Schleicher and Schuell, No. 903 or Whatman 3 MM filter paper (PKU cards).*
2. *Shandon-Panglas Model 30 Chromatography Tank (8 × 12 × 22-inches).*
3. *Whatman 3 MM Chromatography Paper:* Wearing disposable plastic gloves to prevent "finger printing" of amino acids from the hands, trim sheets to 8 1/2 × 12 1/2-inches, draw a light pencil line 2 1/4-inches below the top of the narrow

dimension and dot at 2 cm intervals (3/4-inch) the position of nine origins, leaving 2 1/2-cm (7/8-inch) margins at either side. Fold the sheet twice between the top and the line, spaced so that the sheet can be punched and later anchored in the solvent trough. With a 1/4-inch punch, punch a hole at each pencilled dot for blood samples (see Figure 2).

4. *Butanol:Acetic Acid:Water Solvent:(12:3:5):* For three to four sheets, in a hood, mix 300 ml of the following volumes in an Erlenmeyer flask: 180 ml n-butanol, 45 ml glacial acetic acid, and 75 ml demineralized water.

5. *Ninhydrin-Isatin Stain:* For three to four sheets, in a hood, dissolve 0.5 g ninhydrin and 20 mg isatin in 200 ml acetone in an Erlenmeyer flask. Add 2 ml 2,6-lutidene.

6. *Sodium Nitrite Solution, 5%:* Dissolve 5 g sodium nitrite in 50 ml demineralized water and dilute to the mark in 100 ml volumetric flask.

7. *Sodium Carbonate Solution, 10%:* Dissolve 11.7 g sodium carbonate monohydrate ($Na_2CO_3 \cdot H_2O$) in 50 ml demineralized water and dilute to the mark in 100 ml volumetric flask. Store in plastic bottle.

8. *Sulfanilic Acid Solution, 10%:* Dissolve 900 mg sulfanilic acid in 9 ml concentrated HCl and 90 ml demineralized water, heating gently. Cool and dilute to the mark in a 100 ml volumetric flask.

9. *Pauly Reagent (fresh):* Immediately before use, combine 4 ml 10% sulfanilic acid solution and 4 ml 5% sodium nitrite in an Erlenmeyer flask. Mix well, cover, and let stand five minutes at 4°C. Add slowly 8 ml 10% sodium carbonate solution; mix well and pour into petri plate.

10. *Ehrlich Reagent:* Dissolve 10 g p-dimethylamine benzaldehyde in 50 ml concentrated HCl and dilute to the mark in a 100 ml volumetric flask. Store at room temperature. Immediately before use, dilute 5 ml with 25 ml acetone; mix and pour into petri plate.

11. *Artificial Urine:* Dissolve 3 g urea, 2.5 g sodium chloride, 0.15 g ammonium sulfate, 0.25 g potassium phosphate, and 0.1 g creatinine in 80 ml demineralized water and bring to volume in 100 ml volumetric flask.

12. *Amino Acid Stock Standard, 300 mg%:* Dissolve 600 mg or weights corrected for water of hydration or salt content of the appropriate amino acids in 150 ml N HCl, stirring with heat (50°C). Add 3 N HCl for solution, if necessary. Dilute to volume with artificial urine in 200 ml volumetric flasks. Dispense and store at -20°C in screw-capped tubes.

13. *Amino Acid Working Standards:* Make dilutions of the stock standard with 1 N HCl monthly, as indicated below:

Stock Standard Conc. (Mg%)	ml	Artificial Urine ml	Working Standard Volume (ml)	Conc. (mg%)
300	4	16	20	60
300	4	26	30	40
60	5	5	10	30
40	5	5	10	20
40	5	15	20	10
10	5	5	10	5
40	1	9	10	4
30	1	9	10	3
20	1	9	10	2

Dispense in 1 ml volumes and store at -20°C.

REFERENCES

Bradley, G., and Benson, S.: Examination of the urine. In Davidsohn, I., and Henry, J. (Eds.): *Todd-Sanford Clinical Diagnosis by Laboratory Methods,* 14th ed. Philadelphia, Saunders, 1969, pp. 31-32.

Efron, M. L., Young, D., Moser, H. W., and MacCready, R. A.: A simple chromatographic screening test for the detection of disorders of amino acid metabolism. *N Engl J Med, 270:*1378, 1964.

CREATININE IN URINE

Principle

Creatinine in urine is measured by a colorimetric method based on the tautomeric nature of the compound creatinine forms with picric acid. In the alkaline conditions of the Jaffe test, the dominant tautomers of the mixture are the red, unstable forms.

In a preparative step, creatine in the sample, if any, is dehydrated to creatinine.

Procedure

1. Dilute aliquots of catch urine sample 1:2, 1:10, and 1:20-fold with demineralized water to give volumes of 10 ml.
2. Add 4.0 ml picrate buffer to duplicate 1 ml aliquots of diluted samples, creatinine working standards, and demineralized water (blank) in respective 150 × 20 mm screw-cap tubes. Cap tubes and mix on Vortex.
3. Autoclave tubes thirty minutes at 120°C to dehydrate creatine to creatinine, especially the large amounts in urine from infants under two years of age.
4. Add 0.3 ml 2.5 N sodium hydroxide and let stand twenty minutes at room temperature. Add 15 ml demineralized water and mix on Vortex.
5. Measure optical density $(O.D.)_{520nm}$ of standards and urine sample in duplicate in the *one* dilution which matches the range of the standards.

Calculations

1. Plot standard curve of creatinine concentration versus optical density.
2. Estimate creatinine concentrations of urine dilutions from standard curve. Multiply by dilution factor and express as mg creatinine/100 ml urine.

Interpretation

The creatinine concentration is used as an arbitrary measure of the solute mass of urine when one of its components is measured, i.e. is the unit of urine mass.

Reagents

1. *Sodium Picrate Buffer, 1.17%, pH 2.0*: Dissolve 11.7 g picric acid in 900 ml demineralized water. Adjust to pH 2.0±0.05 with 2.5 N NaOH (about 15 ml). Bring to 1 liter volume.

Readjust pH after several hours. Store at 4°C.

2. *Sodium Hydroxide, 2.5N:* Add gradually 50 g sodium hydroxide pellets to 400 ml demineralized water. Stir until dissolved and bring to volume in 500 ml volumetric flask.
3. *Creatinine Stock Standard Solution, 100 mg/100 ml:* Dissolve 100 mg creatinine in 50 ml demineralized water and bring to volume in 100 ml volumetric flask.
4. *Creatinine Working Standard Solutions:* Dilute 1 ml aliquots of stock standard solution with 19.0 ml and 9 ml aliquots demineralized water to give working standards of 5 and 10 mg/100 ml, respectively. Dilute 1.5 ml stock standard solution with 8.5 ml demineralized water to give working standard of 15 mg/100 ml.

REFERENCES

Clark, L. C., Jr., and Thompson, H. L.: Determination of creatine and creatinine in urine. *Anal Chem, 21*:1218, 1949.

Hunter, Andrew: *Creatine and Creatinine.* New York, Longmans, Green, 1928, p. 26.

OTHER FORMS OF CHROMATOGRAPHY

Chromatography in one-dimensional forms other than on paper are applicable to a variety of tasks. Two-dimensional chromatograms or fingerprints, for example, are more discriminatory than one-dimensional patterns. They require more time and space, however, are not quantitative, and are not convenient for screening large numbers of samples. Now employed when more expensive, automated procedures are unavailable, they are most useful in the identification of aminoacidopathies in individual patients.

Chromatography on silica gel or synthetic polymer matrices is faster than on paper but more expensive. The greater preparation of the sample that they require, furthermore, makes them less popular as a screening method. When applied in two-dimensional chromatography, however, they provide a simple, rapid method for the identifcation of certain amino acids.

The finest separations and most precise estimates of quantity are achieved through automated chromatography on columns of ion exchange resin. Buffers pumped at high pressures elute the amino acids at different times, according to individual structures and properties. A graph records optical densities of the eluted amino acids after reaction with ninhydrin; the resulting peaks are analogous to the fingerprint on two-dimensional chromatograms. The separations and identifications are completed in hours rather than days. Speed, precision, and resolution are features of the procedure which have made it so valuable for the identification of aminoacidopathies and variant forms; the discovery of these aminoacidopathies may depend on relatively minor distinctions in excretory or serum amino acid pattern.

SCREENING BY BACTERIAL-INHIBITION ASSAYS

Principle

Abnormally high concentrations of certain amino acids can be detected in blood or serum through a series of microbiological assays for specific amino acids developed by Dr. Robert Guthrie (1966). For the most part, the assays depend on the principle that limiting the microorganism's supply of particular amino acid limits its growth; an antimetabolite specific for the amino acid is added to the growth medium to counteract the amount present in normal blood samples. Growth occurs, then, only when the sample contains excessive amounts of the amino acid.

In practice, the antimetabolite inhibits the germination of bacterial spores dispersed in agar, the surface of which supports samples of dried blood on discs of filter paper (see Table III). Bacterial growth encircles samples only if they contain excessive amounts of the amino acid which diffuses from the disc with sufficient speed to neutralize the antimetabolite. The diameter of the growth zone corresponds to the concentration of amino acid and, if compared with zones produced by known amounts of amino acid, is a measure of amino acid concentration in the sample.

The assays are sensitive to the levels of excess in homozygous

Table III

BACTERIAL-INHIBITION ASSAYS FOR THE AMINOACIDEMIAS*

Aminoacidemia	Bacillus subtilis BBL Spore No.	Spore Suspension/ 150 ml Agar	Inhibitor or Substrate	Molecular Weight	Composition of Substrate Molar Concentration	Inhibitor or Solution Gms/100 ml Water	Vol. (ml) Inhibitor or Substrate Solution/ 150 ml Agar
Phenylketonuria (Phenylalanine)	6633	1.0	β-2-Thienylalanine	171.0	5.9×10^{-3}	0.100	0.50
Maple syrup urine disease (Leucine)	6051	0.25	4-AZA-leucine	206	10^{-2}	0.206	0.90
Homocystinuria (Methionine)	6633	0.1	DL-Methionine DL-Sulfoximine	180.2	10^{-3}	0.018	0.17
Tyrosinemia	6051	0.3	D-Tyrosine	181.2	10^{-3}	0.018	0.50
Histidinemia	6633	0.1	1, 2, 4-Triazole-3-alanine	156.0	10^{-3}	0.016	0.45
Argininosuccinic aciduria	J_3	0.2	Arginosuccinic acid, Barium salt	425.6	10^{-1}	4.256	0.20

*Data from "Laboratory Screening for Congenital Defects," a conference and demonstration by Dr. Robert Guthrie, February 19, 1971, Buffalo, N.Y. Methods are in use by the N. Y. State Department of Health, Division of Laboratories and Research.

patients but not those in carriers.

The principle involved in the assay for red cell argininosuccinate lyase differs from the above, in that bacterial growth encircles only normal samples: They contain the lyase, which frees arginine from the substrate, thereby providing the bacterium dispersed in agar, an arginine-dependent strain, with an amino acid essential for growth. No growth zones encircle lyase-deficient samples.

Procedure

1. Clean, disinfect, let dry and prick surface of finger or heel with disposable lancet. Collect blood on PKU filter paper card (#903). Saturate card, i.e. collect until circles on under surface are filled also. Air-dry for at least an hour.
2. Suspend Baltimore Biologics PKU test agar base in 150 ml demineralized water, in amounts indicated on container.
3. Boil to dissolve and let simmer five minutes, or autoclave with flowing steam for ten minutes.
4. Add specific antimetabolite (see Table III).
5. Cool in water bath to 50 to 55°C and add spore suspension. Mix well. Pour into Baltimore Biologics plastic trays (10 1/2 × 7 1/2 × 3/4-inches) on level table.
6. Deflate bubbles by skimming agar surface with a small bunsen burner. Leave trays uncovered until gelled.
7. Place numbered Baltimore Biologics template under plastic tray, ready to receive samples.
8. Using 1/4-inch punch with a barrel, punch and position on agar surface blood-saturated filter paper discs and several Difco standards, guiding them into the template pattern with forceps, avoiding corners where agar layer is thin.
9. Cover, invert, and incubate plates for twelve to sixteen hours at 35 to 37°C. Plates can be stored inverted for up to twenty-four hours at 4°C before incubation, if necessary.
10. Examine for circular zones of turbidity, indicating bacterial growth (see Figure 3).
11. Measure diameters of growth zone (mm), compare with those of standands and estimate concentration of amino acid in mg per 100 ml blood.

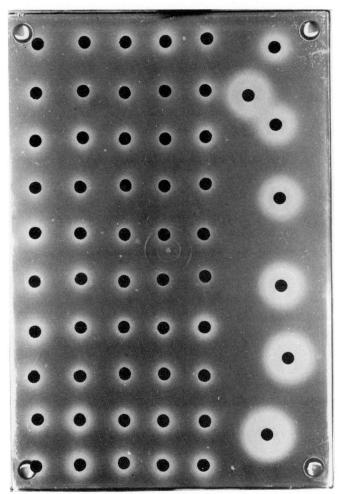

Figure 3. Bacterial-inhibition test showing bacterial growth zone around blood sample from boy with untreated phenylketonuria (lower left, isolated). Growth around samples from fifty normal newborns is minimal. Control samples (bottom row) contain from 2 to 20 mg phenylalanine per 100 ml. Plate from the New York State Department of Health's Division of Laboratories and Research PKU newborn screening laboratory.

Interpretation

Phenylalanine and leucine levels in normal serum are less than 4, methionine less than 2, and tyrosine less than 8 mg per 100 ml blood.

REFERENCES

Guthrie, R. and Susi, A.: A simple phenylalanine method for detecting phenylketonuria in large populations of newborn infants. *Pediatrics,* *32*:338-343, 1963.

Guthrie, R.: Personal communication, MSUD Test, Progress Report, Appendix 1, October, 1966.

Difco Supplementary Literature, Difco Laboratories, Detroit, Michigan: MSUD Test, November, 1968, p. 214.

CHEMICAL ASSAYS FOR INDIVIDUAL AMINO ACIDS

One chooses the chemical tests for a specific aminoacidopathy with the expectation of revealing excessive amounts of the amino acid in question or its derivatives. Taken into consideration are the particular disease suspected, its biochemical expressions, and the fluids or tissues in which they appear (see Table IV).

Derivatives, rather than the amino acid itself, are generally easier to test for since their mere presence is abnormal. The properties of derivatives are distinctive, furthermore, compared to those of amino acids. Nor need they be separated from mixtures before identification, as amino acids in biological fluids often must be. On the whole, finding the derivative(s) implies a greater depth of metabolic derangement. They are more pathognomonic, also, since they form in significant amounts only when the normal metabolic channel closes and an alternative pathway opens. In PKU, for example, the disease named for its amino acid derivatives, the derivatives appear only when blood levels of phenylalanine reach a concentration of about 15 mg per 100 ml or more. They seldom, if ever, appear in variant forms, e.g. hyperphenylalaninemia, in which blood levels are only slightly elevated.

Conversely, the presence of normal metabolites suggests the

Table IV

CHEMICAL TESTS FOR AMINO ACIDS AND DERIVATIVES IN THE AMINOACIDOPATHIES

Metabolite	Test	Disease	Sample
Cystine Homocystine	Nitroprusside Borohydride	Cystinuria Homocystinuria	Urine
Homocystine	Silver nitroprusside	Homocystinuria	Urine
Glycine	Chloramine T	The hyperglycinemias	Serum
Histidine	Cuprizone	Histidinemia	Urine
Tyrosine	1-Nitroso, 2-naphthol	Tyrosinemia	Urine
α-Keto acids	Dinitrophenylhydrazine	Maple syrup urine disease	Urine
Phenylketones	Ferric chloride	Phenylketonuria	Urine
Urocanic acid	Pauly reagent	Histidinemia	Urine Blood
Sulfite	Ferrocyanide-nitroprusside	Sulfite oxidase deficiency	Urine
Homogentisic Acid	Reducing properties	Alkaptonuria	Urine

integrity of the pathway. The demonstration of urocanic acid, for example, indicates that histidine deamination has occurred, the metabolic step blocked in histidinemia.

Details of particular chemical assays are given in the appropriate sections under the heading "Specific Aminoacidopathies."

ENZYME ASSAYS FOR THE AMINOACIDOPATHIES

Specific enzyme defects have been recognized in many of the aminoacidopathies. While they are more certain evidence of an aminoacidopathy than demonstration of excess amino acid substrate or derivative, the less direct measures of abnormality in body fluids are, for the most part, more practical. Demonstrating substrate excesses in blood or derivatives in urine are more expeditious ways of identifying homozygous patients than, for example, measuring enzyme in excised liver tissue.

Other deterrents to the routine use of enzyme assays are their technical difficulty, instability, or paucity of the proper tissue for sampling (see Table V). Microtechniques for white cells and culture of skin tissues, however, are making the definitive enzyme assays a more commonplace undertaking.

Details of particular enzyme assays are given in the appropriate sections under "Specific Aminoacidopathies."

PHENYLKETONURIA

PKU is the most common of the aminoacidemias causing mental retardation. Fortunately, its ravages can be prevented if recognized soon after birth. Children treated from early infancy with a low-phenylalanine diet have relatively normal intelligence; if treated only later in life, the brain damage cannot be reversed.

The gene governing production of the liver enzyme, phenylalanine hydroxylase, is at fault. Infants homozygous for the mutant gene form no hydroxylase, develop phenylalaninemia, and excrete phenylalanine derivatives. The cause of the retardation is not clear, however, beyond the inferences from studies suggesting that the high levels in blood and cerebrospinal fluid interfere with brain cell metabolism.

The disease is inherited in an autosomal recessive pattern: Both parents are obligate carriers; siblings may be affected, carriers, or normal.

Patients with classical PKU have phenylalaninemia of 20 mg per 100 ml or more. Newborns whose blood levels in the perinatal period, before ingesting much protein, are 6 mg per 100 ml or higher, are followed closely. If the level continues to rise and approaches that of classical PKU, a phenylalanine-restricted diet is begun. The treated infant is retested periodically to avoid extremes in the concentration of blood phenylalanine.

Phenylalanine levels may also be high in tyrosinemia of prematurity and nonphenylketonuric hyperphenylalaninemia; these diseases should be excluded before starting treatment for PKU. Tyrosine levels in classical PKU, for example, are extremely low in proportion to the phenylalanine, and the phenylalanine concentration in hyperphenylalaninemia is usually less than 15 mg

Table V

SAMPLING SITES FOR THE DEMONSTRATION OF ENZYME
DEFECTS IN THE AMINOACIDOPATHIES

Disease	*Enzyme Defect*	*Site(s)*
Albinism	Tyrosinase	Hair bulbs
Argininosuccinicaciduria	Argininosuccinic acid lyase	Red cells
Cystathioninuria	Cystathionase	Liver Leukocytes Fibroblasts
Histidinemia	Histidase	Nail scrapings
Homocystinuria	Cystathionine synthetase	Liver Leukocytes Fibroblasts
Ketotic hyperglycinemia	Propionyl-CoA carboxylase	Liver Leukocytes Fibroblasts
	Methylmalonyl-CoA mutase	Liver Fibroblasts
	Methylmalonyl-CoA racemase	Liver Fibroblasts
	5'-deoxyadenosyl cobalamin synthesis	Liver Fibroblasts
	Isovaleryl-CoA dehydrogenase	Leukocytes Fibroblasts
Maple syrup urine disease	Branched chain keto acid decarboxylase(s)	Liver Leukocytes Fibroblasts
Phenylketonuria	Phenylalanine hydroxylase	Liver
Tyrosinemia I	p-hydroxyphenylpyruvate hydroxylase?	Liver Kidney
Tyrosinemia II	Tyrosine aminotransferase	Liver

per 100 ml.

Carriers can be identified through phenylalanine tolerance tests or, in high risk families, through ratios of the concentrations of phenylalanine and tyrosine in blood after an overnight fast.

Phenylketones in the urine are pathognomonic of classical PKU. Demonstrating high levels of phenylalanine in blood samples, however, is a more efficient means of finding homozygous newborns, as the urinary derivatives may not appear until several weeks after birth or when phenylalaninemia reaches 15 mg per 100 ml or more.

Newborns worldwide are now screened for PKU by bacterial-inhibition assays (p. 28). Indeed, the technique was developed with treatment of PKU in mind. Spectrophotofluorometric methods have been devised for blood phenylalanine and tyrosine and, when automated, are appropriate for screening programs. Paper chromatography, while applicable to dried blood samples, is less sensitive, requiring phenylalanine concentrations of 8 mg per 100 ml or greater.

When screening newborns for PKU, take the blood sample a few days after normal feeding has begun. Cord blood is unsatisfactory, as it reflects maternal rather than infantile control of the phenylalanine level.

The screening test result is usually verified and the treatment monitored biochemically by spectrophotofluorometric or column chromatographic methods, both of which are more precise means of estimating blood phenylalanine concentrations than the bacterial-inhibition assays.

Phenylalanine derivatives in urine are demonstrable by Phenistix® or the ferric chloride text, (p. 36), when serum concentrations of phenylalanine are over 15 mg per 100 ml.

FERRIC CHLORIDE TEST

Principle

Ferric ions form a green complex with the phenol groups of urinary phenylalanine and its ketone derivatives, phenylpyruvic acid, p-hydroxyphenylpyruvic acid, and o-hydroxyphenylpyruvic acid.

Procedure

1. Combine 1 drop of the urine sample with 1 drop of ferric chloride reagent in a 75 × 12-mm test tube. Mix by shaking and observe color immediately.
2. Note color change, if any, until color is stable.

Interpretation

The color changes with ferric chloride reagent are variable and best interpreted in combination with Phenistix color (see Table VI). Normal urine remains yellow. Samples containing the phenylketones change briefly to a green or blue-green color and fade gradually to hues of grey, yellow, or red.

Reagents

1. *Ferric Chloride Solution, 0.6 N:* Dissolve 16.2 g $FeCl_3 \cdot 6 H_2O$ in demineralized water and bring to volume in a 100 ml volumetric flask.

REFERENCE

Hsia, David Y.-Y., and Tohru, Inouye: *Inborn Errors of Metabolism, Part 2,* Chicago, Year Bk Med, 1966.

SERUM TYROSINE

Principle

The fluorescent complex tyrosine forms with 1-nitroso-2-naphthol in the presence of nitric acid and sodium nitrite is a sensitive measure of tyrosine levels in serum and, in a ratio with phenylalanine, is used to discriminate among phenotypes of PKU.

Procedure

1. Add 0.3 ml 0.6 N trichloroacetic acid (TCA) to 0.3 ml sample of serum after an overnight fast, mix thoroughly, and let stand ten minutes.
2. Centrifuge at 3000 R.P.M. ten minutes, save supernatant fluid,

Table VI

URINARY FERRIC CHLORIDE AND PHENISTIX REACTIONS

Condition	Metabolite tested	ferric chloride	Phenistix
Phenylketonuria	Phenylpyruvic acid	Green or blue-green, maximum 1 minute, fading slowly to grey-green or yellow in minutes	Grey-green or blue-green, max. 1 minute, fades slowly
	p-hydroxyphenylpyruvic acid	Blue-green	Green, fading to grey to blue few seconds
	o-hydroxyphenylpyruvic acid	Initial d-brown, turns green or blue, fades to mauve	Green, maximum 1 minute
	o-hydroxyphenylacetic acid	Mauve	Very pale mauve
Tyrosinemia	p-hydroxyphenylpyruvic acid	Green, fades rapidly	
Histidinemia	Imidazolepyruvic acid	Green or blue-green, develops slowly; does not fade	Grey-green or blue-green
	Urocanic acid	Green	
Oasthouse disease	α-ketobutyric acid	Intense purple, fading to red-brown in 1-2 seconds	Faint brown-purple

Condition	Substance		
Maple syrup urine disease	Branched chain keto acids	Green, stable. Grey with green tinge	No change
Alkaptonuria	Homogentisic acid	Transient blue or green Brown with stronger solution	No change Brown with stronger solution
Pyridoxine disorders	Xanthurenic acid	Deep green, later brown	No change
Tumors	Melanin	Grey ppt, turning black	
Acidosis (diabetes, organic acid defects)	Acetoacetic acid	Red-brown Cherry red	Red to purple or No change
Increase in direct bilirubin (hepatitis)	Bilirubin	Blue-green (stable)	
Others	3-hydroxyanthranilic acid	Immediate deep brown	Immediate yellow, turns green 1 minute, later brown
	Vanillic acid, 4-amino-5-imidazole carboxamide, and 3-hydroxyanthranilic acid	Deep brown	Brown
Drugs or poisons	Several	Red or purple	
Normal urine	Normal	No reaction; brown or milky white ppt.	No change, grey-green, purple

and recentrifuge to clarify.
3. Prepare reagent mixture immediately before use. (Stable thirty minutes).
4. Add 0.020 ml clarified supernatant fluid or working standards to 0.5 ml reagent mixture in 10 ml tubes. (Assay in triplicate.) Mix.
5. Place all tubes in a boiling water bath for five minutes.
6. Remove tubes from bath, add 3.0 ml demineralized water, and mix.
7. Transfer to fluorometer cuvettes. Read samples and standards against zero standard (blank), using primary filters 2-A and 47-B, secondary filter No. 16 (sharp cut, >535), and No. 10 aperture.

Calculations

Plot fluorescence (F units) of standards and blank against concentration. Estimate concentration of tyrosine from the standard curve, multiply by 2, and express as mg/100 ml serum.

Interpretation

Tyrosine levels in serum from normal persons and in carriers of PKU range from about 1 to 2.3 mg per 100 ml serum and are lower in patients with PKU.

Reagents

1. *Nitric Acid, 0.3 N*: Carefully add 2 ml concentrated nitric acid to approximately 50 ml demineralized water in a 100 ml volumetric flask. Bring to volume with water.
2. *Sodium Nitrite, 1%*: Dissolve 100 mg $NaNO_2$ in 10 ml demineralized water.
3. *1-Nitroso-2-Naphthol, Alcoholic, 0.1%*: Dissolve 50 mg 1-nitroso-2-naphthol in 50 ml 95% ethanol.
4. *Reagent Mixture*: Just prior to use, mix 20 ml 0.3 N nitric acid, 100λ 1% sodium nitrite and 2 ml 1-nitroso-2-naphthol. (Stable for thirty minutes only.)
5. *TCA 0.6 N*: Dissolve 9.8 g TCA in about 80 ml water; dilute to

100 ml with demineralized water in a volumetric flask.
6. *TCA 0.3 N:* Dilute 50 ml 0.6 N TCA with demineralized water in a 100 ml volumetric flask.
7. *Tyrosine Stock Standard Solution, 2.5 mg%:* Sigma tyrosine standard solution (Stock No. 70-5) in 0.2 N TCA; store in the dark at 0-5°C. Before using, add 81.5 mg TCA per 5.0 ml to make TCA concentration 0.3 N.
8. *Tyrosine Working Standards:* Combine the following volumes of 2.5 mg% tyrosine stock standard solution:

Tyrosine (mg/100 ml)	Stock Standard (ml)	0.3 N TCA (ml)
0	0.0	0.5
0.5	0.2	0.8
1.0	0.4	0.6
1.5	0.6	0.4
2.0	0.8	0.2
2.5	0.5	0

The solutions are stable two months at 4°C.

REFERENCES

1. Phillips, R. E.: Tyrosine in serum. In *Manual of Fluorometric Clinical Procedures.* G. K. Turner Associates, Palo Alto, 1967.
2. Perry, T. L., Tischler, B., Hansen, S., and MacDougall, L.: A simple test for heterozygosity for phenylketonuria. *Clin Chim Acta, 15*:45, 1967.
3. Kelly, S., and Rose, F.: Detection of phenylketonuria carriers. *Public Health Reports, 84*:144, 1969.

HISTIDINEMIA

Histidinemia might well be called "an inborn error in search of clinical signs," as both healthy and affected persons have it. Indeed, recent data from newborn screening programs raise the question of the need for treatment, even if recognized in infancy. Clinical signs, when present, are variable. Affected children often are small, develop slowly, articulate poorly. Many have seizures and may be retarded. Some have frequent infections.

The need for and the effects of treatment are less certain than with other inborn errors. The frequency also is unknown, as few populations have been screened. Limited data, however, suggest an incidence at birth similar to that of biochemical PKU.

The high blood levels are usually associated with a deficiency of histidine α-deaminase, or histidase, an enzyme of liver and skin. Its absence blocks the normal metabolic path to urocanic acid, whereby histidine accumulates in the blood and overflows in the urine. The relation to clinical signs, however, is not clear.

The histidinuria is gross and must be distinguished by clinical or biochemical means from that in Hartnup disease, Lowe syndrome, carnosinemia, cerebromacular degeneration, generalized aminoaciduria, and treated galactosemia.

Excretion of urocanic acid, the metabolic product of normal histidine metabolism, is low.

The disease apparently follows an autosomal recessive pattern of inheritance. Obligate carriers are identifiable by one or more, but not necessarily all, of the following: low skin histidase, raised histidine tolerance curve, and high ratios of urinary histidine to intermediary metabolites. The values of these indices, furthermore, may overlap those in the low normal range.

Excessive blood or serum levels of histidine are readily detected by a bacterial-inhibition assay, (p. 28). Paper chromatographic indications may be confused with those from other basic aminoacidemias and should be confirmed by two-dimensional or thin layer chromatography, or other procedures. Histidine and its methyl derivatives in serum are separated and measured by gas or column chromatography.

The urinary excesses of histidinemia are demonstrable with ferric chloride or Phenistix through reaction of the imidazole derivatives, in a manner analogous to the ferric chloride reaction with derivatives of phenylalanine (p. 36). Quantitation is by colorimetric assay, p. 42, automatic method, or column chromatography.

Urocanic acid, the product of normal histidine metabolism, is detected by paper or thin-layer chromatography, (p. 45).

Histidase is demonstrable in liver tissue and the stratum corneum of cuticles, heel, and toes.

URINARY HISTIDINE

Principle

Copper forms a blue complex with bis-cyclohexanone oxaldihydrazone (cuprizone), a reaction which strong concentrations of histidine (20 mg per 100 ml urine or more) will prevent. The lack of complex formation is the basis of a method for measuring histidine in urine, exclusive of 1-methyl histidine, which does not react.

Procedure

1. If catch urine sample has been acidified, raise to pH 2 or higher with solid sodium carbonate.
2. Add 0.2 ml of standard solutions, sample or blank (normal urine), to 4.0 ml 4×10^{-5} M cupric sulfate reagent in 15×125-mm test tubes.
3. Add 0.25 ml demineralized water to blank. Add 0.25 ml cuprizone to other tubes at one-minute intervals. Mix immediately by inverting several times and transfer to cuvette.
4. Exactly six minutes after adding cuprizone to first tube, measure optical density of that tube at 610 mμ. Time measurements accurately, as color development is continuous. Measure O.D. of successive tubes at one-minute intervals.

Calculations

1. Plot standard curve of histidine concentrations versus O.D.
2. Estimate histidine concentration in sample from standard curve.
3. Express excretion rate as mg hist/24 hrs:

$$\frac{\text{mg}/100 \text{ ml} \times 24 \text{ hr vol}}{100}$$

4. Express concentration as mg hist/g creatinine:

$$\frac{\text{mg}/100 \text{ ml} \times 1000}{\text{mg creat}/100 \text{ ml}}$$

Interpretation

Excretion rates of histidine normally range up to 400 mg per day in active adults and to 300 mg per day in children. Catch samples from normal infants and children may contain up to 400 mg/g Cr; those from adults usually contain less than 300 mg/g Cr.

Reagents

1. *Cupric Sulfate Solution, 0.02 M*: Dissolve 249.7 mg $CuSO_4 \cdot 5$ H_2O in 35 ml demineralized water and dilute to volume in a 50 ml volumetric flask.
2. *Sodium Citrate, 1.0 M*: Dissolve 14.7 g $Na_3 C_6 H_5 O_7 \cdot 2 H_2O$ in 35 ml demineralized water and dilute to volume in a 50 ml volumetric flask.
3. *TRIS Buffer, 0.1 M*: Dissolve 6.06 g TRIS (hydroxymethyl) aminomethane in 400 ml demineralized water. Adjust to pH 7.4 with concentrated HCl and dilute to volume in a 500 ml volumetric flask.
4. *Cupric Sulfate Reagent, 4.0×10^{-5} M*: Combine 1.0 ml 0.02 M $CuSO_4$ solution, 3.12 ml 1.0 M sodium citrate solution and 500 ml 0.1 M TRIS (hydroxymethyl) aminomethane solution. Stable at room temperature for six months.
5. *Cuprizone Solution 0.1%*: Dissolve 30 mg bis-cyclohexanone oxaldihydrazone (cuprizone) in 15 ml ethanol and 15 ml demineralized water. Stable at room temperature for two months.
6. *Stock Standard in Urine 100 mg%*: Dissolve 10 mg histidine in 10 ml artificial urine.
7. *Standard Solutions:* Dilute the 100 mg% stock standard with artificial urine as follows:

Standard Solution (mg%)	Diluent (ml)	100 mg% Standard (ml)
5	4.75	0.25
10	4.50	0.5
20	4.00	1.0
30	3.50	1.5
40	3.00	2.0

Dispense in 0.3 ml quantities in small stoppered tubes and

freeze at -15°C until used.

REFERENCE

Gerber, M. G. and Gerber, D. A.: A simple screening test for histidinuria, *Pediatrics, 43*:40-43, 1969.

PAPER CHROMATOGRAPHY OF URINARY UROCANIC ACID

Principle

Urocanic acid, the deamination product of histidine, is present in normal urine and can be detected on the same chromatography sheet as the amino acids by specific staining. Patients with histidinemia form no urocanic acid, because they lack the enzyme which catalyzes the deamination.

Procedure

1. Spot on sheets of Whatman No. 1 chromatography paper, 20 1/2 × 8 1/2 inches, 30 µl aliquots of reconstituted, lyophilized sample and control (normal urine) and 10 µl aliquots of standard solutions. Prepare samples and sheets and chromatograph as described in "Paper Chromatography of Amino Acids," (p. 17).
2. Dip sheet in Pauly reagent and examine immediately.

Interpretation

Urocanic acid in control urine and standards appears as an orange-brown spot slightly below the solvent front.

Reagents

1. *Butanol-Acetic Acid-Water Solvent*: Refer to "Paper Chromatography of Amino Acids," (p. 24).
2. *Pauly Reagent*: Refer to "Paper Chromatography of Amino

Acids."

3. *Urocanic Acid Stock Standard Solution (100 mg%)*: Dissolve 100 mg urocanic acid in 100 ml artificial urine (refer to "Paper Chromatography of Amino Acids").

4. *Urocanic Acid Working Solutions*: Dilute the 100 mg% stock standard solution with artificial urine as follows:

Stock Standard (ml)	Diluent (ml)	Standard (mg%)
40	60	40
20	80	20
10	90	10
5	95	5

REFERENCES

Middleton, J. E.: Detection by paper chromatography of imidazoles in urine after histidine dosage. *J Clin Pathol, 18*:605, 1965.

Smith, Ivor (Ed.): *Chromatographic and Electrophoretic Techniques*, 3rd Ed. New York, Wiley, 1969, Vol. I, pp. 274-285.

TYROSINEMIA

Hereditary tyrosinemia (tyrosinemia I) is a fatal liver disease of infants and young children. The acute form was first recognized in French-Canadian newborns who failed to thrive, had fever, were irritable and lethargic, and died with signs of severe hepatic cirrhosis a few weeks after onset. A chronic form begins in infancy and runs its course through early childhood. Rickets and cirrhosis appear, and later changes are related to liver and renal tubular dysfunction. Patients may benefit from treatment with a diet restricted in phenylalanine and tyrosine.

Liver p-hydroxyphenylpyruvic acid oxidase is thought to be defective, as p-hydroxyphenylpyruvic acid, the enzyme's substrate, and the reduction product, p-hydroxyphenyllactic acid, are excreted. Tyrosine, the substrate's precursor, accumulates in the serum and "overflows" into the urine. Methionine and other amino acids of the serum increase as the liver fails, and distinction from hypermethioninemia is difficult, if not impossible. A generalized aminoaciduria results from the tubular defect.

The disease follows an autosomal recessive pattern of inheritance.

A few patients with other forms of hereditary tyrosinemia have been described. Patients with tyrosinemia II have normal liver and kidney function, but are retarded and may have skin lesions or other clinical findings. Hepatic cytosol tyrosine aminotransferase is probably the defective enzyme.

Physiological tyrosinemia develops in newborns receiving high protein formula without adequate vitamin C, when the liver enzyme systems are immature. Although resembling the hereditary tyrosinemias biochemically, the condition disappears in a few months, has no major sequelae, and improves with large doses of the vitamin.

Excessive tyrosine in serum or blood is detected by the bacterial-inhibition assay (p. 28), or quantitated by column chromatography.

Tyrosyluria is detected by the colorimetric method for the hydroxyl derivatives of tyrosine (p. 47), or quantitated by column chromatography.

URINARY TYROSINE BY NITROSONAPHTHOL

Principle

Tyrosine, tyramine, and other p-alkylated phenol derivatives in urine form soluble red complexes stoichiometrically with nitrosonaphthol in nitric acid.

Procedure

1. Combine, in four test tubes, 1 ml 2.63 N nitric acid, 1 drop 2.5% sodium nitrite and 10 drops nitrosonaphthol reagent.
2. Add immediately 3 drops standard solutions or urine sample. Mix by shaking.
3. Match color in sample five minutes later with those of standard solutions.

Interpretation

Normal urine contains 25 mg or less tyrosine or tyrosine derivatives per 100 ml.

Reagents

1. *Nitric Acid, 2.63 N:* Dilute 17 ml concentrated HNO_3 (15.4 N) to volume with demineralized water in a 100 ml volumetric flask. Store at room temperature.
2. *Sodium Nitrite, 2.5%:* Dissolve 2.5 gm $NaNO_2$ in 100 ml of demineralized water. Store at 4° C.
3. *1-Nitroso-2-Naphthol Reagent, 0.1%:* Dissolve 0.1 g 1-nitroso-2-naphthol in 100 ml of 95% ethanol. Store at 4° C.
4. *Tyrosine Standard Solutions:* Dissolve 100 mg tyrosine in demineralized water and bring to volume in a 100 ml volumetric flask (100 mg percent standard). Dilute 50 ml of the 100 mg% standard 1:1 with demineralized water (50 mg percent standard). Repeat with the 50 mg percent standard (25 percent standard). Store at 4° C.

REFERENCES

Perry, T. L.: Urinary screening tests in the prevention of mental deficiency, *Canad Med Assoc J, 95:*89, 1966.

Udenfriend, S., and Cooper, J. R.: The chemical estimation of tyrosine and tyramine, *J Biol Chem, 196:*227, 1952.

SULFITE OXIDASE DEFICIENCY

A deficiency in sulfite oxidation has been found in a single patient, a two and one-half-year-old retarded boy with severe neurological signs, including spasticity, hyperextension and decerebrate posturing, dislocated lenses, and frequent respiratory infections.

Tissues from the liver, brain, and kidneys obtained at autopsy were unable to oxidize sulfites to sulfates, a major step in the metabolism of organic sulfate. The patient's urine, furthermore, contained large volumes of sulfite and sulfite metabolites (sulfocysteine, thiosulfate) instead of inorganic sulfate.

The inheritance pattern is uncertain and the disease is apparently very rare.

No measures of the carrier state were demonstrated, although three older siblings had died soon after birth with central nervous system signs.

Excess sulfite is demonstrable by means of a spot test of freshly-voided urine (p. 49). Urinary sulfocysteine can be detected by thin-layer chromatography (p. 50). The enzyme defect appears in liver, brain, and kidney tissue.

URINARY SULFITES

Principle

Labile excretory products of sulfite oxidase deficiency, in the form of sulfites, are detectable in freshly voided urine by means of a color reaction with sodium nitroprusside. The color deepens on addition of zinc sulfate and ferrocyanide solution.

Procedure

1. To one drop of zinc sulfate solution on a spot plate add one drop 1 N potassium ferrocyanide. Rotate plate to mix.
2. Add one drop 1% sodium nitroprusside. Rotate plate to mix and disperse resulting white precipitate of zinc ferrocyanide.
3. Add one drop of fresh neutralized urine sample and observe color change.

Interpretation

Sulfite is present if precipitate turns red.

Reagents

1. *Sodium Nitroprusside, 1%*: Dissolve 0.1 g in 10 ml demineralized water on day of test.
2. *Potassium Ferrocyanide, 1 N*: Dissolve 4.2 g in 10 ml demineralized water; can be stored at 4°C for one month.

3 *Zinc Sulfate, Cold Saturated Solution:* Dissolve 9 g $ZnSO_4 \cdot 7$ H_2O in 10 ml demineralized water. Can be stored at 4°C for one month.

4. *Positive Sulfite Control:* Dissolve 10 mg Na_2SO_3 in 10 ml demineralized water on the day of test.

5. *Neutral Urine:* Adjust sample to pH 7 with either 0.1 N NaOH (4 g/l) or 0.1 N HCl (8 ml conc. HCl/1).

REFERENCES

Feigl, Fritz and Anger, Vinzenz: *Spot Tests in Inorganic Analysis,* 6th Ed. Amsterdam, Elsevier, 1972, pp. 444-445.

Kutter, D., and Humbel, R.: Screening for sulfite oxidase deficiency. *Clin Chim Acta,* 24:211, 1969.

THIN-LAYER CHROMATOGRAPHY OF S-SULFO-L-CYSTEINE

Principle

Patients with sulfite oxidase deficiency excrete S-sulfo-L-cysteine and excessive sulfite ions. Since S-sulfo-L-cysteine is more stable than sulfite, a test based on its demonstration is a more reliable means of identifying patients with the disease, especially if there is a delay between sampling and testing.

S-sulfo-L-cysteine is identified by position and color on two dimensional thin-layer cellulose chromatograms.

Procedure

1. Spot 5λ aliquot sample of urine on 20 × 10 cm Kodak 13255 Chromagram® sheet of cellulose.

2. Develop in sandwich chamber in phenol-water solvent, 75:25, until front rises 9.5 cm.

3. Dry sheet in 70°C vented oven for ten minutes.

4. Develop same distance in other dimension in acetone-acetic acid-water solvent, 70:10:20. Dry in 70°C oven ten minutes.

5. Spray with 0.25% ninhydrin in acetone; heat in 95°C oven

until spots appear (~15 minutes).

Interpretation

S-sulfo-L-cysteine in excess appears as a dense purple spot 1 cm from origin.

Reagent

1. *Phenol-Water Solvent, 75:25*: Measure 75 ml phenol (COR-ROSIVE) in a graduated cylinder, and pour into Erlenmeyer flask. Add 25 ml demineralized water. Mix carefully by gentle swirling.
2. *Acetone-Acetic Acid-Water Solvent, 70:10:20*: Combine and mix: 70 ml acetone, 10 ml acetic acid, and 20 ml demineralized water.
3. *Ninhydrin, 0.25%, in Acetone:* Dissolve 0.25 gm ninhydrin in 100 ml acetone. Mix by swirling.

REFERENCES

Kutter, D., and Humbel, R.: Screening for sulfite oxidase deficiency. *Clin Chim Acta, 24*:211, 1969.

Irreverre, F., Mudd, S. H., Heizer, W. D., and Laster, L.: Sulfite oxidase deficiency: Studies of a patient with mental retardation, dislocated ocular lenses, and abnormal urinary excretion of S-sulfo-L-cysteine, sulfite, and thiosulfate. *Biochem Med, 1*:187, 1967.

CYSTINURIA

Cystinuria, a rare cause of stone formation, usually comes to light in childhood or adolescence. Once recognized, the disease can often be controlled by hydration, alkalinization, or complexing with chelating agents. In some instances, stones, or the kidney itself, must be removed. Recently, treatment has included kidney transplantation, if the patient's kidneys fail.

The basic defect is apparently one of amino acid transport across membranes. In particular, the renal tubules fail to reabsorb cystine and the dibasic amino acids. Three types of cystinuria, and combinations thereof, have been recognized. Dr. Harry Harris and coworkers (1953, 1955) recognized early completely recessive and incompletely recessive forms, based on differences in the carriers' excretion patterns. Later, Dr. Leon Rosenberg (1966) delineated three forms, Type I, in which the carrier's excretion pattern was normal, i.e. completely recessive, and Types II and III which represent Harris' incompletely recessive group. These carriers are biochemically cystinuric, the Type II carriers more so than Type III. The homozygous stone formers of the three types and their combinations, so far, appear more or less alike.

The renal tubular defects in patients homozygous for Types I and II cystinuria are accompanied by absorption defects in intestinal epithelium, the clinical effects of which, apparently, are negligible.

Cystinuric patients and Types II and III carriers also excrete excesses of the dibasic amino acids — lysine, arginine, and ornithine. They excrete about twice as much lysine as cystine, only the latter of which crystallizes because of its low solubility and forms stones.

Biochemical cystinuria occurs also in Hartnup and Wilson's diseases and in Lowe syndrome. Found commonly among mental retardates, it may merely be an expression of the nonrecessive cystinuric carrier states in a population more frequently screened than the general population. Biochemical cystinuria in cystinosis, on the other hand, is a manifestation of systemic cystine excess.

The biochemical diagnosis of cystinuria is made by observing typical microscopic crystalluria, positive reaction of urine with nitroprusside (p. 52), or excessive urinary excretion rates of cystine, lysine, arginine, and ornithine. Therapeutic progress can also be followed biochemically through column chromatographic estimates of residual cystine and chelated cystine complexes.

The zygosity and genetic form in a family, furthermore, are postulated from biochemical data derived from excretion rates of the family's obligate carriers.

CYSTINE IN URINE

Principle

Nitroprusside reacts with the urinary disulfides, cystine, and homocystine, following their reduction to sulfhydryl compounds by cyanide.

Procedure

1. Add 4.8 ml aliquots of catch urine sample and control solution to 20 × 125 ml screw-capped test tubes containing 0.2 ml aliquots of saturated sodium carbonate solution.
2. Mix and test with pH paper. If sample is still acid (below pH 2.5), add 3 drops 10 N sodium hydroxide (40 g/100 ml).
3. In a hood or well-ventilated room add 2.0 ml sodium cyanide with bulb pipette.
4. Cap tubes, mix by shaking (in hood), and let stand ten minutes.
5. Add 5 drops fresh sodium nitroprusside solution, mix, and examine immediately.

Interpretation

Samples with excessive amounts of cystine (10 mg/100 ml or more) or homocystine (5 mg/100 ml or more) are purplish-red; normal samples remain yellow or orange. (See Color Illustration 4.)

Reagents

1. *Saturated Sodium Carbonate (Na₂CO₃):* Saturate demineralized water with Na_2CO_3. Store in a plastic bottle at room temperature.
2. *Sodium Cyanide, 5%:* In a hood, dissolve 0.50 g sodium cyanide in 10 ml demineralized water in screw-cap tube just before use.
3. *Sodium Nitroprusside, 5%:* Dissolve 0.25 g sodium nitroprusside in 5 ml demineralized water in screw-cap tube just before use.
4. *Positive Control:* Dispense catch urine sample from a known

cystinuric patient (or urine containing 10 mg cystine per 100 ml) in 5 ml amounts and store at -20°C until used.

REFERENCES

Harris, H. and Warren, F. L.: Quantitative studies on the urinary cystine in patients with cystive stone formation and their relatives. *Ann Eugenics,* *18*:125, 1953.

Harris, H., Mittwock, U., Robson, E. B., and Warren, F. L.: Phenotypes and genotypes in cystinuria. *Ann Hum Genet, 20*:57, 1955.

Levy, H. L., Shih, V. E., Madigan, P. M., Karolkewicz, V. and MacCready, R. A.: Results of a screening method for free amino acids in urine, *Clin Biochem, 1*:208, 1968.

Rosenberg, L. E.: Cystinuria: Genetic heterogeneity and allelism. *Science,* *154*:1341, 1966.

Rosenberg, L. E., Downing, S., Durant, J. L. and Segal, S.: Cystinuria: Biochemical evidence for three genetically distinct diseases. *J Clin Invest,* *45*:365, 1966.

NITROPRUSSIDE SPOT TEST FOR CYSTINE AND HOMOCYSTINE

Principle

The nitroprusside spot test is an adaptation of Brand's cyanide-nitroprusside test for cystine for small volumes.

Procedure (In Hood)

1. Saturate strips of Whatman No. 3 filter paper with urine samples and let dry.
2. Place 1/4-inch discs punched from dried samples in depressions of porcelain spot plate.
3. Wet discs with 1 drop 5% sodium cyanide. Cover plate with plastic sheet and let stand three to five minutes.
4. Wet discs with 1 drop 5% sodium nitroprusside. Observe immediately.

Interpretation

Pink or purple discs indicate cystinuria or homocystinuria.

Reagents

1. *Sodium Cyanide, 5%*: Dissolve 125 mg sodium cyanide in 0.5 ml demineralized water and add 2.0 ml of 95% ethanol.
2. *Sodium Nitroprusside, 5%*: Dissolve 125 mg sodium nitroprusside in 0.5 ml demineralized water and add 2.0 ml 95% ethanol.
3. *Positive Control Urine*: As in Brand's nitroprusside-cyanide method (p. 53).

REFERENCE

Brand, E., Harris, M. M., and Biloon, S.: The excretion of a cystine complex which decomposes in the urine with the liberation of free cystine, *J Biol Chem, 86*:315, 1930.

BOROHYDRIDE SPOT PLATE METHOD FOR CYSTINE AND HOMOCYSTINE

Principle

Borohydride replaces cyanide in the reduction of urinary disulfides reacting with nitroprusside. The method is performed on a microscale, as end points are visible in a spot plate.

Procedure

1. Add potassium borohydride powder in 20 mg portions to alternate depressions in a spot plate. Add 0.2 ml aliquots of catch or control urine.
2. Ten minutes later add 1 drop concentrated HCl. When evolution of gas has stopped, add another small drop. Continue until evolution is complete.
3. Add 4 drops 12.5 N NaOH. Add more, in drops, until solution is strongly basic (pH 9 or greater).
4. Add 12 drops saturated NH_4Cl and 1 drop 1% sodium nitroprusside.
5. Observe immediately.

Interpretation

Cystinuria of 10 mg per 100 ml or more gives a purple color lasting more than one minute. Urine samples containing cystine in concentrations of 5 mg per 100 ml or less are clear, yellow, or slightly orange. If the color is deep yellow, repeat the test, adding one extra drop of concentrated HCl.

Reagents

1. *Potassium Borohydride Powder.*
2. *Hydrochloric Acid, Concentrated.*
3. *Sodium Hydroxide, 12.5 M*: Dissolve 50 g sodium hydroxide in 75 ml demineralized water. Dilute to 100 ml with demineralized water in a volumetric flask.
4. *Ammonium Chloride, Saturated Solution*: Dissolve approximately 110 grams of ammonium chloride in 200 ml demineralized water until saturated.
5. *Sodium Nitroprusside, 1%*: Dissolve 50 mg sodium nitroprusside in 5 ml demineralized water.
6. *Normal Control*: Catch sample of normal urine.
7. *Positive Control*: As in Brand's nitroprusside-cyanide method (p. 53).

REFERENCES

Rosenthal, A. F. and Yaseen, A.: Improved qualitative screening test for cystinuria and homocystinuria, *Clin Chim Acta, 26*:363-364, 1969.
Kelly, S., Leikhim, E. and Desjardins, L.: A qualitative spot test for cystinuria, *Clin Chim Acta, 39*:469-471, 1972.

HOMOCYSTINURIA

The clinical picture of homocystinuria, a recessively inherited aminoacidopathy, mimics that of a disease with dominant inheritance and no specific biochemical markers, Marfan syndrome. Both kinds of patients are tall and thin for their age, have long fingers (arachnodactyly), and dislocated lenses. Children with homocystinuria often present with thromboembolic events, have seizures, and may be retarded. The young patient with Marfan syndrome, on the other hand, usually presents with poor vision or heart failure.

The clinical signs of homocystinuria can be prevented by treating infants with special diets. Older children also benefit by restricting methionine-containing protein; many, but not all, improve with vitamin B_6 therapy.

Patients with classical homocystinuria have little or no cystathionine synthetase, an enzyme found in liver. The enzyme's substrate, homocystine, is an intermediate in the metabolism of methionine and is normally absent from the body fluids. In the absence of synthetase, however, homocystine and methionine accumulate in the blood and overflow in urine. Some homocystinuric patients have little or no enzyme; others have synthetase which requires priming by the coenzyme, vitamin B_6.

A few patients excrete homocystine because of defects in other steps of methionine metabolism, those involving the remethylation of homocystine. Vitamin B_{12} metabolism is faulty in some, and others have a deficiency of the enzyme, $N^{5,10}$-methylene tetrahydrofolate reductase. Clinical signs in these patients differ, for the most part, from those in classical homocystinuria.

Some obligate carriers of classical homocystinuria can be identified through the persistence of high serum methionine levels after a loading dose. Their leukocytes, furthermore, can be induced to form only small amounts of synthetase in response to stimulation by phytohemagglutinin, and their liver synthetase levels are also less than normal.

Homocystinuria is demonstrable in urine by Brand's nitroprusside-cyanide reaction (p. 52). A silver ion modification of the reaction is specific (p. 58). Homocystine separates in one-dimensional paper chromatography but must be distinguished from glutamine. Homocysteine and its stabler oxidation product, homocystine, are measured precisely by column chromatography, a procedure especially valuable when following the effects of dietary or vitamin therapy. Also measurable by column chromatography is the mixed disulfide of homocysteine and cysteine, an equilibrium product of the monomeric forms.

Methionine levels in blood are measurable by a bacterial-inhibition test (p. 29). Like the procedure for PKU, the assay is well-suited to screening newborns. More precise estimates, however, are made by column chromatography.

The synthetase defect can be demonstrated in liver or short-term cultures of leukocytes stimulated by phytohemagglutinin (p. 59).

HOMOCYSTINE IN URINE

Principle

Brand's cyanide-nitroprusside reagent for sulfhydryl compounds, modified by the addition of ammoniacal silver nitrate, invests the test with specificity for urinary homocystine. The dismutative action of silver reduces homocystine to the thiol form faster than it does cystine; with cyanide as an ion-binder, homocysteine's sulfhydryl group reacts immediately with nitroprusside well before that of cysteine's slower reactive group.

Procedure

1. Add 5 ml aliquots of catch urine sample and control in 16 × 100 ml test tubes containing approximately 2.0 gms of solid sodium chloride. Mix and let settle.
2. Remove and add 2.5 ml aliquots of supernatant fluids to clean 16 × 100 ml test tubes. Add 0.25 ml 1% silver nitrate-3% ammonium hydroxide solution.
3. Mix and let stand one minute. Add 0.25 ml 1% sodium nitroprusside.
4. Mix and in a hood add 0.25 ml 0.7% sodium cyanide with bulb pipette. Mix each tube immediately after adding cyanide and observe immediately.

Interpretation

Samples containing homocystine turn pink or purple immediately, the color lasting at least one minute.

Reagents

1. *Ammonium Hydroxide, 3%*: Add 2.5 ml ammonium hy-

droxide to 22.5 ml demineralized water in 50 ml Erlenmeyer flask.

2. *Silver Nitrate, 1% in 3% Ammonium Hydroxide*: Dissolve 100 mg AgNO₃ in 10 ml 3% ammonium hydroxide. Prepare fresh in amount needed.

3. *Sodium Nitroprusside, 1%*. Dissolve 100 mg sodium nitroprusside in 10 ml demineralized water. Prepare fresh in amount needed.

4. *Sodium Cyanide 0.7%*. In a hood, dissolve 70 mg NaCN in 10 ml demineralized water. Prepare fresh in amount needed.

5. *Positive Control*: Dispense catch urine sample from a known homocystinuric patient (or urine containing 5 mg of homocystine per 100 ml) in 5.0 ml amounts and store at -20° C until used.

REFERENCE

Spaeth, L. and Barber, G.: Prevalence of homocystinuria among the mentally retarded: Evaluation of a specific screening test, *Pediatrics, 40*:586, 1967.

CYSTATHIONINE SYNTHETASE IN PHA-STIMULATED LYMPHOCYTES

Principle

Cystathionine synthetase, an enzyme which catalyzes the condensation of homocysteine and serine to cystathionine in the liver, is normally not found in peripheral leukocytes. Some can be induced, however, by culturing leukocytes with the mitogen, phytohemagglutinin (PHA), for a few days.

Activity is measured as the amount of ^{14}C-labeled product formed by extracts of PHA-stimulated lymphocytes during incubation with labeled substrate. The ^{14}C-labeled cystathionine is separated from labeled serine by paper chromatography before measurement of radioactivity.

Procedure

1. Let red cells in 10 ml fresh heparinized blood settle at 37° C for

two hours under aseptic conditions.

2. Add 2.5 ml sterile plasma-leukocyte suspension to 75 ml Falcon culture flask, add 22.5 ml McCoy's media, 0.5 ml Difco PHA M and incubate at 37° C for four days.

3. On the day of harvest, shake culture flask gently, but thoroughly, dispersing cultured cells.

4. Remove two 0.5 ml aliquots of cultured cells, shaking flask between time, and save in 3 ml glass Sorvall tubes at 0 to 5°C for estimates of protein concentration.

5. Pour remainder of culture into a 50 ml Nalgene Sorvall tube, centrifuge at 1000 R.P.M. at 4° C for ten minutes, and decant supernatant fluid into a 50 ml graduated cylinder, removing by pipette all the liquid which collects on the lip. Do not disturb pellet during this step.

6. Record volume of all the supernatant fluid as *total volume of culture used in assay* and discard.

7. Suspend pellet in 1.0 ml saline, centrifuge at 1000 R.P.M. at 4° C for ten minutes, decant supernatant fluid, and resuspend pellet in 0.1 ml 30 mM TRIS-HCl lysate buffer, pH 8.3.

8. Freeze and thaw cells in CO_2-ethanol bath three times, centrifuge at 12,000 R.P.M. at 4° C for five minutes, remove all supernatant fluid carefully with 100λ and 50λ micropipettes, recording volume as *cell-free lysate,* and use for enzyme assay.

9. Combine 40λ substrate mixture (50λ syringe) and 10λ serine-3-^{14}C (6.8 nanomoles/10λ) in three 10 × 75 mm tubes, adding 50λ cell lysate to two and 50λ of 30 mM TRIS-HCl lysate buffer to the third (blank).

10. Incubate all tubes in 37° C water bath for four hours.

11. Assay cultured cells for protein during incubation period above, as in steps 19 through 24 below.

12. Remove tubes from water bath and freeze in CO_2-ethanol bath to stop reaction. Store overnight at this step, if necessary.

13. Spot 25λ of 60 mg% cystathionine/serine standard solution 2.5 cm in from left edge and 6.5 cm from bottom of sheet of #3 MM chromatography paper, 17 1/2 × 7-inch. Spot 50λ of the three reaction mixtures at 3 cm intervals, beginning 3 cm

from the application of the cystathionine/serine standard solution.

14. Develop by descending chromatography overnight in Bu:Ac:H$_2$O solvent.
15. Remove papers from tank, air-dry for thirty minutes, and in 60°C explosion-proof oven for fifteen minutes.
16. Cut strip containing 60 mg% cystathionine/serine standard solution from chromatography sheet, stain with ninhydrin for fifteen minutes, as described in the section, "Paper Chromatography of Amino Acids" (p. 20), and examine.
17. Locate positions of labeled cystathionine and serine-3-^{14}C on unstained chromatogram by comparing with respective positions on ninhydrin-stained strip.
18. Cut out the corresponding spots with scissors, attach to planchettes, and count ^{14}C in planchette counter.
19. Begin protein estimation in the two 0.5 ml aliquots of cultured cells saved at 4°C by centrifuging at 1000 R.P.M. at 4°C for ten minutes. Discard supernatant fluids, suspend pellets in 0.5 ml 0.9% NaCl, add 2.0 ml 0.83% NH$_4$Cl, and leave at room temperature for thirty minutes during lysis of red cells.
20. Centrifuge immediately at 1000 R.P.M. at 4°C for ten minutes, remove supernatant fluids carefully, and discard.
21. Suspend pellets of white cells in 100λ demineralized water, and lyse by freezing and thawing in a CO$_2$-ethanol bath three times. Add 2.0 ml working alkaline copper reagent. Mix by inversion and let stand fifteen minutes.
22. To 100λ protein standards in 10 × 75 mm cuvettes add 2.0 ml working alkaline copper reagent. Mix by inversion and let stand at room temperature for fifteen minutes.
23. Add rapidly 0.2 ml diluted phenol reagent to tubes containing lysed white cells and cuvettes containing protein standards, and let stand thirty minutes.
24. Transfer lysed white cell solution to cuvettes. Measure optical density in all cuvettes at 750 nm.

Calculations

1. Since the conversion of labelled serine to cystathionine is mea-

sured in counts per minute (c.p.m.), c.p.m. for each sample must be related to the molar concentration of the reactants. This is accomplished by deriving the factor (F) from the c.p.m. given by known concentration of the substrate, as follows:

$$\frac{V_c}{CPM_c} \times nmoles/V \times 1000 = picomoles/c.p.m.$$

where V_c and c.p.m.$_c$ are the volume and counts per minute, respectively, of serine ^{14}C measured; and nmoles/V is the concentration of serine ^{14}C in the reaction mixture. For example:

$$\frac{5\lambda}{20,854} \times 6.8 \ nmoles/10\lambda \times 1000 = picomoles/c.p.m.$$

2. Calculate picomoles cystathionine formed, as follows:
   a. Subtract c.p.m. of blank from sample c.p.m., multiply by F (picomoles/c.p.m.) and again by 2 for picomoles cystathionine formed in 100λ reaction mixture or 50λ cell lysate.
   b. Multiply by measured volume of cell-free lysate (λ), divide by 50 for picomoles cystathionine formed by total culture used in assay, divide by measured *total volume of culture used in assay* (ml), and multiply by 100 for picomoles cystathionine formed per 100 ml culture per four hours at 37° C.
3. Calculate mg protein from curve and O.D. of mg protein per 100 ml concentrated cell suspension; divide by concentration factor of 5 (from 0.5 ml to 0.1 ml) for mg protein per 100 ml culture.
4. Calculate picomoles cystathionine/mg protein/four hours from the formula:

$$\frac{Picomoles \ cystathionine}{100 \ ml \ culture} \times \frac{100 \ ml \ culture}{mg \ protein}$$

Interpretation

Mean activities ± standard error in leukocytes from normal persons were 666.9 ± 70.2 units (picomoles cystathionin formed per mg protein per four hours at 37° C); those from patients with homocystinuria were 2.0 ± 1.6 units or less and from obligate carriers, 114.4 ± 27.3 units.

Reagents for Enzyme Assay

1. *Culture Media*: Add 20 ml sterile fetal calf serum and 10,000 units each of penicillin-streptomycin solution to 100 ml McCoy's 5A medium (modified) with HEPES buffer (from Grand Island Biological Co. [GIBCO]).
2. *Phytohemagglutinin M*: Reconstitute vial of lyophilized GIBCO phytohemagglutin M with 10 ml of sterile demineralized water. (Stable for one month at 4° C.)
3. *TRIS · HCl, 30 mM, and Pyridoxal-Phosphate, 1.3 mM, Lysate Buffer, pH 8.3*: Dissolve 0.363 g Trizma® Base and 0.032 g pyridoxal phosphate in 80 ml demineralized water. Adjust to pH 8.3 with 1 N HCl and bring to volume in 100 ml volumetric flask.
4. *TRIS · HCl, Substrate Buffer, 375 mM, pH 8.3*: Dissolve 4.54 g Trizma Base in 80 ml demineralized water. Adjust to pH 8.3 with 4 N HCl and bring to volume in a 100 ml volumetric flask.
5. *Substrate Base*: Dissolve the following: 23.2 mg disodium ethylenediamine tetraacetic acid-(EDTA), 4.03 mg pyridoxal phosphate, 0.002 ml L (+) cystathionine (9 mg/0.2 ml 1 N HCl in 10.0 ml 375 mM TRIS · HCl substrate buffer).
6. *Substrate*; Dissolve 3.4 mg L (+) homocysteine in 1.0 ml substrate base.
7. *Serine-3-^{14}C (6.8 nanomoles/10λ; 100 μC/2.0 ml):* In radioactive hood, combine 100λ serine 3-^{14}C stock (3.2 nmoles/10λ; 100 μC/2.0 ml) and 2λ serine (cold) (3.78 mg/2.0 ml).
8. *Chromatography Solvent (Bu:Ac:H$_2$O; 12:3:5):* Combine 60 ml butanol, 15 ml acetic acid, and 25 ml demineralized water.
9. *Ninhydrin Stain*: Dissolve 250 mg ninhydrin in 200 ml acetone.
10. *Cystathionine/Serine Standard Solution, 60 mg%*: Dissolve 30 mg L (+) cystathionine and 30 mg L (+) serine in 25 ml

demineralized water. Bring to volume in 50 ml volumetric flask.

Reagents for Protein Assay

1. *Ammonium Chloride, 0.83%*: Dissolve 415 mg NH_4Cl in 50 ml demineralized water.
2. *Alkaline Tartrate Reagent*: Dissolve 2.0 g Na_2CO_3, 50 mg Na or K tartrate in 100 ml 0.1 N NaOH (0.8g/200 ml).
3. *Copper Sulfate, 0.1%*: Dissolve 100 mg $CuSO_4 \cdot 5\ H_2O$ in 100 ml demineralized water.
4. *Working Alkaline Copper Reagent*: On the day of test, combine 18 ml alkaline tartrate reagent and 2 ml 0.1% $CuSO_4$.
5. *Dilute Phenol Reagent*: On the day of test, combine 2 ml phenol reagent 2N (Fisher) and 2 ml demineralized water.
6. *Protein Standard Stock Solution, 600 mg% Bovine Serum Albumin:* Combine 1 ml 30% bovine albumin (Armour Pharmaceutical Co.) and 49 ml demineralized water.
7. *Protein Standard Working Solutions*: Combine the following volumes of the protein standard stock solution with the following volumes of demineralized water:

Protein (mg)	Protein 600 mg% Stock Solution (ml)	Water (ml)
0	0	2
25	0.25	5.75
50	0.25	2.75
100	0.50	2.50
200	1.0	2.0
300	1.0	1.0

REFERENCES

Lowry, O. H., Rosebrough, N. J., Farr, A. L., and Randall, R. J.: Protein measurement with the Folin phenol reagent, *J Biol Chem, 193*:265, 1951.

Goldstein, J. L., Campbell, B. K., and Gartler, S. M.: Cystathionine synthase activity in human lymphocytes: Induction by phytohemagglutinin, *J Clin Invest, 51*:1034, 1972.

Goldstein, J. L., Campbell, B. K. and Gartler, S. M.: Homocystinuria: Heterozygote detection using phytohemagglutinin-stimulated lymphocytes, *J Clin Invest, 52*:218, 1973.

ARGININOSUCCINICACIDURIA

Early-onset argininosuccinicaciduria affects newborns who die a few days after birth. Some live a few months, but fail to thrive and develop hepatomegaly before death. Late-onset disease, on the other hand, appears in childhood. Affected children are ataxic, convulsive, retarded, and episodically comatose from ammonia toxicity. Hair may be dry and breakable. The biochemical abnormalities in either form appear early in the newborn period, after several days of feeding. Prompt institution of a low protein diet prevents or lessens the clinical signs.

The basic biochemical lesion is lack of red cell and liver argininosuccinase, an enzyme of the urea cycle. Argininosuccinic acid (ASA) accumulates in the cerebral spinal fluid as unused substrate and, along with citrulline, is excreted by the kidney, especially after protein meals. Serum contains only trace amounts, however, as the kidneys clear ASA readily.

The disease is recessively inherited. Carriers can be detected biochemically by half-normal levels of enzyme; they usually do not excrete ASA.

The defect in red cell enzyme is detected by a microbiologic assay with an ASA-sensitive mutant, (p. 29). The urinary abnormalities of homozygous persons are visible on paper chromatograms as excessive arginine and citrulline (p. 18, 22). ASA excretion is measured by column chromatography as its anhydride.

MAPLE SYRUP URINE DISEASE (MSUD)

Infants with classical maple syrup urine disease or branched-chain ketoaciduria emit an odor resembling maple syrup a few days after birth; vomiting, hypertonicity, convulsions, and death ensue. A milder, intermittent form may appear in older infants; they become lethargic, vomit, and emit the typical odor when subjected to stress from infections, surgery, or excessive protein intake. Both forms of the disease can be treated by a protein-restricted diet.

The metabolic block is due to a failure in oxidative decarboxylation of the α-keto acids to fatty acids by a series of enzymes.

The α-keto acids and their antecedent amino acids, valine, leucine, and isoleucine, accumulate in the blood with "overflow" in urine. In the intermittent form, the abnormalities are found only during exacerbations.

The classical form is detectable soon after birth by a bacterial-inhibition assay for excessive leucine levels in dried blood spots (p. 29), similar to that for screening newborns for PKU. Leucine, isoleucine, and valine concentrations in serum are measured quantitatively by column chromatography. α-Keto aciduria is detected by the dinitrophenylhydrazine reaction (p. 66), and the individual α-keto acids are identified by paper chromatography (p. 67).

SCREENING TEST FOR α-KETO ACIDS IN URINE

Principle

The α-keto derivatives of the branched chain amino acids and ketones form insoluble colored hydrazones in acidified urine by reaction of the carbonyl groups with dinitrophenylhydrazine.

Procedure

1. To 1.0 ml aliquots filtered urine sample and standard solutions, in respective 12 × 75 mm test tubes, add 0.2 ml 0.5% 2,4-dinitrophenylhydrazine in 2 N HCl, in drops. Leave at room temperature for twenty minutes.
2. Examine for fine yellow precipitate against a light background. Swirl to mix. Compare samples with standards.

Interpretation

Precipitate equivalent to 25 mg per 100 ml standard α-ketoglutaric dinitrophenylhydrazone or greater is abnormal.

Reagents

1. *2,4-Dinitrophenylhydrazine in 2 N HCl, 0.5%:* Dissolve 1.25 g 2,4-dinitrophenylhydrazine in 125 ml 4 N HCl (use magnetic

stirrer). Dilute to 250 ml with demineralized water.

2. *α-Keto Acid Stock Standard, 50 mg%:* Dissolve 25.0 mg α-ketoglutaric acid in 40 ml normal urine. Dilute to volume in 50 ml volumetric flask with normal urine.

3. *Standard α-Keto Acid Solutions:* Dilute the 50 mg% stock standard with the following volumes of normal urine:

Concentration of Standard (mg%)	Normal Urine (ml)	50 mg% Stock Standard (ml)
0	25	0
15	17.5	7.5
25	12.5	12.5
50	0	25

Dispense standard solutions in 1.7 ml quantities in 12 × 75 mm tubes. Store stoppered tubes at -20°C.

REFERENCE

Menkes, John H.: Biochemical methods in the diagnosis of neurological disorders. In Plum, Fred and McDowell, Fletcher H. (Eds.): *Recent Advances in Neurology.* Philadelphia, Davis, 1969, p. 8.

THIN-LAYER CHROMATOGRAPHY OF DNP HYDRAZONES OF α-KETO ACIDS

Principle

The dinitrophenyl (DNP) hydrazones formed by reaction of 2,4-dinitrophenylhydrazine with the urinary α-keto acids in maple syrup urine disease are concentrated and identified by thin layer chromatography on silica gel.

Procedure

1. Add 2 ml 2.0% 2,4-dinitrophenylhydrazine in 2 N HCl to 10 ml catch urine sample, (or proportionally less with smaller sample volumes) and 10 ml aliquots of normal urine containing 1.5 mg amounts of α-ketoglutaric acid (control) and the following standards: α-keto isovaleric, α-keto isocaproic and α-keto-β-methylvaleric acids. Let precipitates form

(yellow) thirty minutes at room temperature.

2. Add suspension to 50 ml separatory funnel and shake with three 15 ml portions of chloroform-ethanol solution. Centrifuge suspensions if emulsions form. Save bottom layers and combine.
3. Shake combined extracts with 15 ml 10% Na_2CO_3 in 50 ml separatory funnel. Discard lower layer.
4. Wash with 10 ml chloroform-ethanol solution in 50 ml separatory funnel. Discard lower layer.
5. Acidify to pH 1 with 5 NHCl (pH paper) (about 5ml).
6. Shake three times with 10, 5, and 5 ml portions, respectively, of chloroform-ethanol solution. Save bottom layers and combine.
7. Dry combined extracts with solid, anhydrous Na_2SO_4, added from a spatula.
8. Filter through Whatman No. 1 filter paper. Save filtrate and dry in an evaporating dish in a stream of filtered air (thirty minutes).
9. Add 0.2 ml ethanol to dried, extracted precipitates.
10. On 20 × 20 cm Eastman Kodak Silica Gel Chromatogram sheet Type K, 301R, spot from 1 to 5 μl aliquots sample precipitates, according to amount of precipitate formed in screening test, and 5 μl aliquots of control and standard precipitates.
11. Develop in butanol, ethanol, ammonium hydroxide solvent, 84:7:7 until front reaches 15 cm (six hours).
12. Air dry and compare with mobilities of DNP hydrazones and standard α-keto acids.

Interpretation

The DNP hydrazones of the α-keto acids form yellow precipitates which separate on silica gel according to their respective mobilities. The DNP hydrazones of the α-keto acids found in urine from patients with maple syrup urine disease, (isovaleric, isocaproic, and β-methyl valeric) appear about midway on the chromatogram and move much faster than those of normally occurring, α-keto glutaric acid.

Reagents

1. *Chloroform-Ethanol Extraction Solution, 80:20*: Combine 80 ml chloroform with 20 ml absolute ethanol in 300 ml Erlenmeyer flask. Mix.
2. *Butanol:Ethanol:Ammonium Hydroxide Developing Solvent, 84:7:7*: Combine 84 ml butanol, 7 ml ethanol, and 7 ml ammonium hydroxide in 300 ml Erlenmeyer flask. Mix.

REFERENCES

Menkes, J. H.: The pattern of urinary alpha keto acids in various neurological diseases. *A.M.A. J of Diseases of Child, 99*:130, 1960.

Seligson, D., and Shapiro, B.: α-Keto acids in urine, *Anal Chem, 24*:754, 1952.

Tocci, Paul M., Ruiz, Eva, and Aquero, Graciella: Chemical Detection of Inherited Disorders. In Farrell, Gordon (Ed.): *International Symposium in Mental Science, Advances in Mental Science I, Congenital Mental Retardation.* Austin, U of Tex Pr, 1969, pp. 182-183.

THE HYPERGLYCINEMIAS

Hyperglycinemia occurs in three or more severe ketoacidotic diseases of infancy, including propionicacidemia, methylmalonicacidemia (MMA) and isovalericacidemia (IVA). Certain dietary proteins, and even infections, precipitate episodes of vomiting and seizures in the newborn, culminating in coma and death. Not tolerated are proteins containing isoleucine, valine, threonine and methionine, nor, in propionicacidemia, leucine. Several infants, saved by early treatment with special low-protein diets, are now developing normally.

The enzyme defects in two of the ketotic hyperglycinemias — propionicacidemia and MMA — cause blocks in the succinate-tricarboxylic acid cycle, through which propionicacid is oxidized to carbon dioxide. They are, respectively, deficiency of propionyl coenzyme A carboxylase and absence of the subsequent catalyst, methylmalonyl coenzyme A mutase, an enzyme requiring cobolamide coenzyme (vitamin B_{12}). In IVA, the pathway of leucine degradation is involved, and the defect interferes with the conversion of isovaleric acid to β-methylcrotonyllic acid. In none is the relationship of hyperglycinemia clear.

Some affected infants, but not all, respond to vitamin therapy. The coenzyme, biotin, for example, primes the defective enzyme system of propionicacidemia, and vitamin B_{12} primes that in MMA.

Other infants have nonketotic forms of hyperglycinemia. These newborns are lethargic, convulsive, and irritable; survivors are retarded. A specific enzyme defect has not yet been identified, although the defect of propionicacidemia has been found in one patient. Infants with nonketotic hyperglycinemia are less responsive to dietary treatment than those with ketotic forms.

The degree of hyperglycinemia and rate of glycine excretion differ according to the etiology. The greatest, for example, occur in propionicacidemia. Hyperglycinemia in MMA and IVA, conversely, may be intermittent.

The specific enzyme defects of the ketotic forms are demonstrated by isotopic assays of enzyme in leukocytes, liver, or cultured cells.

Hyperglycinemia and hyperglycinuria are revealed by paper chromatograms (p. 17) and measured by column chromatography. Serum levels can be measured colorimetrically (p. 70).

The organic acids from which the diseases derive their names accumulate in serum and are demonstrable by gas chromatography. They or their derivatives may be excreted. Urinary methylmalonic acid, for example, is detected in a screening test (p. 73) and quantitated (p. 76). Urinary isovalerylglycine, a metabolic conjugate of isovaleric acid, on the other hand, is detected by thin layer chromatography, as are a number of other organic acids or derivatives (p. 78).

GLYCINE IN SERUM BY COLORIMETRY

Principle

Glycine in serum is degraded to formaldehyde through decarboxylation and deamination by Chloramine T in an acid medium. Glycine is measured as formaldehyde, which condenses stoichiometrically with acetylacetone and ammonia to form the colored pyridine derivative, dihydrodiacetyllutedine.

Procedure

1. Prepare oil bath: Add paraffin oil to a metal container on a hot plate deep enough to cover levels of reaction volume. Immerse thermometer in oil, avoiding bottom. Heat oil bath one hour before use and check temperature frequently before and during use to assure temperature equilibrium of 135 to 140° C.
2. Deproteinize 0.5 ml aliquot of serum or blood sample in 15 ml Sorvall centrifuge tube with 4 ml 0.08 N sulfuric acid and 0.5 ml 10% sodium tungstate. (If only 0.1 ml serum is available, use 1/5 amounts of reactants in 4 ml Sorvall tube). Mix and centrifuge at 2000 R.P.M. at 4° C for ten minutes. Remove supernatant fluid by pipette and save as deproteinized serum.
3. Combine 0.5 ml aliquots deproteinized serum, standards, and demineralized water (blank) with 0.1 ml 1% Chloramine T solution and 0.5 ml 0.2 N sulfuric acid in respective 100 × 16 mm test tubes (eight). Mix well and place in previously heated oil bath (metal) at 135 to 140° C for exactly one minute.
4. Drain rack on absorbent paper after removing from bath.
5. Add 0.9 ml demineralized water and 2 ml acetylacetone reagent to all tubes. Mix well and incubate in water bath at 58° C for ten minutes. Be sure level in water bath is higher than that in tubes.
6. Cool tubes to room temperature.
7. Measure absorbance of sample and standards at 412 nm.

Calculations

1. Plot optical density versus concentration glycine in μg/ml.
2. Estimate μg glycine per ml deproteinized serum from standard curve and express glycine concentration in mg/100 ml serum sample.

Interpretation

Glycine concentration ranges from 2.0 through 5.3 mg per 100 ml normal serum.

Reagents

1. *Sulfuric Acid, 0.2N:* Add slowly and cautiously 0.57 ml concentrated sulfuric acid to 80 ml demineralized water in 300 ml Erlenmeyer flask. Mix by swirling. Bring to volume in 100 ml volumetric flask.
2. *Sulfuric Acid, 0.08N:* Bring to volume 40 ml 0.2 N sulfuric acid in 100 ml volumetric flask with demineralized water.
3. *Sodium Tungstate, 10%:* Dissolve 10 g sodium tungstate in 80 ml demineralized water in 300 ml Erlenmeyer flask. Bring to volume in 100 ml volumetric flask.
4. *Chloramine T, 1%.* Weigh cautiously, avoiding inhalation, and dissolve carefully, avoiding contact with skin and eyes, 100 mg in 10 ml demineralized water in 15 $\times$ 125 mm screw-capped tube. Prepare fresh daily.
5. *Acetyl Acetone Reagent, pH 6.0.* Mix 7.5 g ammonium acetate, about 0.5 ml glacial acetic acid and 0.1 ml acetyl acetone in 40 ml demineralized water in 125 ml beaker. Adjust to pH 6.0 and dilute to 50 ml in Erlenmeyer flask. Stable two weeks at 4°C.
6. *Glycine Stock Standard Solution, 10 mg/ml.* Dissolve 250 mg glycine in demineralized water and bring to volume in 25 ml volumetric flask with demineralized water. Stable at least one month at 4°C.
7. *Glycine Working Standards:* Prepare working standards for standard curve on the day of test: Dilute 10 mg/ml glycine stock standard solution one-hundred fold with demineralized water to give solution containing 100 μg glycine/ml. Dilute 100 μg glycine/ml standard solution as follows:

Glycine Standard (μg/ml)	Volume Standard (ml)	Volume Diluent (ml)
20	2.0	8.0
10	1.0	9.0
7.5	0.75	9.25
5	0.5	9.5
2.5	0.25	9.75
1.0	2.0 ml 5 μg/ml	8.0

REFERENCE

Sardesai, V. M. and Provido, H. S.: The determination of glycine in biological fluids. *Clin Chim Acta, 29*:67, 1970.

METHYLMALONIC ACIDURIA SCREENING TEST

Principle

The gross excesses of methylmalonic acid excreted in hereditary methylmalonic aciduria are detected by reaction with the diazonium salt of para-nitroaniline in alkaline solution, with which it forms an emerald green chromogen.

Procedure

1. Add single drops of test sample, positive and negative controls in respective 10 ml test tubes.
2. Add 15 drops of 0.1% p-nitroaniline and 5 drops of 0.5% sodium nitrite, in that order, to each tube.
3. Mix by swirling and observe partial decoloration.
4. Add 1 ml 1M sodium acetate buffer (pH 4.3), mix, and place immediately in boiling water bath for from one to three minutes. Be sure water level of bath is higher than level of liquid in tubes.
5. Remove tubes from bath and immediately add 5 drops of 8 N sodium hydroxide. Mix.
6. Compare test sample with positive control and record results.

Interpretation

Excessive methylmalonic acid in urine (600 mg/l or more) forms an immediate emerald green color. Malonic and ethylmalonic acids form green chromogens also, but usually are present in trace amounts only. Creatinine, uric acid, vitamin K, ampicillin, penicillin G, diphenylhydantoin, and a variety of amino acids, on the other hand, form brown chromogens which may mask the color from methylmalonic acid, unless the latter is present in concentrations of 1000 mg/l or more. (See Color Illustration 5.)

Reagents

1. *Para-nitroaniline, 0.1%*: Dissolve 0.1 g p-nitroaniline in final volume of 100 ml 0.16 N HCl. Stable in dark glass bottle at room temperature for six months or longer. Dispense in small, colored, dropping bottle for daily use.
2. *Sodium Nitrite (Certified Reagent), 5%*: Dissolve 0.25 g NaNO$_2$ in demineralized water to final volume of 50 ml. Stable at 4°C for two months or longer. Dispense in small, colored, dropping bottle for daily use.
3. *Sodium Acetate Buffer (Trihydrate), 1M, pH 4.3*: Dissolve 13.6 g sodium acetate in demineralized water to final volume of 100 ml. Add 158 ml of 1 M acetic acid to give pH 4.3±0.02. Adjust pH, if necessary. Stable at 4°C for two to three months.
4. *Sodium Hydroxide, 8N*: Dissolve 33.4 g sodium hydroxide (reagent pellets) in demineralized water to final volume of 100 ml. Dispense in small dropping bottle for daily use.
5. *Positive Control: Methylmalonic Acid Standard (Grade A) 0.025M*: Dissolve 147.5 mg methylmalonic acid in 50 ml demineralized water; add a drop of 6 N HCl. Stable at 4°C for six months or longer.
6. *Negative Control; Reagent Blank*: Normal urine.

REFERENCE:

Giorgio, J. and Luhby, A. L.: A rapid screening test for the detection of congenital methylmalonic aciduria in infancy. *Am J Clin Pathol, 52*:374, 1969.

PAPER CHROMATOGRAPHY OF URINARY METHYLMALONIC ACID

Principle

MMA is detectable by overstaining with tetrazotizedodianisidine the paper chromatograms developed and stained for amino acids. The chromatography method is a valuable adjunct to the MMA screening test (p. 73), which is sometimes difficult to interpret because of interference by chromatogens.

Procedure

1. Proceed as described for paper chromatography of amino acids (p. 17). Include a 50 mg% standard of methylmalonic acid on the test sheet and mark the position of the ninhydrin-stained spot of leucine-isoleucine.
2. Develop overnight but not longer than sixteen hours.
3. Stain sheet from tyrosine spot to solvent front by dipping in freshly prepared 0.5% Sigma o-dianisidine.
4. Match with standard fifteen to twenty minutes later (after color deepens) to estimate concentration.

Interpretation

1. Methylmalonic acid forms a purple spot beyond the fastest-moving urinary amino acids, leucine-isoleucine.
2. Pyruvic acid appears instantly as a reddish-purple spot in the marked position of glutamic acid, if the entire sheet is stained.

Reagents

1. *Chromatography Reagents*: As described for paper chromatography of amino acids, on p. 23.
2. *o-Dianisidine, 0.5%:* Dissolve 0.5 gm Sigma o-dianisidine in 100 ml absolute ethanol. Avoid contact or inhalation, as compound irritates the mucous membranes. Add 4 ml glacial acetic acid and let stand at least twenty minutes but not more than one hour before using.

REFERENCE

Personal communication. J. Thomas Coulombe, 1974.

METHYLMALONIC ACIDURIA QUANTITATIVE TEST

Principle

Methylmalonic acid is extracted from urine, concentrated, and coupled with diazotized p-nitroaniline to form a colored complex.

Procedure

1. Measure and record volume of twenty-four-hour collection of urine in liters (A).
2. Adjust 10 ml aliquots of sample and positive control to pH 2 or less with 1 N sulfuric acid, using narrow range indicator paper.
3. Add ammonium sulfate ($\pm$ 7 g) to sample and control until saturated.
4. Shake with 15 ml portion of ether-ethanol solution, 3.1, in 50 ml separatory funnel. Save both layers. Repeat extraction of bottom layer twice, combining top layers. Discard bottom layer after third extraction.
5. Pass combined ether-ethanol extracts through Dowex 1 resin, 100 to 200 mesh, $\times$ 10, regenerated to Cl^- form with 0.1N HCl, in separate 5 cm x 1.2 cm columns.
6. Wash columns with 50 ml demineralized water and elute with 20 ml portions of 0.1 N HCl. Measure and record eluate volumes(V_E).
7. Mix eluates thoroughly. Place 1.0 ml aliquots of 0.1N HCl (reagent blank), working standards and eluates in respective 100 $\times$ 16 mm test tubes. Add 1.5 ml 1.0 M acetate buffer, pH 4.3, and 1.5 ml cold diazo reagent. Mix. Heat in water bath at 95° C for three minutes.
8. Remove tubes from bath, add 1.0 ml 3 N NaOH, mix gently and stopper immediately.
9. Cool to room temperature for ten minutes, in water bath at 25° C.
10. Measure optical densities at 620 mμ, zeroing instrument with reagent blank.

Calculations

1. Plot optical density at 620 mμ against concentration of standard solutions (mg/ 1).

2. Estimate methylmalonic acid concentrations in eluates directly from standard curve (mg/1 eluate) and multiply by dilution factor:

$$\frac{V_E}{\text{Vol Sample}} \quad \text{or} \quad \frac{V_E}{10}$$

and express as mg methylmalonic acid per liter urine sample (B).
3. Calculate twenty-four-hour methylmalonic acid excretion rate as follows: mg/24 hr. = B X A

Interpretation

The normal methylmalonic acid excretion rate is usually less than 10 mg/24 hr.

Reagents

1. *Hydrochloric Acid, 0.1 N:* Dilute 1.7 ml concentrated HCl to 200 ml with demineralized water.
2. *Sodium Nitrite, 0.5%:* Dissolve 5.0 gm $NaNO_3$ in 1 liter demineralized water.
3. *p-Nitroaniline, 0.075%:* Dissolve 375 mg in 500 ml 0.2 N HCl (17.2 ml concentrated HCl/1).
4. *Sodium Acetate, 0.2 M:* Dissolve 13.6 g $NaC_2H_3O_2 \cdot 3\ H_2O$ in 500 ml demineralized water in volumetric flask.
5. *Acetate Buffer, 1.0 M, pH 4.3:* Dissolve 13.6 g $NaC_2H_3O_2$ in 100 ml demineralized water. Adjust to pH 4.3 with 1 M acetic acid (5.75 glacial acetic acid/1).
6. *Sodium Hydroxide, 3 N:* Dissolve 12 g in 100 ml demineralized water.
7. *Standard Methylmalonic Acid, Stock Solution, 1000 mg/1:* Dissolve 100 mg methylmalonic acid in 100 ml demineralized water and dilute to volume in liter volumetric flask. Store at 4° C.
8. *Standard Methylmalonic Acid, Dilute Solution:* Dilute 1 ml standard methylmalonic acid stock solution to 20 ml with

0.1 N HCl.

9. *Working Standards:* Combine the following volumes of stock or diluted stock standard with 0.1N HCl:

Concentration of Standard (mg/1)	Vol. Stock (ml)	Vol. Diluted Standard (ml)	Vol. of 0.1 N HCl (ml)
0	—	—	5
10	—	1	4
20	—	2	3
30	—	3	2
40	—	4	1
50	—	5	0
60	0.6	—	9.4
100	1.0	—	9.0

10. *Diazo Reagent:* Mix 4.0 ml 0.5% sodium nitrite with 15 ml p-nitroaniline solution. Cool in an ice bath to 4° C. Add 4.0 ml 0.2 M sodium acetate. Stable for twenty-four hours at 4°C.
11. *Positive Control:* Dissolve 3 mg methylmalonic acid in 15 ml normal urine.

REFERENCES

Green, A.: Colorimetric method for estimating methylmalonic acid in urine. *J Clin Path, 21*:221, 1968.

Giorgio, A. J., and Plaut, G. W. E.: A method for the colorimetric determination of urinary methylmalonic acid in pernicious anemia. *J Lab Clin Med, 66*:667, 1965.

ISOVALERYLGLYCINE IN URINE

Principle

Isovalerylglycine, the conjugation product of isovaleric acid, is distinguished from the normal urinary organic acid, hippuric, by thin-layer chromatography on silica gel.

Procedure (In Hood)

1. Add 1/5 volume 5 M H_2SO_4 to aliquot of twenty-four hour urine collection containing 0.7 mg creatinine (usually from 0.5 to 2.0 ml) in a 15 ml screw-capped centrifuge tube.

2. Add 5 ml butanol-chloroform extraction fluid and shake vigorously by hand or rotator for two minutes.
3. Centrifuge at 1500 R.P.M. for ten minutes, remove upper, aqueous layer and discard.
4. Evaporate 2 ml lower, chloroform layer to dryness in a stream of air.
5. Dissolve 10 µl residue in 0.2 ml extraction fluid, and spot on Silica Gel G or Eastman Kodak Silica Gel 13179 chromatography sheet or plate (TLC).
6. Spot 10 µl of hippuric acid standard on the same sheet.
7. Develop with benzene-isoamylalcohol-formic acid solvent until front rises 10 cm (approximately two hours).
8. Remove volatile solvents by drying sheet in explosion-proof oven at 75°C for thirty minutes. Remove formic acid by drying at 100°C for thirty minutes.
9. Spray sheet evenly with bromocresol purple stain. Observe immediately, as background fades after several minutes.
10. If a spot appears below that of hippuric acid, chromatograph residue and hippuric acid standard on fresh TLC plate with butanol-acetic acid-water solvent until front rises 10 cm.
11. Dry in explosion-proof oven at 75°C for an hour, stain as above, and observe immediately.
12. Verify isovalerylglycine spot by rechromatographing sample residue to which hippuric acid has been added. Develop in benzene-isoamylalcohol-formic acid solvent and observe for presence of two discrete spots.

Interpretation

The nonvolatile organic acids, including hippuric acid and isovalerylglycine and others, appear as yellow spots against a blue-purple background. The respective mobilities in benzene-isoamylalcohol-formic acid solution are represented in Figure 4. Both hippuric acid and isovalerylglycine have the same mobility when developed in the second, butanol-acetic acid solvent. Verification with known standards added to the sample residue is helpful in distinguishing among organic acids with mobilities more or less alike.

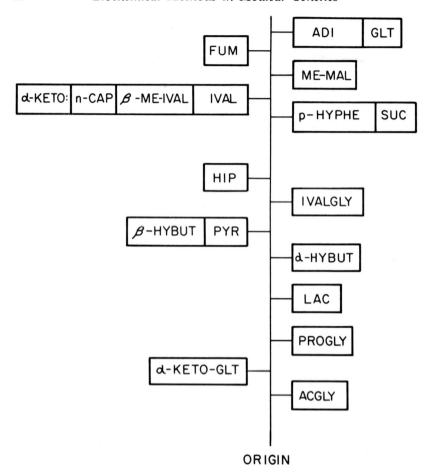

Figure 4. One-dimensional thin-layer silica gel chromatographic separation of the urinary organic acids and derivatives likely to be found in the ketotic hyperglycinemias.

Hippuric acid is the only organic acid normally excreted in amounts detectable by this method.

Reagents
1. H_2SO_4, *5.0 M:* Add slowly, with gentle mixing, 27.7 ml concentrated H_2SO_4 to 100 ml demineralized water.
2. *n-Butanol-Chloroform Extraction Fluid, 1:5:* Add 2 ml n-butanol to 10 ml chloroform. Mix well.

3. *Benzene-Isoamylalcohol-Formic acid Solvent 70:25:5:* Add 25 ml isoamylalcohol and 5 ml formic acid to 70 ml benzene in 300 ml Erlenmeyer flask, swirling to mix.

4. *Bromocresol purple (5, 5'-dibromo-c-cresolsulfonphthalein) Stain:* Dissolve 0.1 g bromocresol purple in 100 ml ethanol, add a few drops dilute NH_4OH solution (approximately 3%) until red-purple solution becomes purple (pH 10).

5. *Hippuric acid, 30μg/10 μl:* Dissolve 3 mg hippuric acid in 1 ml extraction fluid.

6. *Butanol-Acetic Acid-Water Solvent, 5:1:1:* Add 20 ml glacial acetic acid and 20 ml demineralized water to 100 ml butanol in 300 ml Erlenmeyer flask. Mix by swirling.

REFERENCE

Ando, T., and Nyhan, W. L.: A simple screening method for detecting isovalerylglycine in urine of patients with isovaleric acidemia. *Clin Chem,* *16*:420, 1970.

GENERALIZED OCULOCUTANEOUS ALBINISM

The clinical signs of the various hereditary oculocutaneous forms of albinism refer primarily to the lack of melanin, the skin and eye pigment. Two forms of generalized albinism have been recognized biochemically: one in which tyrosinase is demonstrable, and the other in which it is not. Melanin forms in the tissues of tyrosinase-positive albino patients when induced; no melanin forms under the same conditions in tyrosinase-negative tissues. Patients with the tyrosinase-positive form may be slightly less affected. The distinction, furthermore, applies in predicting phenotypes, as the children of parents with different forms of albinism are heterozygous for the different mutant genes i.e. are doubly heterozygous and, therefore, will not be albino, while children of parents with similar forms are homozygous for the same mutant gene and will be albino.

HAIR BULB TEST

Principle

Tyrosine is detected histochemically in hair bulbs by observing the formation of melanin during incubation with tyrosine.

Procedure

1. Pluck several scalp hairs with bulbs intact.
2. Trim hairs and immerse in 3 ml tyrosine substrate or buffer (control) solutions in 10 ml stoppered test tubes.
3. Incubate eighteen hours at 37°C.
4. Drain and add 3 ml 10% formalin. Fix thirty minutes.
5. Mount hair bulbs on slide in 50% glycerol, examine at magnification of 100 or 200x in either transmitted or reflected light. Compare pigment formation in the two tubes.

Interpretation

Hair bulbs from tyrosinase-negative albinos fail to form melanin during incubation with tyrosine, while those from tyrosinase-positive albinos form the pigment. Thus, the tyrosinase-negative bulbs are relatively unchanged by the incubation, while the tyrosinase-positive bulbs darken. Bulbs from normal persons are variably pigmented and may or may not darken with incubation.

Reagents

1. *Phosphate Buffer, 0.1N, pH 6.8*: Dissolve 7.0 g Na_2HPO_4 anhydrous and 7.05 g $NaH_2PO_4 \cdot H_2O$ in 800 ml demineralized water. Adjust to pH 6.8 and dilute to a liter. Store at 4°C.
2. *L-Tyrosine Substrate, 100 mg%*: Dissolve 100 mg L-tyrosine in 10 ml 1 N HCl. Add to 70 ml 0.1 N phosphate buffer and adjust to pH 6.8 with 10 N NaOH. Dilute to 100 ml with phosphate buffer.
3. *Formalin, 10%*: Add 10 ml formaldehyde (40%) to 90 ml demineralized water.

REFERENCE

Nance, Walter E.: Genetic and biochemical evidence for two forms of oculocutaneous albinism in man. In Bergsma, Daniel, (Ed.): *The Second Conference on the Clinical Delineation of Birth Defects, Part VII, EYE.* Baltimore, Williams and Wilkins, 1971, p. 126.

DISORDERS OF TRYPTOPHANE METABOLISM

The clinical signs of the heritable disorders of tryptophane metabolism often parade in the guise of a vitamin B deficiency. A pellagra-like skin rash, for example, and sensitivity to sunlight are common to several forms. They may or may not be accompanied by convulsions, dwarfism, or mental retardation.

Some types of tryptophane disorders involve transport mechanisms, the clinical signs of which relate to malabsorption in the intestinal tract or abnormal excretion by the kidneys. Both functions are affected in Hartnup disease. In "blue-diaper syndrome," on the other hand, an isolated malabsorption of tryptophane is the defect, strikingly revealed by the excretion of indigo blue, an enterobacterial product of indole metabolism.

Other types of tryptophane disorders arise from errors in intracellular mechanisms. Enzymes catalyzing the conversion of tryptophane through the kynurenine pathway, for example, are defective in at least three diseases, tryptophanuria, xanthurenicaciduria and hydroxykynureninuria. Kynureninase is inactive in the latter two diseases, a defect responsive to vitamin B$_6$ in xanthurenicaciduria, but unresponsive to hydroxykynureninuria.

The inheritance patterns of Hartnup disease and tryptophanuria are clearly autosomal recessive. Pedigree data, although incomplete, support a similar mode of inheritance in "blue diaper syndrome" and hydroxykynureninuria. An unequal sex ratio and a linear pedigree, however, obscure the definition of an autosomal recessive pattern in xanthurenicaciduria.

Distinctive patterns of urinary tryptophane metabolites can be seen in the various disorders by paper chromatography in two dimensions (p. 83).

PAPER CHROMATOGRAPHY OF URINARY METABOLITES OF TRYPTOPHANE

Principle

Kynurenine and hydroxykynurenine, the intermediary metabolites of tryptophane normally converted by enzymic action to anthranilic acid and hydroxykynurenine, respectively, are detected as fluorescent and Ehrlich-reactive spots by two-dimensional paper chromatography of urine.

Procedure

1. Overlay 10 μl aliquots of the standard metabolite solutions and urea in one corner of a 18 1/2 $\times$ 8 1/2-inch Whatman No. 1 sheet, folded as described for amino acid paper chromatography (p. 23). Apply 20 μl aliquots of a twenty-four-hour collection of urine sample and normal urine (control) to the corners of additional Whatman No. 1 sheets.
2. Develop the three sheets in vertical dimension by descending chromatography overnight in butanol-acetic acid-water solvent.
3. Dry sheets in hood one hour and at 70° C in explosion-proof oven five minutes.
4. Observe color and location of fluorescent spots under short wave ultraviolet light.
5. Develop in second dimension by ascending chromatography, with 20% KCl solvent covering bottom of tank. Curl sheets to fit tank, stapling top and bottom of sheets loosely so edges do not touch; immerse sheets to a depth of about 1/8-inch. Remove when solvent front is one inch from top (about two hours).
6. Dry sheets at room temperature one hour (in hood) and examine under shortwave ultraviolet. Mark and identify spots by comparing with standard metabolites.
7. Stain with Ehrlich solution for further definition. Note immediate color change and intensity and reexamine the following morning.

Interpretation

Hydroxykynurenine appears as a light blue fluorescent spot near tryptophane (See Figure 5 and Color Illustration 6.) Color reactions are listed in Table VII.

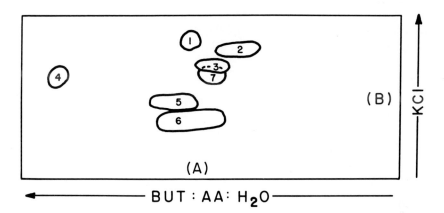

Figure 5. Two dimensional paper chromatographic separation of tryptophane (3) and urinary derivatives excreted in hydroxykynureninuria: kynurenine (2), kynurenic acid (5), xanthurenic acid (6) and hydroxykynurenine (7). The latter two are excreted in greatest excess. Anthranilic acid (4) is *not* excreted. Urea (1) serves as position control.

Table VII

FLUORESCENCE OF TRYPTOPHANE METABOLITES AND REACTION
WITH EHRLICH SOLUTION

Metabolite	Fluorescence	Ehrlich
Tryptophane	Dull purple	Pink
Kynurenic acid	Blue-green to green	No color (overnight)
Xanthurenic acid	Bright blue-white	Weakly yellow
Anthranilic acid	Bright violet	Yellow
Kynurenine	Light blue	Orange (overnight)
Urea	None	Yellow
Hydroxykynurenine	Light blue	Pink-orange

Reagents

1. *Standard Metabolite Solutions, 1 mg/ml*: Dissolve 10 mg amounts of the following in 10 ml portions 50% acetone: tryptophane, kynurenic acid, xanthurenic acid, anthranilic acid, kynurenine, and urea. Add a few drops 1 N NaOH to dissolve kynurenine and kynurenic acid.
2. *Butanol-Acetic Acid-Water Solvent System, 12-3-5*: Mix 120 ml butanol and 30 ml acetic acid in 500 ml Erlenmeyer flask. Add 50 ml distilled water; mix.
3. *Potassium Chloride Solution, 20%*: Dissolve 200 grams KCl in 800 ml distilled water; dilute to volume in one liter volumetric flask.
4. *Ehrlich Reagent*: As described in amino acid chromatography (p. 24). For immediate use dilute 5 ml Ehrlich reagent with 25 ml acetone.

REFERENCES

Dalgliesh, C. E.: Two dimensional chromatography of urinary indoles and related substances. *Biochem J, 64*:481, 1956.

Komrower, G. M., Wilson, V., Clamp, J. R., and Westall, R. G.: Hydroxykynureninuria: A case of abnormal tryptophan metabolism probably due to a deficiency of kynureninase. *Arch Dis Child, 39*:250, 1964.

Smith, Ivor (Ed.): *Chromatography and Electrophoresis Techniques,* 3rd Ed. New York, Wiley, 1969, Vol. I, pp. 793-799.

ALKAPTONURIA

The early clinical signs of alkaptonuria, darkening of urine and pigment deposition (ochronosis), may be missed in children and young adults. By middle age, however, arthritis of the spine and large joints develop, usually severe enough to require medical attention.

The nature of the basic defect, a defect in liver homogentisic acid oxidase, was recognized seventy years ago by Dr. Archibald

Garrod who included alkaptonuria in his original concepts of inborn errors. Later investigations supported his viewpoint and revealed a similar defect in the kidney. The defect causes the accumulation in tissues and excretion of homogentisic acid, an intermediate of phenylalanine and tyrosine metabolism. The pigment formed, a polymerized derivative of the acid, is bound to collagen. Its deposition in articular cartilage lessens the tissue's resilience. The arthritic changes relate to the brittle, abnormal cartilage, fragments of which erode and penetrate the joint.

The disease is rare and inherited in an autosomal recessive pattern. A very few obligate carriers are known to excrete slight excesses of homogentisic acid; for the most part, however, they have not been identified by biochemical means.

Biochemical tests for the disease depend chiefly on the identification of homogentisic acid in the urine by means of its reducing properties (p. 87) and chromatographic mobility (p. 90).

SCREENING TESTS FOR HOMOGENTISIC ACID

Principle

Homogentisic acid is detected by a series of simple tests for compounds with reducing properties. It reduces ferric chloride, for example, turning the solution blue or green. Red cuprous oxide forms in reaction with copper sulfate. Homogentisic acid immediately reduces an ammoniacal solution of silver nitrate to a black precipitate of silver. Finally, and more specifically, homogentisic acid causes darkening of urine-made alkaline, as it gradually oxidizes to a melanin-like product.

Procedure

1. Add 2 drops 10% ferric chloride reagent to 2 ml urine sample. Observe color changes.
2. Add 5 drops urine sample to 16 × 100 mm test tube. Rinse

dropper with water and add 10 drops water. Add Ames Clini-test® tablet. Observe color changes.
3. Add 5 ml 3% silver nitrate to 0.5 ml urine sample. Mix. Add a few drops 10% ammonium hydroxide. Observe.
4. Add 1.0 N sodium hydroxide, dropwise, to 2 ml urine sample until alkaline. Observe.

Interpretation

Homogentisic acid reacts with any or all of the reagents above. Similar reactions, however, occur with urine from patients with other diseases or conditions and should be recognized: Ferric chloride changes in PKU and histidinemia; Clinitest and silver nitrate reactions in glycosuria; darkening of urine from patients who received the X-ray contrast medium, sodium diatrizoate.

Reagents

1. *Ferric Chloride, 10%:* Dissolve 16.7 g $FeCl_3 \cdot 6 H_2O$ in 60 ml demineralized water and bring to volume in 100 ml volumetric flask.
2. *Sodium Hydroxide, 1.0 N:* Dissolve 4.0 g NaOH in 80 ml demineralized water and bring to volume in 100 ml volumetric flask.
3. *Silver Nitrate, 3%:* Dissolve 0.3 g in 9.7 ml demineralized water.
4. *Ammonium Hydroxide, 10%:* Dilute 35.7 ml concentrated ammonium hydroxide to volume in 100 ml volumetric flask.

REFERENCE

Henry, Richard J., Cannon, Donald C., and Winkelman, James W. (Eds.): *Clinical Chemistry, Principles and Technics,* 2nd ed., Hagerstown, Harper, 1974, pp. 622-625.

CONFIRMATORY TEST FOR HOMOGENTISIC ACID

Principle

Homogentisic acid, when separated from urinary pigments

and other interfering substances by butanol and water extractions, forms a pink-brown color complex with alkaline copper sulfate. The reactants are similar to those in the screening tests (p. 87), and the color complex is probably caused by a mixture of products formed by the oxidation of homogentisic acid.

Procedure

1. Concentrate 15 ml urine sample to about 3 ml in 22 ml evaporating dish on warm hot plate (in hood).
2. Transfer concentrated sample and 3 ml aliquots normal urine (negative control) and normal urine containing 15 mg homogentisic acid (positive control) to respective 10 ml screw-cap tubes, add 3 ml n-butanol, invert tubes five times, and let stand. Discard bottom (aqueous) layers.
3. Transfer butanol extracts to clean screw-cap tubes, add 5 ml demineralized water, invert five times, and let stand. Discard top (butanol) layers.
4. Transfer 0.05 ml aqueous extracts to 100×15 mm tubes, add 0.5 ml 0.1% copper sulfate, 5 ml demineralized water, and 0.5 ml 0.1 N sodium hydroxide. Mix (Vortex), let stand twenty minutes, and compare color in sample with positive and negative controls.

Interpretation

A pinkish-brown color forms when homogentisic acid is present.

Reagents

1. *Copper Sulfate, 0.1%:* Dissolve 156 mg $CuSO_4 \cdot 5\ H_2O$ in 50 ml demineralized water and bring to volume in 100 ml volumetric flask.
2. *Sodium Hydroxide, 0.1 N:* Dissolve 400 mg NaOH in 80 ml demineralized water and bring to volume in 100 ml volumetric flask.

REFERENCES

Winsten, Seymour and Dalal, Fram R.: *Manual of Clinical Laboratory Procedures for Non-Routine Problems.* Cleveland, Chemical Rubber, 1972, p. 97.

Valmikinathan, K., and Verghese, N.: Simple colour reaction for alkaptonuria. *J Clin Pathol, 19*:200, 1966.

THIN-LAYER CHROMATOGRAPHY OF HOMOGENTISIC ACID

Principle

An ethyl acetate extract of urine is chromatographed on thin-layer sheets of silica gel.

Procedure

1. Acidify with concentrated HCl to pH 1 (pH paper) 2.5 ml catch urine sample (or twenty-four-hour collection) and standard solutions of gentisic and homogentisic acid. Add 0.7 g NaCl and mix.
2. In hood, add 4.0 ml ethyl acetate to 2.0 ml aliquots acidified sample and standards in respective 16 × 125 mm screw cap tubes and shake for 2.5 minutes.
3. Spot 20 μl aliquots of upper layers (ethyl acetate) on Eastman Chromagram silica gel sheet for thin-layer chromatography.
4. Develop with upper (benzene) layer of solvent until front rises 15 cm (~ two hour).
5. Air-dry sheet in hood fifteen minutes at room temperature.
6. In hood, spray with 1 N phenol reagent, followed by 10% sodium carbonate solution.
7. Compare mobilities of sample urine with those of standard solutions of gentisic and homogentisic acid.

Interpretation

Homogentisic acid is excreted by persons affected with alkaptonuria. Not present in normal urine, it is distinguished from gentisic acid by its slightly slower mobility. Gentisic acid, a salicylate derivative, may be excreted when taking aspirin, as, for example, by the patient with arthritis, one of the clinical signs of alkaptonuria.

Reagents

1. *Benzene: Acetic Acid: Water Solvent, 2:3:1:* On the day of test, combine 100 ml benzene, 150 ml acetic acid, 50 ml demineralized water. Mix well and let layers separate. Use upper (benzene) layer.
2. *Sodium Carbonate, 10%:* Dissolve 10 g Na_2CO_3 in 80 ml demineralized water. Dilute to 100 ml.
3. *Homogentisic Acid Standard Solution, 50 mg%:* Dissolve 5.0 mg homogentisic acid in 10 ml urine from a healthy adult.
4. *Homogentisic Acid Standard Solution, 100 mg%:* Dissolve 10.0 mg homgentisic acid in 10 ml urine from a healthy adult.
5. *Gentisic Acid Standard Solution, 50 mg%:* Dissolve 5 mg gentisic acid in 10 ml normal urine, as above.
6. *Gentisic Acid Standard Solution, 100 mg%:* Dissolve 10 mg gentisic acid in 10 ml normal urine, as above.
7. *Phenol Reagent, 1 N:* Add 15 ml Fisher phenol reagent 2 N to 15 ml demineralized water and mix.

REFERENCE

Feldman, J. M., and Bowman, J.: Urinary homogentisic acid: Determination by thin-layer chromatography. *Clin Chem, 19*:459, 1973.

CHAPTER 3

ORGANIC ACIDURIAS

PRIMARY HYPEROXALURIA

SOME patients with the rare, recessively inherited disease of primary hyperoxaluria form calcium oxalate kidney stones. Stones form early in life in Type I disease, glycolic aciduria, and patients die young from chronic renal failure and oxalate deposits in the tissues. A second type, L-glyceric aciduria, is less severe.

Glyoxylate accumulates, in the Type I form, is converted to oxalate and glycolate and excreted. The likely site of the defect is a block in the synergistic decarboxylation of glyoxylate to CO_2 and α-hydroxy-β-ketoadipate in the presence of α-ketoglutarate, i.e. deficiency of α-ketoglutarate: carboligase, an enzyme of liver, kidney, and spleen.

The origin of the hyperoxaluria is not clear in the Type II form. D-glyceric acid dehydrogenase, a leukocyte enzyme catalyzing serine metabolism, is defective, causing the accumulation of hydroxypyruvate, which, in turn, is converted to L-glyceric acid and excreted.

The two forms of primary hyperoxaluria can be distinguished by the excretory products and respective enzyme defects. Patients with Type I hyperoxaluria excrete glyoxylate and glycolic acid; those with Type II disease excrete L-glyceric acid. The hyperoxaluria of both types can be demonstrated by a screening method (p. 92) or by quantitation (p. 94, 97).

OXALIC ACID SCREENING

Principle

Oxalic acid in urine is distinguished from other organic acids by its relative immobility on one-dimensional paper chromatograms, developed with organic-acidic or organic-basic solvent systems, and bright Prussian blue staining reaction with ferrocyanide.

Procedure

1. Lyophilize 1.0 ml aliquots of catch urine and oxalic acid standards in concentrations of 10, 20, 40, and 60 mg% in 50% artificial urine.
2. Reconstitute and dissolve in 0.2 ml ethanol.
3. Apply total volumes to a sheet of Whatman No. 1 chromatography paper in 25λ aliquots, drying sheet between applications for about ten minutes and for one hour after final application at room temperature.
4. Equilibrate chromatography tank for thirty minutes with butanol-acetic acid-water solvent (in glass dish on tank floor). Saturate sheet with solvent by placing in equilibrated tank for thirty minutes. Add solvent to reservoir and develop overnight.
5. Remove sheet from tank, air-dry for an hour, and place in 70°C explosion-proof oven for five minutes.
6. Dip in potassium ferrocyanide reagent and air-dry on rack until sheet is stiff.
7. Dip in ferric ammonium sulfate reagent and air-dry on rack.
8. Note development of a blue spot or streak near origin within twenty minutes. Compare with standards. Color fades gradually.

Interpretation

Normal urine contains less than 10 mg oxalic acid per 100 ml.

Reagents

1. *Butanol:Acetic Acid:Water Solvent, 12:3:5:* Prepare as described on page 24.
2. *Potassium Ferrocyanide, 10%:* Dissolve 10 g potassium ferrocyanide in 100 ml demineralized water.
3. *Ferric Ammonium Sulfate in 70% Ethanol, 0.5%:* Dissolve 1

gram ferric ammonium sulfate in 40 ml demineralized water.
Add 147 ml ethanol (95%) and bring to 200 ml with demineralized water.

4. *Artificial Urine, 50%:* Combine 10 ml artificial urine, (p. 24) with 10 ml demineralized water.

5. *Oxalic Acid Stock Standard Solution, 4000 mg%:* Dissolve 40 mg oxalic acid in 1 ml demineralized water.

6. *Oxalic Acid Standard Solutions, 10, 20, 40, and 60 mg%:* Dilute the stock standard solution with 1 ml 50% artificial urine in aliquots of 15, 10, 5, and 2 1/2λ for concentrations of 60, 40, 20, and 10 mg%, respectively.

REFERENCE

Nordmann, J., and Nordmann, R.: Organic Acids. In Smith, Ivor (Ed.): *Chromatography and Electrophoretic Techniques,* 3rd Ed. New York, Wiley, 1969, Vol. I, pp. 342-363.

URINARY OXALATE

Principle

Urinary oxalic acid is measured as calcium oxalate, which is formed by precipitation with calcium chloride, dissolved in sulfuric acid, and titrated with potassium permanganate solution.

Procedure

1. Measure and record total volume of a twenty-four-hour urine sample, which has been preserved with 5 ml of concentrated HCl/1. Filter and pipette exactly 50 ml into 100 ml centrifuge tube.

2. Add 1 ml of brom-cresol purple aqueous solution and neutralize excess acid with 7.5 N ammonium hydroxide until solution becomes alkaline (changes from yellow to purple).

3. Acidify slightly with 6 N acetic acid to pH 5.0 to 5.2, using pH paper.

4. Precipitate oxalates with 2 ml 5% calcium chloride solution.

5. Mix thoroughly and let stand overnight at room temperature.
6. Centrifuge suspension twenty minutes at 3300 R.P.M.
7. Transfer precipitate to 5.0 ml centrifuge tube. Rinse tube with multiple small portions 0.35 N ammonium hydroxide. Combine rinsings with precipitate.
8. Centrifuge, remove supernatant fluid by pipette, and resuspend precipitate in 4 ml 0.35 N ammonium hydroxide.
9. Centrifuge as before, pipette off supernatant fluid and discard, invert tubes, and let drain several minutes.
10. Dissolve sedimented precipitate in 2 ml 1 N sulfuric acid and bring to 70°C in water bath.
11. Titrate with standardized $KMnO_4$ in 5 ml buret until solution remains pink for at least fifteen seconds. Titrate also blank tube containing 2.0 ml 1 N H_2SO_4 and standard tube containing 1 ml 0.01 N oxalic acid and 2 ml 1 N H_2SO_4. Subtract blank from standard and test sample volumes to obtain net volumes consumed. Calculate and record normality of standardized potassium permanganate. Compare normality with previous normality. If they differ by more than 0.0003, repeat standardization, using 5.0 ml 0.010 N oxalate.
12. Determine oxalic acid excretion by comparing amount of $KMnO_4$ required to oxidize equivalent weights of oxalic acid in sample with that of a known solution, as indicated next.

Calculations

1. Calculate normality of 0.01 N potassium permanganate standard from the equation:

$$N \times V = N_{ox} \times V_{ox} \text{ oxalic acid,}$$

substituting known values,

$$N_{ox} \times V_{ox} = 0.05 \text{ and } V = \text{volume titrated.}$$

2. Calculate weight of oxalic acid in urine sample titrated, from the equation:

$$\text{mg oxalic acid} = V \times N \ KMnO_4 \times 63.05 \text{ mg (equivalent weight}$$
$$\text{oxalic acid).}$$

3. Calculate daily excretion rate of oxalic acid from the formula:

$$\text{mg oxalic/day} = \text{mg oxalic acid/50 ml urine} \times 24 \text{ hr volume}$$

Reagents

1. *Hydrochloric Acid, Concentrated.*
2. *Brom-Cresol Purple Aqueous Solution, 0.04% w/v:* Dissolve 40 mg brom-cresol purple, sodium salt, in 100 ml demineralized water.
3. *Calcium Chloride, 5% w/v:* Dissolve 10 gm $CaCl_2 \cdot 2 H_2O$ in demineralized water and bring to volume in 200 ml volumetric flask.
4. *Ammonium Hydroxide, 0.35 N:* Add 2.3 ml concentrated ammonium hydroxide to 50 ml demineralized water in 100 ml volumetric flask and dilute to mark.
5. *Sulfuric Acid, 1 N:* Add 5.4 ml concentrated H_2SO_4 to 150 ml demineralized water in 500 ml Erlenmeyer flask and dilute to 200 ml in volumetric flask.
6. *Standard Oxalic Acid, 0.01N:* Dry sodium oxalate in oven at 100-105°C for twelve hours and equilibrate at room temperature in desiccator. Dissolve *exactly* 0.670 gm in demineralized water, add 5 ml concentrated sulfuric acid, and dilute to final volume in 1 liter volumetric flask. Store at 1 to 4°C.
7. *Potassium Permanganate, 0.01 N:* Dilute 0.1 N potassium permanganate tenfold with demineralized water. Let stand several days at room temperature in amber bottle before standardizing.
8. *Potassium Permanganate, Standardized:* Pipette (volumetric) exactly 5.0 ml 0.010 N oxalic acid standard into 50 ml Erlenmeyer flask; add 5 ml 1 N sulfuric acid. Heat to 70°C and titrate in water bath with 0.01 N potassium permanganate until solution remains pink for at least fifteen seconds. Also titrate blank composed of 5 ml 1 N sulfuric acid and 5 ml demineralized water. Subtract blank from standard to obtain net volume consumed.

REFERENCE

Archer, H. E., Dormer, A. E., Scowen, E. F. and Watts, R. W. E.: Studies on the urinary excretion of oxalate by normal subjects. *Clin Sci, 16*:405, 1957.

COLORIMETRIC METHOD FOR URINARY OXALATE

Principle

Urinary oxalate is precipitated as calcium oxalate, corrected for incomplete precipitation and measured indirectly by the extent of its interference with formation of the red complex, uranium (IV)-4-(2-pyridylazo) resorcinol.

Procedure

1. Record volume of twenty-four-hour urine collection preserved with 10 ml concentrated HCl (V_u). Freeze sample until assay, if necessary.
2. Filter 50 ml through Whatman No. 1 filter paper, adjust to pH 5.0 with concentrated and 4 M ammonium hydroxide solutions, and add 8 ml aliquots to three 12 ml graduated conical centrifuge tubes. If urine sample failed to give positive paper chromatographic screening test result (p. 92) (contained less than 0.6 mmole/1.) and oxalic acid level is still desired, add 0.4 ml 10 mmole/1 disodium oxalate solution (V_{Ox}).
3. Bring to 9 ml mark in graduated centrifuge tube with demineralized water.
4. Place tubes in boiling water bath; quickly add 1 ml 2.0% calcium chloride solution, using 1 ml syringe and 25-gauge needle to form jet stream (promotes mixing).
5. Heat ten minutes in bath, cool five minutes in tap water and one hour in ice water bath.
6. Centrifuge tubes fifteen minutes at 500 g.
7. Decant supernatant fluids and dry tube walls with cotton

swab.
8. Add 1.0 ml 1.0 M HCl and heat tubes ten minutes at 65°C to dissolve calcium oxalate precipitates.
9. Cool in tap water and adjust to original 9.0 ml volumes with demineralized water.
10. Add 0.1 ml portions of samples and standards to 3.0 ml working PAR reagent in 16 × 100 mm test tubes. Mix, transfer to cuvettes, and read fifteen minutes later at 515 nm.

Calculations

1. Plot standard curve of concentration of oxalate standards (mmoles) against absorption at 515 nm.
2. Obtain mmoles oxalate in total (8 ml) sample directly from standard curve (Ox_m).
3. Estimate mmoles oxalate excreted per twenty-four hours (Ox_t) from the regression formula for Ox_m (mx+b):

$$Ox_t = (Mx+b)_{Ox_m} \times \frac{V_u}{1000}, \text{ substituting}$$

from **Baadenhuijsen and Jansen's data:**

$$Ox_t = (1.14\ Ox_m + 0.156) \times \frac{V_u}{1000}$$

4. If V_{OX} is used (see Procedure step 2), subtract regression formula factor for V_{OX} (1.25), as follows:

$$Ox_t = (1.14\ Ox_m + 0.156 - 1.25\ V_{OX}) \times \frac{V_u}{1000}$$

Interpretation

Up to 0.53 mmoles or 46.6 mg oxalate are normally excreted per twenty-four hours. Patients who form stones, however, do no necessarily excrete oxalate in excess during the sampling period.

Reagents

1. *Ammonium Hydroxide, 4 M*: Dilute 50 ml concentrated

NH₄OH with demineralized water and bring to 100 ml in volumetric flask.

2. *Calcium Chloride, 2.0%*: Dissolve 2.0 gms $CaCl_2 \cdot 2 H_2O$ with demineralized water and dilute to 100 ml.

3. *HCl, 1 M*: Dilute 8.3 ml concentrated HCl with demineralized water in 100 ml volumetric flask.

4. *Formate Buffer, 0.100 M*: Combine 0.86 ml 88% formic acid and 90 ml demineralized water. Adjust to pH 3.7 with 10 N NaOH, added in drops. Bring to volume in 100 ml volumetric flask.

5. *Perchloric Acid, 1 M*: Dilute 14.3 ml 70% $HClO_4$ with demineralized water and bring to volume in 100 ml volumetric flask.

6. *Uranylnitrate, 1 mM*: Combine 5.02 g of $UO_2(NO_3) \cdot 6 H_2O$ with 10 ml 1 M perchloric acid. Bring to volume in 100 ml volumetric flask with demineralized water. Dilute 1:100 with demineralized water (1 mM).

7. *PAR-Reagent, 1 mM*: Dissolve 0.0215 g 4-(2-pyridylazo) resorcinol (PAR) and bring to 100 ml volume with dimethylformamide (DMF).

8. *Working PAR reagent*: Combine 1 part 1 mM uranylnitrate solution, 2 parts PAR-reagent, 5 parts formate buffer, 10 parts DMF, and 10 parts demineralized water.

9. *HCl, 0.11 M*: Dilute 0.91 ml concentrated HCl with demineralized water and bring to 100 ml in volumetric flask.

10. *Disodium Oxalate Standard Stock Solution, 10.0 mM*: Dissolve 0.134 g in 90 demineralized water and bring to 100 ml in volumetric flask. Mix.

11. *Disodium Oxalate Working Standard Solutions:* Combine the following:

Concentration (mM)	Stock Standard (ml)	0.11 M HCl (ml)
0.15	0.15	9.85 ml
0.30	0.30	9.7 ml
0.60	0.60	9.4 ml
0.90	0.90	9.1 ml
1.20	1.20	8.8 ml

REFERENCES

Baadenhuijsen, H., and Jansen, A. P.: Colorimetric determination of urinary oxalate recovered as calcium oxalate. *Clin Chim Acta, 62*:315, 1975.

Neas, R. E., and Guyon, J. C.: Indirect spectrophotometric determination of oxalate using uranium and 4-(2-pyridylazo) resorcinol. *Anal Chem, 44*:799, 1972.

OROTICACIDURIA

A few infants with primary hereditary oroticaciduria have been described. The clinical findings are physical and mental retardation, severe megaloblastic anemia which resists treatment with Vitamin B_{12} or folic acid, and gross excretion of orotic acid with crystalluria. Two of the patients survived and were maintained with oral uridine therapy.

There are two primary defects in red cell enzymes: deficiencies of orotidylic pyrophosphorylase and orotidylic decarboxylase. The enzymic blocks interfere with the formation of pyrimidine nucleotides, and thus cell functions requiring a continual supply of pyrimidine nucleotide products, e.g. myelination (lecithin), cell division (nucleic acids), and red cell maturation. Secondarily, high concentrations of orotic acid in the tissues depress the formation of the low density lipoproteins required for myelination.

The oroticaciduria is detected in a screening test (p. 100) and quantitited (p. 100). It should be distinguished from acquired oroticaciduria produced by 6-azauridine and the oroticaciduria in ornithine carbamyl transferase deficiency.

The enzyme defects are demonstrable in red cells and cultured fibroblasts.

SCREENING AND QUANTITATIVE TESTS FOR URINARY OROTIC ACID

Principle

Urinary orotic acid is brominated, reduced to barbituric acid by ascorbic acid, and complexed with p-dimethyl-aminobenzaldehyde (Ehrlich's reagent). The interference by urinary pigments is minimized by dilution in samples from homozygous persons (quantitative) and by comparing absorption at two wave lengths in samples from carriers and persons of unknown phenotype (screening).

Screening Procedure

1. Mix 0.5 ml aliquot catch urine sample (fresh or frozen) with 2.5 ml 0.2 M potassium citrate buffer, pH 2.5, in 10 ml screw capped test tube. Add 3.0 ml citrate buffer (alone) to blank tube.
2. In hood, add 0.5 ml saturated bromine water to both tubes, mix by inversion, and let stand one minute.
3. Add 1.0 ml 5% ascorbic acid, mix, and let stand two minutes.
4. Add 2.0 ml 2.5% p-dimethylaminobenzaldehyde solution, mix, and let stand ninety minutes. Measure optical densities at 412 mμ and 480 mμ.
5. Express orotic acid as the ratio, O.D. $\frac{480}{412}$ nm.

Quantitative Procedure

1. Bring 0.01, 0.05, and 0.10 ml aliquots of the urine sample and orotic acid standard to 3.0 ml volumes with citrate buffer. Prepare blank as above.
2. Add bromine water, ascorbic acid, etc., as above.
3. Plot O.D. of standard solutions against orotic acid concentration. Estimate concentration of orotic acid in samples from the standard curve and express in mg/ml.

Interpretation

Urinary orotic acid ratio, O.D. $\frac{480}{412}$, is 0.6 or less in normal persons, at least 0.6 in heterozygous, and greater in homozygous persons. Orotic acid concentrations in homozygous persons range from 1 to 3.6 mg/ml urine.

Reagents

1. *Potassium Citrate Buffer, 0.2 M, pH 2.5:* Dissolve 16.2 g potassium citrate (monohydrate) in 225 ml demineralized water. Adjust to pH 2.5 with concentrated HC1, and bring to volume in 250 ml volumetric flask with demineralized water. Store in plastic bottle at room temperature.
2. *Bromine Water (Saturated at Room Temperature):* Add 5 ml bromine to 250 ml demineralized water. Store in brown bottle at room temperature.
3. *Ascorbic acid, 5%:* Dissolve 2.50 g ascorbic acid in demineralized water and bring to volume in 50 ml volumetric flask. Store frozen in 7 ml aliquots in brown plastic bottles.
4. *2.5% P-Dimethyl Aminobenzaldehyde in N-Propanol:* Dissolve 6.25 g p-dimethyl aminobenzaldehyde in 225 ml N-propanol. Dilute to 250 ml in volumetric flask with N-propanol.
5. *Normal Control:* Catch sample of urine from healthy person, freeze and store at -20°C in aliquots of 1.0 ml.
6. *Screening Control:* 4 mg orotic acid in 100 ml of normal urine. Store at -20°C in aliquots of 1.0 ml.
7. *Orotic Acid Standard, 1.0 mg/ml:* Dissolve 50.0 mg orotic acid in 40 ml demineralized water. Dilute to 50 ml in volumetric flask with demineralized water. Store at -20°C in 2 ml quantities in stoppered 12×75 mm test tubes.

REFERENCES

Rogers, L. E., and Porter, F. S.: Hereditary orotic aciduria II. A urinary screening test, *Pediatrics, 42*:423, 1968.
MacLoed, P., Mackenzie, S., and Scriver, C. R.: Partial ornithine carbamyl transferase deficiency: an inborn error of the urea cycle presenting as orotic aciduria in a male infant. *Can Med Assoc J, 107*:405, 1972.

CHAPTER 4

THE GALACTOSEMIAS

NEWBORNS with "classical" galactosemia are usually intolerant to milk. They fail to thrive, form cataracts, and die from liver failure or overwhelming infection. Occasional survivors are blind and retarded. A less catastrophic form of galactosemia causes early blindness from congenital cataract. The various clinical signs recede when the infant is given a galactose-free diet, usually by means of a milk substitute.

Both diseases reflect heritable defects in the ability to metabolize galactose, which accumulates in blood and overflows in urine. Galactose-1-phosphate uridyl transferase is deficient in the classical form of galactosemia, and galactokinase is missing in the milder disease.

Many normal persons, furthermore, carry a different, less active form of the transferase. The variant enzyme in itself is usually harmless. In combination with the mutant gene for the classical form of galactosemia, however, the infant who also carries the Duarte variant of enzyme may have serious clinical signs.

Carriers are identified biochemically by subnormal activities of the respective enzymes.

Galactosuria occurs when the renal threshold for galactose in blood is reached. Glucosuria may be present also, although the vomiting, poorly-nourished infant often displays neither.

Newborns with the transferase-deficient form of galactosemia are now easily found through screening programs for the transferase defect, as described on p. 109. Carriers and infants homozygous for the Duarte variant are not dependably detected by the method, however. Absolute levels of the enzyme are measured by fluorometric methods (p. 110) and are carried out to confirm screening test results. Quantitative methods are also needed to identify the carriers and distinguish variants (p. 113).

An additional means of distinguishing variant forms and their mixtures is by electrophoretic demonstration of multiple forms of the transferase, or isozymes, as described on p. 115.

The galactokinase-deficient form of galactosemia is detected by an isotopic assay for the kinase in whole blood (p. 126). A new screening test for the specific enzyme defect is described within; otherwise screening tests rely on demonstrating excessive blood galactose.

Urinary reducing sugar that is Ames Clinitest positive and Ames Clinistix® negative is assumed to be galactose. Galactosuria is identifiable by paper chromatography (p. 104) and recently by Ames Galactostix®. Urinary galactose concentrations are measured by an assay with galactose dehydrogenase (p. 106).

GALACTOSE-1-PHOSPHATE URIDYL TRANSFERASE DEFICIENCY

PAPER CHROMATOGRAPHY OF SUGARS FOR GALACTOSURIA

Principle

Galactose and other sugars in serum, plasma, or urine can be identified by paper chromatography in an ethyl acetate, pyridine, and water solvent system, stained with silver nitrate.

Procedure

1. Label chromatography sheet at origins for eight test samples (blood or urine) or respective standards, 3/4 inches apart.
2. Apply 10 μl aliquots of reconstituted urine samples and urine standards at alternate origins.
3. Punch blood samples and blood standards with 1/4-inch punch, corresponding to size of origin hole.
4. Insert blood sample and blood standard discs with forceps in alternate origin holes. Firm them into position by rubbing briskly with a forceps' handle on a plastic ruler held against them.
5. Place solvent in beakers or glass dishes in chromatography tank and equilibrate for two to three hours.

6. Slip glass rod under second fold of chromatography sheet, clip edges to rod, hang in chromatography tank, and dip folded ends into trough.
7. Pour 90 to 100 ml solvent into trough, saturating folded ends. Weight folded ends below solvent surface with glass bar.
8. Seal lid with silicone grease and develop overnight (sixteen to seventeen hours).
9. Dry sheets in hood one hour.
10. Pass sheets through silver nitrate stain in glass dish three to five times. Dry in hood thirty minutes.
11. Rinse and fix by passing sheets three to five times through (1) sodium hydroxide in ethanol, (2) water, (3) Ansco Surefix,® and (4) water.
12. Suspend papers and read while wet.
13. Identify sugars and estimate concentrations by matching spots and densities with those of sugar standards.

Reagents

1. *Battery Jar or Chromatography Tank, 23 x 11-inches*
2. *Whatman 3MM Chromatography Paper, 22 1/2 x 7-inches*: Crease sheet across width by folding 3/8-inches and 1 1/4-inches from top edge. Draw line across sheet, 1 inch below second fold, and mark positions for eight samples, 3/4-inch apart, with outer samples 7/8-inch in from the side edges. Punch holes at marked positions with 1/4-inch punch.
3. *Ethyl Acetate, Pyridine, Water Solvent; 60:25:20 V/V*: At the time of use mix the following for three to four chromatography sheets: 180 ml ethyl acetate; 75 ml pyridine, 60 ml demineralized water.
4. *Silver Nitrate Stain*: 0.1 ml saturated $AgNO_2$ in water and 100 ml acetone.
5. *0.5% Sodium Hydroxide in Ethanol*: Dissolve 0.5 gm NaOH in 100 ml ethanol overnight in Erlenmeyer flask in hood. (100 ml for each sheet)
6. *Reducing Agent*: Ansco Surefix, or similar photographic fixer, 200 ml. May reuse until it becomes turbid and darkens.
7. *Whole Blood, Plasma, or Serum Samples*: Spot Schleicher

and Schuell paper 903 with *fresh* sample until area is saturated. Dry for at least an hour.

8. *Urine Samples*: Estimate creatinine concentration in 1 ml aliquot by Jaffe reaction (p. 25). Lyophilize 2 ml aliquot to dryness (approximately one hour), reconstitute with 2 ml or less demineralized water, so that 10 μl sample contains 15 μg creatinine, as indicated below:

$$\text{ml} = \frac{\text{creatinine concentration (mg/100 ml)} \times 2}{150}$$

9. *Blood Standards*; Saturate 3 MM filter paper cards with fresh normal whole blood only, for glucose standard; whole blood containing 50 mg per 100 ml galactose (5 μl 10 mg galactose per 100 μl demineralized water solution in 1 ml whole blood) for galactose standard; whole blood containing 50 mg per 100 ml fructose blood, for fructose standard. Dry and store at -20°C.

10. *Urine Standards*: Dissolve 25 mg amounts of galactose, glucose, and their respective amines in 25 ml aliquots of normal urine (100 mg per 100 ml). Dilute 1:1, 1:1.5, and 1:4 with normal urine to give working standard solutions of 50, 40, and 20 mg per 100 ml, respectively. Dispense in 0.5 ml aliquots and store at -20°C until used. Do not refreeze.

Interpretation

Normal blood contains undetectable amounts of galactose by this method, and urine normally contains trace amounts only.

REFERENCE

Haworth, J. C.: A simple chromatographic screening test for the detection of galactosemia in newborn infants. *Pediatrics, 39*:608, 1967.

QUANTITATION OF GALACTOSURIA BY GALACTOSE DEHYDROGENASE

Principle

Urinary galactose is oxidized when galactose dehydrogenase is added to the sample, catalyzing the transfer of hydrogen ions to the nicotinamide adenine dinucleotide (NAD-NADH) system. The reaction:

$$\beta\text{-D-Galactose} + \text{NAD} \rightleftharpoons \gamma\text{-D-galactonolactone} + \text{NADH} + \text{H}^+$$

proceeds to completion under alkaline conditions as the lactone is hydrolyzed. The oxidation of galactose is measured as the increase in optical density at 340 mμ during reduction of NAD to NADH.

Procedure

1. Add 2 ml TRIS HCl buffer to pH 8.6 and 0.1 ml NAD solution to 0.2 ml of urine sample and control (25 mg per 100 ml) (galactose standard) in respective 10 x 75 mm round cuvettes. Mix.
2. Measure absorption at 340 mμ several times during a two-minute period to assure stability. Record on arithmetical graph as zero time O.D.
3. Begin oxidation by adding 10λ galactose dehydrogenase to both tubes. Mix by inverting and immediately start measuring and recording optical densities. Measure O.D. for twelve minutes at one minute intervals.
4. Subtract zero time from final (plateau) optical densities. If O.D. difference of the sample is less than 0.15, galactose is absent or present in trace amounts only.
5. If O.D. difference of sample is more than 1.0, dilute sample at least 1:1 with demineralized water and repeat incubation.
6. If O.D. difference of sample or diluted sample is less than 1.0, but greater than 0.15, incubate the entire series of galactose standards and obtain O.D. differences.
7. Plot arithmetic graph showing increase in O.D. with increasing concentrations of galactose.

Calculation

Estimate concentration of galactose in sample by comparing O.D. difference with those of standards. Express as mg galactose/100 ml urine.

Interpretation

Normal infants two weeks old or less may excrete up to 25 mg galactose per 100 ml; otherwise the normal concentration does not exceed 10 mg per 100 ml.

Reagents

1. *β-Galactose Dehydrogenase (D-galactose:NAD oxidoreductase) (E. C. No. 1.1.1.48), 2mg/ml.*
2. *NAD, 10 mg/ml:* Prepare 1 ml suspension in demineralized water just before use.
3. *TRIS-HCl Buffer, 0.1 M TRIS, pH 8.6:* On the day of test, dissolve 2.42 gm TRIS in 80 ml demineralized water, adjust to pH 8.6 with 1 N HCl, and bring to 100 ml volume in volumetric flask.
4. *Galactose Standard Solution, 100 mg/100 ml:* Dissolve 100 mg galactose in demineralized water and bring to volume in 100 ml volumetric flask. Age for at least four hours at 37°C or for three to four days at 4°C to promote equilibrium between reacting and nonreacting forms. On the day of test, prepare control by diluting stock standard to give 25 mg per 100 ml solution.
5. *Galactose Working Standards:* If necessary, on the day of test dilute the stock standard to give a series of solutions containing 50, 25, 12.5, and 6.25 mg galactose per 100 ml.

REFERENCES

Wallenfels, K., and Kurz, G.: β-D-galactose dehydrogenase from *Pseudomonas saccharophilia,* in Wood, Willis A. (Ed.): *Methods in Enzymology Carbohydrate Metabolism,* Vol. IX. New York, Acad Pr, 1966, p. 112.
Beutler, Ernest: *Red Cell Metabolism.* New York, Grune, 1971, pp. 86-87.
Bickel, H.: Mellituria. *J Pediatr, 59:*641, 1961.
Dahlquist, A., Gamstrop, I., and Madsen, H.: A patient with hereditary galactokinase deficiency. *Acta Pediatr Scand, 59:*669, 1970.

ASSAYS FOR GALACTOSE-1-PHOSPHATE URIDYL TRANSFERASE: FLUORESCENT SPOT TEST

Principle

The reaction catalyzed by the transferase:

Uridine diphosphoglucose (UDPG) + Galactose-1-P-$\rightarrow$ UDPGalactose + Glucose-1-P

is observed indirectly by observing the development of fluorescence in dried aliquots of reaction mixture. During incubation with transferase the nonfluorescing coenzyme, nicotinamide adenine dinucleotide phosphate (NADP), is reduced to the fluorescent form, NADPH, during a series of conversions in which the transferase reaction is coupled to the indicator through enzymic transformations of the phosphogluconate pathway.

Procedure

1. Spot Schleicher and Schuell 903 filter paper (PKU card) with blood from finger or heel pricks until areas are saturated. Air dry.
2. Punch 1/4 inch discs from test and control samples and place in cups of a Linbro Disposo Tray.
3. Overlay with 0.2 ml reaction mixture, mix gently with plain microhematocrit tube, remove aliquot, and drop on prelined and prenumbered No. 1 Whatman filter paper sheet.
4. Incubate tray in 37°C water bath or incubator.
5. Remove aliquots and spot at three hours and again at eighteen hours, if necessary.
6. Dry spots for ten minutes or longer at room temperature and observe fluorescence with Ultra Violet Products' long-wave ultra violet lamp. Record degree of fluorescence as bright, dull, or black (see Color Illustration 1).

Interpretation

Brightly fluorescing aliquots of reaction mixtures after three hours' incubation indicate normal transferase activity. Dull fluorescence suggests subnormal levels or partial inactivation of transferase by artifact. Black spots indicate no activity; if clinical signs have appeared, treatment should be begun immediately and confirmatory studies completed as soon as possible.

Reagents

1. *TRIS Buffer, 0.75 M, pH 8.0*: Dissolve 9.1 g TRIS (hydroxymethyl) aminomethane in 75 ml demineralized water. Adjust to pH 8.0 with acetic acid and bring to volume in 100 ml volumetric flask.
2. *Reaction Mixture*: (for 300 tests — 60 ml). Dissolve the following anhydrous weights (mg) in 20 ml demineralized water:

Uridine-5′-diphosphoglucose (UDPG)	11.6
α-D-Galactose-1-phosphate	36.3
NADP	30.3
EDTA	3.0

   Add 8 ml saturated digitonin and 20 ml TRIS buffer, 0.75 M, pH 8.0. Dispense in 3 ml amounts (enough for fifteen tests) in 10 ml screw-capped test tubes and store at -20°C.
3. *Negative Control*: Normal blood spotted on PKU card.
4. *Positive Control*: Normal blood spotted on PKU card and autoclaved to destroy enzyme activity.

REFERENCE

Beutler, E., and Baluda, M.: A simple spot screening test for galactosemia. *J Lab Clin Med, 68*:137, 1966.

ASSAYS FOR GALACTOSE-1-PHOSPHATE URIDYL TRANSFERASE: FLUOROMETRY

Principle

As in the fluorescent spot test (p. 109), transferase activity is indicated by the development of fluorescence during reduction of NADP to NADPH in reactions coupled through enzymic conversions of the phosphogluconate pathway.

Procedure

1. Turn on fluorometer and spectrophotometer at least one hour before use.
2. Lyse red cells in about 0.1 ml of whole blood by freezing and thawing three times in a dry ice-alcohol bath. Samples collected in ACD (acid-citrate-dextrose solution) may be stored for up to four weeks before lysis; if collected in heparin or EDTA, store for up to one week only.
3. Add 0.1 ml reaction mixture to four 100 x 6 mm tubes and equilibrate in a 37°C water bath for three to five minutes. (Add 10λ working G-6-PD (glucose-6-phosphate dehydrogenase) solution to tubes containing samples from G-6-PD deficient patients.)
4. Add 10λ saline to blank, note the time and, at thirty-second intervals, add 10λ of hemolyzed sample to remaining tubes. Mix by gentle tapping and incubate at 37°C.
5. Stop reactions exactly thirty minutes later by diluting 20λ aliquots incubation mixtures in 4 ml phosphate buffer. Mix.
6. Measure fluorescence (F) in Turner 110 fluorometer in 10 mm round Turner cuvettes against blank set at zero, with Corning 7-60 primary filter and No. 2A Turner secondary filter. Record F or No. 1 aperture. The diluted hemolysates are stable for several hours.
7. Obtain hemoglobin concentrations from optical densities of the same solutions at 410 mμ in 12 by 75 mm tubes with blank set at zero.

Calculations

1. Express enzyme activity (E) in units from the formula:

$$E = \frac{\text{fluorescence (F)} \times \text{calibration factor (C)}}{\text{Absorbance (A)}}$$

2. Calibrate the fluorometer for NADPH fluorescence every six months as follows:
   a. Establish concentration of NADPH in a solution containing approximately 1 mg/ml by measuring optical density at

340 nm in a Beckman DU-2 spectrophotometer, as follows:
1) Measure O.D. of blank in a 1 ml cuvette containing 0.85 ml TRIS-HCl buffer and 0.10 ml water against an air blank. Record as A_O.
2) Measure O.D. again after adding 0.050 ml NADPH solution and inverting to mix. Record as A_1.
3) Calculate molarity (mM) of NADPH solution as

$$mM = \frac{A_1 - A_O}{0.311}$$

b. Establish fluorescence constant for a standard solution of NADPH (1 μM), as follows:
1) Measure fluorescence of 0.25 μM , 0.50 μM, 0.75 μM, 1.0 μM, and 1.25 μM solutions of NADPH in 0.01 M potassium phosphate buffer in Turner fluorometer against a buffer blank, using primary filter Corning 7-60 and secondary filter Turner No. 2A.
2) Plot curve on arithmetic graph paper. Record fluorescence of a 1 μM solution on the curve as F_1.
3. Calibrate spectrophotometer for hemoglobin absorbance at six-month intervals or less, as follows:
   a. Estimate concentration of hemoglobin in blood by optical density of cyanmethemoglobin at 540 nm, as follows:
   1) Add 0.02 ml frozen and thawed hemolysate from freshly drawn normal blood to two tubes containing 5.0 ml cyanmethemoglobin reagent.
   2) Add 0.02 ml Hycel hemoglobin controls to 5.0 ml cyanmethemoglobin reagent.
   3) Measure $O.D._{540nm}$ of hemolysates, controls, and Hycel cyanmethemoglobin standard. Plot standard curve of O.D. versus hemoglobin concentration. Express hemoglobin concentration of normal hemolysate in g/l.
   b. Establish absorbance constant for a standard solution of hemoglobin, as follows:
   1) Measure $O.D._{410}$ of 1:100, 1:200, and 1:400 dilutions of standardized normal blood (0.1 ml in 1 ml of 0.133% digitonin) in 0.01 M potassium phosphate buffer in Coleman spectrophotometer, using buffer as blank.

2) Plot curve of O.D. versus g/l. Record optical density of 0.1 g/liter solution on the curve as A_1.
3) Calculate calibration factor (C) from the formula:

$$C = \frac{10 \times A_1}{F_1}$$

4) Adjust normal values accordingly.

Interpretation

Normal children and adult blood contains from 19 to 29 units/gm Hgb.

Homozygotes of classical galactosemia usually have no red cell transferase activity. Carriers have half-normal activity and are distinguished by pedigree and isozyme studies from persons homozygous for the variant, who also have about half-normal activity. Carriers of the Duarte variant have about three-fourths normal activity. Carriers of both forms, i.e. genetic compounds of the classical and Duarte variant have less activity than carriers of the classical form. Enzyme levels in infants homozygous for the Duarte variant or with the phenotype of the genetic compound may rise from those at birth.

If low activities are found in patients who might also be deficient in glucose-6-phosphate dehydrogenase, assay the sample for the dehydrogenase. If G-6-PD-deficient, repeat the transferase assay, with reaction mixtures enriched with 10λ of working G-6-PD enzyme solution.

Reagents for Calibrations

1. *TRIS-HCl Buffer, 1M, pH 8.0*: Dissolve 12.1 g Trizma® base in 80 ml demineralized water. Adjust to pH 8.0 with 1 N HCl and bring to volume in 100 ml volumetric flask.
2. *NADPH Solution (fresh)*: Dissolve approximately 2.5 mg NADPH in 2.5 ml demineralized water. Use quickly as NADPH is very unstable. Keep in dark when not in use.
3. *Hycel Cyanmethemoglobin Reagent*: Dilute content of vial to 1000 ml with demineralized water.

4. *Hycel Cyanmethemoglobin Standard*
5. *Hycel Hemoglobin Controls*
6. *Digitonin, 0.133%:* Dissolve 67 mg digitonin in 50 ml demineralized water.
7. *Potassium Phosphate Buffer, 0.01 M, pH 7.4:* Dissolve 1.41 gm K_2HPO_4 and 0.26 gm KH_2PO_4 in 800 ml demineralized water. Adjust to pH 7.4, if necessary, and bring to volume in 1 liter volumetric flask. Store at room temperature.

Reagents for Assay

1. *Potassium Phosphate Buffer, 0.01 M, pH 7.4*: As above.
2. *TRIS-Acetate Buffer, 0.75 M, pH 8*: Dissolve 9.1 g TRIS (hydroxymethyl aminomethane) in 75 ml demineralized water. Adjust to pH 8.0 with glacial acetic acid and dilute to volume in 100 ml volumetric flask. May be stored at 4°C for several weeks. Check pH before use.
3. *Digitonin, Saturated*: Dissolve 10 mg digitonin in 10 ml demineralized water until saturated. Filter and store in 1 ml aliquots at -20°C.
4. *Disodium EDTA, 27 mM:* Dissolve 50 mg EDTA · 2 H_2O in 5 ml demineralized water. Store at 0.5 ml aliquots at -20°C.
5. *Uridine-5′-diphosphoglucose (UDPG), 10 mM*: Dissolve 68.2 mg UDPG · 4 H_2O in 10 ml demineralized water. Store in 1 ml aliquots at -20°C.
6. *Galactose-1-PO₄, 27 mM*: Dissolve 115 mg galactose-1-PO₄ · 5 H_2O in 10 ml demineralized water. Store in 1 ml aliquots at -20°C.
7. *NADP, 6 mM:* Dissolve 24.6 mg NADP · 3 H_2O in 5 ml demineralized water. *Make fresh daily.*
8. *Magnesium Chloride, 0.1 M*: Dissolve 101 mg $MgCl_2$·6 H_2O in 5 ml demineralized water. Store in 0.5 ml aliquots at -20°C.
9. *Reaction Mixture (for sixty tests)*:

Reagent	Volume (ml)
UDPG, 10 mM	0.6
Galactose-1-PO₄, 27 mM	0.6
NADP, 6 mM	0.8

TRIS-acetate Buffer, 0.75 M, pH 8.0	2.0
Saturated digitonin	0.8
Disodium EDTA, 27 mM	0.09
MgCl₂, 0.1 M	0.13
Demineralized water	1.00

The reaction mixture may be stored for up to one week at -20°C.

10. *Control*: Fresh, normal blood, heparinized.
11. *Sodium Citrate Buffer, 0.005 M, pH 7.5*: Dissolve 52.6 mg citric acid · H_2O in 40 ml demineralized water. Adjust to pH 7.5 with 0.3 M Na_2HPO_4 (4.3 g per 100 ml water) and bring to volume in a 50 ml volumetric flask with demineralized water.
12. *G-6-PD Stock Enzyme*: Dissolve 250 units of Sigma® glucose-6-phosphate dehydrogenase (G-6-PD) in 2.5 ml citrate buffer, 0.005 M, pH 7.5, as indicated on the vial.
13. *Working G-6-PD Solution (0.004 Units/10λ)*: Dilute 10λ stock enzyme with 2.5 ml demineralized water.

REFERENCE

Beutler, E., and Mitchell, M.: New rapid method for estimation of red cell galactose-1-phosphate uridyl transferase activity, *J Lab Clin Med,* 72:527, 1968.

ASSAYS FOR GALACTOSE-1-PHOSPHATE URIDYL TRANSFERASE: ISOZYMES BY STARCH GEL ELECTROPHORESIS

Principle

Structural variants of galactose-1-phosphate uridyl transferase, or isozymes, have been identified by electrophoretic mobility. Although the mutation site is not known, apparently molecular changes cause a change in net electric charge of the enzyme protein. The isozymes separate during electrophoresis on horizontal starch gels and are localized by staining. The stain consists of a reaction mixture of substrate, coenzymes, and auxiliary enzymes of the phosphogluconate pathway and an NADP-NADPH "tag." During incubation the indicator is reduced from nonfluorescing NADP to the fluorescent NADPH form.

Procedure

1. Five or six hours before use, prepare gel by adding 250 ml gel buffer to 29 g Connaught starch in 500 ml filtering flask over low heat, stirring at slow speed. When bubbles of approximately 2 to 3 mm diameter form at the bottom, remove flask from heat, reduce pressure with water aspirator until suspension boils, and boil for exactly one minute. Pour starch into tray (15 × 21 cm glass plate with sides made of 6 mm thick plexiglass rods) and cool to room temperature for an hour. Wrap tray tightly with thin plastic and store at 4°C until used (within twelve hours).

2. Remove gel from 4°C storage and unwrap. Add 1 liter electrophoresis buffer to the two buffer compartments of electrophoresis chamber at 4°C, attach leads to power supply, and place a 4 1/2 × 5-inch wick of Whatman 3 MM filter paper in each compartment.

3. Make slots in gel with spatula, one for each sample, 8 mm wide, and 1 1/2-inch from cathode end of gel. Saturate Whatman 3 MM paper, 8 × 4-mm, with sample hemolysate and place in slot with spatula forceps.

4. Place gel plate across buffer compartment at 4°C with the sample origins toward cathode. Connect wick and apply constant current of 35 ma for eighteen hours.

5. After first half hour, blot gel at sample origins. Cover gel with a thin sheet of firm plastic.

6. Prepare solution A and keep in water bath at 40°C until used (in one to two hours).

7. Prepare solution B and keep at 4°C until used.

8. Stop electrophoresis, remove gel from 4°C, uncover, and remove plexiglas rods from sides and cathode end of gel.

9. Cut off cathode end of gel along line of sample origins; cut off same width at anode end.

10. Place long, 3 mm thick, plexiglas rods firmly against both long edges of gel to regulate thickness during slicing. Cover gel with thin plastic sheet. Slice through gel with large kitchen knife, holding knife firmly at both ends, pulling toward body with slow, even motion. Place upper half of gel in a plastic tray adjacent to gel plate by inverting it, end over end,

holding the cut surface in place with knife and supporting plastic-covered surface with hand. Slide gel, cut surface up, onto tray by tilting plastic sheet toward body and pushing gel carefully with knife downward onto tray.

11. Remove 3 mm plexiglas rods and replace with 6 mm rods on both sides and both ends of both gels.

12. Prepare reagent gel by mixing quickly equal volumes (15 ml) of solutions A and B. Immediatley pour over cut surfaces of gels. Place moist paper towels at both ends of the gels, cover with plastic trays taped to bottoms, and let stand five minutes for solidification. Incubate at 37°C for forty-five minutes. Examine for pattern in Ultraviolet Products Chromato-Vue,® using Ultra-violet Products Mineralight® and compare with controls. Leave at room temperature and observe periodically for one hour.

Reagents

1. *Glycine-EDTA Gel Buffer, 0.05 M, pH 8.0*: Dissolve 0.94 g glycine and 0.28 g EDTA in about 200 ml demineralized water, with stirring. Add 0.05 ml β-mercaptoethanol. Adjust to pH 8.0 with 1.0 N sodium hydroxide (about 1.2 ml) and bring to volume in 250 ml volumetric flask.

2. *Hemolysates*: Centrifuge whole blood sample at 3000 R.P.M., 4°C, for ten minutes and discard serum. Wash packed red cells three times with one volume 0.85% NaCl, centrifuging between washes. Freeze final pack of red cells in dry ice-alcohol bath for fifteen minutes. Just before use, thaw and add one volume demineralized water to make 50% hemolysate.

3. *TRIS, 0.5 M, pH 8.0*: Dissolve 121.2 g Trizma base in 2 liters demineralized water. Adjust to pH 8.0 with 1 N HCl (8.6 ml concentrated HCl/100 ml solution). Store at 4°C for up to two months.

4. *Sodium Chloride, 0.5 M*: Dissolve 58.4 g sodium chloride in demineralized water. Dilute to volume in 2 liter volumetric flask. Store at 4°C for up to two months.

5. *EDTA, 0.03M*: Dissolve 22.2 g EDTA, disodium salt, in 1800

ml demineralized water. Adjust to pH 7 with 1 N NaOH (4 g/100 ml). Bring to volume in 2-liter volumetric flask. Store at 4°C for up to two months.

6. *TRIS-EDTA Electrophoresis Buffer, 0.05 M, pH 8.0*: Combine the following: 200 ml each of 0.5 M TRIS, 0.5 M sodium chloride, and 0.03 M EDTA. Add 1200 ml demineralized water and 0.42 ml β-mercaptoethanol. Adjust to pH 8.0 with 1 N HCl or 1 NaOH and bring to volume in 2-liter volumetric flask.

7. *Glycine Buffer, 1.0 M, pH 8.7*: Dissolve 7.5 g glycine in 80 ml demineralized water, with stirring. Adjust to pH 8.7 with 1 N NaOH and bring to volume in 100 ml volumetric flask.

8. *Staining Solution A*: In a 125 ml Erlenmeyer flask, combine 2.7 g Connaught starch, 5.0 ml 1.0 M glycine buffer pH 8.7, and 35 ml demineralized water. Heat with stirring until mixture is uniform in consistency. Hold at 40°C in water until used for reagent gel.

9. *Staining Solution B:* Combine the following in a 50 ml Erlenmeyer flask:

NADP	20.1 mg
Galactose-1-phosphate	10.9 mg
Uridine-5′-diphosphoglucose	8.6 mg
Magnesium chloride	32.5 mg
Phosphoglucomutase*	20 λ (2 mg/1 ml)
Glucose-6-phosphate dehydrogenase*	20 λ (5 mg/ml)
6-Phosphogluconate dehydrogenase*	20 λ (5 mg/ml)
Glucose-1,6-diphosphate	5 λ (10 mg/100λ)

Mix and hold at 4°C. Just before slicing the gel, add 0.8 ml β-mercaptoethanol (0.2 ml/10 ml) and 14.4 ml cold (4°C) demineralized water. Mix well.

10. *Controls*: Fresh human blood of known isozyme pattern.

Interpretation

The electrophoretic pattern of normal transferase consists of a single diffuse band of isozyme anodal to that of hemoglobin A. The Duarte transferase variant moves slightly faster than the normal. Homozygotes of either type have single-banded patterns of isozymes of the respective mobility; heterozygotes of the clas-

*Reagents available from Boehringer-Mannheim Corporation, New York, N.Y.

sical type of galactosemia have normal transferase isozyme but less of it than normal homozygotes; heterozygotes of the Duarte variant have two-banded patterns of normal and Duarte enzymes (see Figure 6); carriers of both the mutant gene for classical galactosemia and the Duarte variant have single-banded patterns

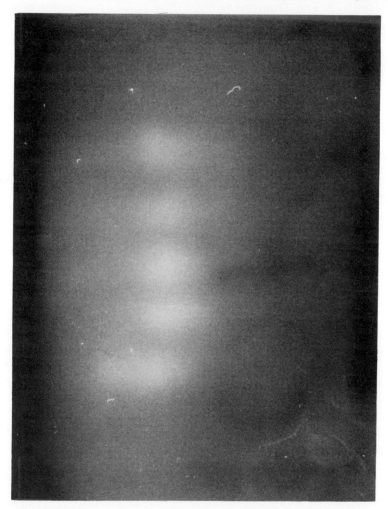

Figure 6. Photograph of fluorescence of red cell galactose-1-phosphate uridyl transferase isozymes on starch gel. Phenotypes are (from top to bottom): normal/Duarte heterozygous; classical galactosemia heterozygous (rows 2, 3 and 4); normal homozygous.

resembling the Duarte homozygote. The homozygote of classical galactosemia, of course, has no isozyme pattern.

The interpretation of isozyme pattern augments the result of the quantitative assay of transferase activity in assessing phenotypes of heterozygotes of the classical form, genetic compounds of the classical, and Duarte variant forms and homozygotes of the Duarte variant.

REFERENCES

Ng, W. G., Bergren, W. R., Fields, M., and Donnell, G. N.: An improved electrophoretic procedure for galactose-1-phosphate uridyl transferase: demonstration of multiple activity bands with the Duarte variant. *Biochem Biophys Res Commun, 37*:354, 1969.

Bissbort, S., and Kömpf, J.: Population genetics of red cell galactose-1-phosphate-uridyl-transferase (EC:2.7.7.12). Gene frequencies in southwestern Germany. *Humangenetik, 17*:79, 1972.

Kompf, J., Personal Communication, 1973.

ASSAYS FOR GALACTOSE-1-PHOSPHATE URIDYL TRANSFERASE: UDPG CONSUMPTION METHOD

Principle

Galactose-1-phosphate uridyl transferase catalyzes the conversion of phosphorylated galactose to phosphorylated glucose through action of the coenzyme, uridine diphosphoglucose (UDP-Glucose):

$$\text{UDPGlucose} + \text{galactose-1-P} \dashrightarrow \text{UDPGalactose} + \text{glucose-1-P}$$

The substrates are added in great excess, so that the conversion rate is limited only by the amount of transferase present.

UDPG not consumed during incubation is measured in a linked reaction with NAD and UDPG dehydrogenase, whereby the amount of NADH formed is inversely related to the transferase activity:

$$\text{UDPG} +, 2\text{NAD}^+ \dashrightarrow \text{UDPGlucuronic acid} + 2\text{NADH} + \text{H}^+$$

Procedure

1. Centrifuge 1 ml or more of heparinized blood, at 3000 R.P.M. for ten minutes at 4°C.
2. Discard plasma and wash red cells three times with 0.85% NaCl. Carefully remove and discard white cells (buffy coat) after second and third washes.
3. Mix equal volumes of packed, washed red cells and cold distilled water. Freeze and thaw quickly in a CO_2-alcohol bath. Incubate at 37°C for ten minutes to inactivate epimerase by destroying endogenous NAD. If samples are from infants less than three months old (in whom epimerase levels are high), additional destructive measures are needed: Add 0.025 volume of solution of NADase (0.63 U/m.) to each volume of hemolysate before incubation.
4. For each sample and fresh normal control add 200 μl UDPG · glycine to three 12 ml Sorvall-Pyrex® tubes, 100 μl galactose-1-P, 8 mM, to two of them (A & B) and 100 μl demineralized water to the third tube (blank).
5. Incubate tubes at 37°C for three to five minutes, add 200 μl hemolysate to all tubes, and incubate at 37°C for exactly fifteen minutes. (Save rest of hemolysate for estimating hemoglobin content.)
6. Remove from 37°C bath and add 1.0 ml ice cold saline (0.85%) to all tubes.
7. Place tubes in a boiling water bath, shaking occasionally, for two minutes.
8. Centrifuge at 7000 R.P.M. at 4°C for twenty minutes.
9. Remove and save supernatant fluid. If not clear, recentrifuge at 7000 R.P.M. for ten minutes.
10. Store supernatant fluid at -20°C overnight, if necessary.
11. Estimate UDPG as follows: Add 200 μl 1 M glycine, pH 8.7, 500 μl 2 mM NAD and 200 μl supernatant fluids, A, B, and blank, to respective 1 ml respective cuvettes.
12. Add 100 μl UDPG-DH (800 ΣUnits/ml) to the blank cuvette, mix by inversion and measure OD_{340} exactly one-half minute after mixing and at one-half minute intervals for five minutes.
13. Repeat Step 12 with cuvettes A and B.

14. Measure OD_{340} in all tubes at five-minute intervals until change in OD_{340} is complete (thirty to forty-five minutes).
15. Measure hemoglobin concentration in 20 μl hemolysates by adding to 5.0 ml Hycel cyanmethemoglobin reagent and compare OD_{540} with those of standard solutions of hemoglobin.

Calculations

1. Plot concentration of hemoglobin in mg/100 ml versus $O.D._{340}$ on linear scale.
2. Obtain mg% hemoglobin in control and test hemolysates from standard curve and multiply by 0.25 for g per 100 ml original sample.
3. Extrapolate $O.D._{340}$ to zero time for blank and test samples from $O.D._{340}$ measurements of the first five minutes.
4. Subtract $O.D._{340}$ at zero time from $O.D._{340}$ of completed reaction.
5. Calculate activity of transferase as micromoles of UDPG consumed per gram of hemoglobin per hour (units):

$$\text{Units} = \frac{(\Delta OD_B - \Delta OD_R \times 1210 \times F_c)}{Hb}$$

where ΔOD_B is O.D. change in blank, ΔOD_R is O. D. change of test samples and Hb is hemoglobin concentration in gram per 100 ml. F_c corrects for departure from linearity when $(\Delta OD_B - \Delta OD_R)$ is greater than 0.200, as given below:

$(\Delta OD_B - \Delta OD_R)$	F_c	$(\Delta OD_B - \Delta OD_R)$	F_c
<0.200	1.000	0.250	1.100
0.200	1.010	0.255	1.110
0.205	1.020	0.260	1.119
0.210	1.029	0.265	1.132
0.215	1.037	0.270	1.144
0.220	1.045	0.275	1.160
0.225	1.053	0.280	1.175
0.230	1.061	0.285	1.189
0.235	1.072	0.290	1.203
0.240	1.083	0.295	1.220
0.245	1.094	0.300	1.243

Interpretation

Red cell galactose-1-phosphate uridyl transferase levels in

phenotypes of galactosemia, as measured by UDPG consumption, are given below:

Galactosemia Phenotype	Range Units
Normal	18.5 - 28.5
Duarte variant carrier	13.5 - 18.5
Classical gene carrier	8.5 - 13.5
Duarte variant homozygote	8.5 - 13.5
Duarte/galactosemia compound heterozygote	3.5 - 8.5
Classical gene homozygote	Not detectable

Reagents

1. *NADase, 0.63 U/ml:* Reconstitute vial of Sigma NADase with demineralized water to contain 0.63 U/ml, e.g. vial containing 0.5 mg with 1.6 U/mg activity would be reconstituted with 1.27 ml water for final concentration of 0.63 U/ml.
2. *Uridine Diphosphoglucose, 7 mM (UDPG):* Dissolve 19.1 mg UDPG · Na · 4 H$_2$O in 4 ml demineralized water. Solution is stable two weeks at -20°C.
3. *Glycine, 1 M, pH 8.7:* Dissolve 7.5 g glycine in 80 ml demineralized water. Adjust to pH 8.7 with 1 N NaOH (40 g/l) and bring to volume in 100 ml volumetric flask.
4. *UDPG-Glycine mixture: Just before use,* combine 2 ml 7 mM UDPG with 8 ml 1 M glycine buffer.
5. *Galactose-1-phosphate, 8 mM:* Dissolve 17.1 mg galactose-1-phosphate-dipotassium · 5 H$_2$O in 50 ml demineralized water.
6. *NAD:* Dissolve 14.7 mg β-NAD · 4 H$_2$O in 10 ml demineralized water.
7. *Uridine diphosphoglucose dehydrogenase (UDPG-DH) (0.032 IU/ml):* Dissolve Sigma UDPG-DH in 10 ml demineralized water, to give a final concentration of 0.032 IU/ml.
8. *Hemoglobin Standards:* Combine the following volumes of cyanmethemoglobin reagent (the contents of one vial reconstituted with 1000 ml demineralized water) and Hycel cyanmethemoglobin standard (80 mg%) to give the following hemoglobin standards:

Hemoglobin (mg%)	Volume Hycel Reagent (ml)	Volume Hycel Standard (ml)
0	6.0	0
20	4.5	1.5
40	3.0	3.0
60	1.5	4.5
80	0	6.0

REFERENCE

Beutler, E.: *Red Cell Metabolism*. New York, Grune & Stratton, 1971.

GALACTOKINASE DEFICIENCY

GALACTOKINASE IN DRIED BLOOD SPOTS: SCREENING TEST

Principle

Galactokinase catalyzes the phosphorylation of galactose to the ester, galactose-1-phosphate, in the initial metabolic conversion of the hexose. Deficiency is demonstrated by a fluorescent spot test for red cell galactokinase, similar to the dried blood spot test for galactose-1-phosphate uridyl transferase. The sample's concomitant hexokinase activity and interference with fluorescent endpoints are inhibited by preincubation with the specific hexokinase inhibitor, N-acetyl-β-D-glucosamine.

Procedure

1. Spot capillary or venous blood on Schleicher and Schuell 903 filter paper cards (PKU card) and dry for at least one hour at room temperature. Samples stored at 4°C retain activity for up to one month.
2. Punch 1/4-inch discs of the test samples, normal control, blank, (blank filter paper), and positive (galactokinase-deficient) control, if available, and place in depressions of plastic Linbro Disposo Tray.

3. Overlay discs with 0.1 ml volumes of preincubation mixture. Mix with a plugged microcapillary tube, cover tray and incubate fifteen minutes in 37°C water bath.
4. Remove tray and add 0.1 ml reaction mixture. Mix and spot on lined Whatman DE-81 paper. Let sample flow smoothly from tube to paper at one spot, causing hemoglobin to diffuse rapidly and minimize quenching of fluorescence. Add 5λ drops demineralized water to maximize dispersion of hemoglobin.
5. Replace cover and continue incubation; remove aliquots one, two, and three hours later and spot on paper as in Step 4.
6. Dry spots at room temperature for at least thirty minutes and examine for fluorescence under long or shortwave ultraviolet in Ultraviolet Products Chromato-vue, using Ultraviolet Products Mineralight (see Color Illustration 2).

Interpretation

Samples with normal levels of galactokinase fluoresce brightly in long-wave ultraviolet after two hours' incubation, while deficient samples remain dull. Similar differences are seen in shortwave ultraviolet, but of lesser brilliance; the changes, however, require three to four hours' incubation.

Reagents

1. *TRIS-Acetate Buffer, 0.75 M, pH 8.0*: Dissolve 9.08 g Trizma base in 75 ml demineralized water. Adjust to pH 8.0 with glacial acetic acid and dilute to 100 ml with water in volumetric flask. May be stored at 0 to 5°C for several weeks.
2. *Preincubation Mixture*: Combine in a 10 ml screw-capped tube on the day of test (for forty samples):

n-Acetyl-β-D-glucosamine	10 mg
Saturated digitonin	0.65 ml
TRIS-acetate buffer, 0.75 M, pH 8.0	1.65 ml
Demineralized water	2.65 ml

3. *Reaction Mixture*: Combine in a 50 ml Erlenmeyer flask on the day of test:

ATP	132.6 mg
NADP	33.2 mg
Galactose	19.4 mg*
Magnesium chloride	85.5 mg
Sodium fluoride	18.1 mg
EDTA	3 mg
Saturated digitonin	4 ml
TRIS-acetate buffer, 0.75 M, pH 8.0	10 ml
Demineralized water	16 ml
	30 ml

REFERENCE

Kelly, S., Desjardins, L., and Leikhim, E.: A fluorescent spot test for the detection of galactokinase deficiency. *Clin Chim Acta, 51*:157, 1974.

GALACTOKINASE ACTIVITY IN RED CELLS: QUANTITATIVE ASSAY

Principle

As in the initial metabolic conversion of galactose in vivo, red cell galactokinase catalyzes the phosphorylation of the hexose to galactose-1-phosphate. The reaction product, galactose-1-phosphate, is recovered on diethylaminoethyl (DEAE) cellulose paper and the amount is measured radiometrically.

Procedure

1. Wash a 0.2 to 0.3 ml slurry of microgranular DEAE (Whatman DE-52) in a small glass column made from a tuberculin syringe barrel, plugged with glass wool, with a few drops of 3.8 mM galactose (3.0 mg/ml), followed by 5 ml demineralized water.
2. Dilute galactose-1-^{14}C stock to contain 10 μC/ml. Example: 0.05 ml stock of 100 μC/0.2 ml diluted with 2.5 ml water

---

*Dissolve galactose (19.4 mg) in 16 ml demineralized water and equilibrate at 37°C for at least four hours before adding other reagents. This step may be done several weeks in advance, provided the galactose solution is stored at -20°C after equilibration.

gives 2.55 ml solution containing 10 μC/ml.

3. Incubate diluted stock (2.55 ml) for one hour at 37°C with the following:

0.005 ml	1 M TRIS-HCl, pH 8
0.0125 ml	0.1 M MgCl$_2$
0.25 ml	Hexokinase (2 units/ml)
0.025 ml	⸳0.06 M Neutralized ATP

4. Pass incubated mixture through column and wash with 10 ml demineralized water.

5. To each ml of cleaned galactose-1-^{14}C solution add 0.66 mg (4.1 μmole) "cold" galactose, giving a solution which contains:

   a. 2 μC/ml of ^{14}C (100 μC/0.2 ml or 500 μC/ml solution was diluted fifty fold to give 10 μC/ml and again five fold to give a final ^{14}C concentration of 2 μC/ml) and

   b. 4.2 μmoles/ml of galactose (20.7 mC/mmole and 100 μC/0.2 ml give 0.024 mmole/ml. A fifty fold dilution gave 0.00048 mmole/ml or 0.48 μmole/ml and a further five fold dilution gave 0.096 μmole/ml. 4.1 μmole/ml were added, giving 4.2 μmole/ml).

   The specific activity of the solution is, therefore, 2 μC/ml per 4.2 μmole/ml or 0.48 μC/μmole..

6. Freeze and thaw 0.2 ml aliquot of whole blood sample twice in a CO_2-alcohol bath to lyse red cells; add 50λ lysate to 200λ substrate mixture in a 10 x 75 mm test tube and mix (reaction mixture).

7. Immediately remove two 50λ aliquots of reaction mixture, add to 20λ aliquots of 1 M galactose in separate depressions of a spot plate, and mix (preincubation controls).

8. Spot 50λ aliquots of the two preincubation controls on 1-inch discs of DEAE paper (Whatman DE-81). Let one disc dry (total ^{14}C control) and rinse the other in 150 ml beaker of demineralized water (zero time control). Only one set of these controls is needed for a series of samples tested.

9. Incubate reaction mixture at 37°C for one hour.

10. Remove two 50λ aliquots, add to 20λ aliquots 1 M galactose in a spot plate, mix, spot 50λ aliquots on DEAE paper, and rinse in a 150 ml beaker of demineralized water (60 minute

samples).

11. Wash zero time control and sixty-minute samples on a sintered glass funnel with 600 to 700 ml demineralized water.

12. Air dry all discs, glue to planchets with rubber cement, and count ^{14}C in Nuclear Chicago planchet counter.

13. Mix whole blood sample under test by inverting and make suspension homogenous. Centrifuge in hematocrit centrifuge for seven minutes and express hematocrit in ml per 100 ml.

14. Prepare a series of standards for the estimation of hemoglobin concentration in blood samples by diluting Hycel standard (80 mg%) with Hycel cyanmethemoglobin reagent as follows:

	Volume	
Hgb	*Standard*	*Reagent*
(mg%)	(ml)	(ml)
0	—	6.0
20	1.5	4.5
40	3.0	3.0
60	4.5	1.5
80	6.0	—

15. Add 0.02 ml aliquots to Hycel controls and whole blood sample to 5.0 ml Hycel cyanmethemoglobin reagent.

16. Measure O.D. of standards, controls, and sample at 540 nm.

Calculations

1. Plot O.D. of Hycel standards against concentration of hemoglobin in mg per 100 ml blood. Obtain concentration of hemoglobin in sample and diluted controls from standard curve. Multiply by 250 for hemoglobin concentration in original sample.

2. Calculate activity (E) in nanomoles galactose phosphorylated per minute per gram hemoglobin* (μunits/Hgb), as follows:

$$E = \frac{(A_{60} - A_o) \times (0.38 + 0.2) \times 1000}{S} \Big/ (A_{100} - bkg) \times 0.01 \; Hb \times 60 \times 0.2$$

*Activity can also be expressed in microunits/ml packed red cells by substituting hematocrit in ml/100 ml blood for Hb in the above formula.

or

$$\frac{8333.33 \ (A_{60} - A_o) \times (0.38 + \frac{0.2}{S})}{(A_{100} - bkg \times Hb}$$

or

$$\frac{6666.7 \ (A_{60} - A_o)}{(A_{100} - bkg) \times Hb} \quad (\text{where } S = 0.48) \ ^*$$

Interpretation

Red cell galactokinase activity in forty normal adults was 29.12 ± 5.97 (S.D.) microunits per gram Hgb.

Reagents

1. *Galactose, 7.6 mM*: Dissolve 13.7 mg D(+) galactose in 10 ml demineralized water. Leave at 4°C for at least twenty-four hours for equilibration.
2. *Sodium Fluoride, 0.1 M*: Dissolve 42.0 mg NaF in 10 ml demineralized water.
3. *Magnesium Chloride, 0.1 M*: Dissolve 203.3 mg $MgCl_2 \cdot 6$ H_2O in 10 ml demineralized water.
4. *TRIS · HCl Buffer, 1 M, pH 7.4*: Dissolve 12.1 g Trizma Base in 80 ml demineralized water. Adjust to pH 7.4 with 1 N HCl and bring to volume in 100 ml volumetric flask. (Dilute 8.6 ml concentrated hydrochloric acid to 100 ml for 1 N HCl).
5. *Saponin, 1%*: Dissolve 100 mg saponin in 9.9 ml demineralized water.
6. *Adenosine Triphosphate (ATP), Neutralized, 0.12 M*: Dissolve 304 mg ATP in 4 ml demineralized water. Adjust to pH

---

[*] Key: A_{60} = c.p.m. of sixty-minute sample

A_o = c.p.m. of 0 time control

A_{100} = c.p.m. of total ^{14}C control

Hb = hemoglobin concentration in grams per 100 ml

S = specific activity of C^{14} in microcuries per micromole

bkg = c.p.m. of background

7.0 with 1N NaOH (4 g NaOH per 100 ml solution) and bring to final volume of 5 ml.

7. *Galactose-1-C^{14}* (2μCi/ml; 4.2 μmole/ml): Prepare as described in "Procedure," (p. 126).

8. *Substrate Mixture*: Combine the following

Saponin, 1%	1.0 ml
Sodium fluoride, 0.1 M	0.25 ml
Magnesium chloride, 0.1 M	0.5 ml
TRIS · HCl, 1 M, pH 7.4	1.0 ml
Galactose, 7.6 mM	0.25 ml
Galactose-1-^{14}C, 2 μCi/ml	0.5 ml
ATP, 0.12 M, pH 7.0	0.25 ml
Demineralized water	0.25 ml
	4.0 ml

9. *Galactose, 1 M*: Dissolve 1.8 g galactose in 10 ml demineralized water. Leave at room temperature for twenty-four hours for equilibration. Store at -20°C.

REFERENCE

Beutler, E., and Matsumoto, F.: A rapid simplified assay for galactokinase activity in whole blood. *J Lab Clin Med, 82*:818, 1973.

CHAPTER 5

THE MUCOPOLYSACCHARIDOSES

COARSE facies and dwarfism with skeletal abnormalities characterize the mucopolysaccharidoses (MPS), a group of diseases with variable clinical and biochemical features. The discoveries of "corrective factors" in complementary tissues cultured together and, recently, specific defects in lysosomal enzymes have helped clarify the confusing taxonomy. At least seven mucopolysaccharidoses are now recognized (Table VIII). The clinical signs of three differ chiefly in degree: The facies and dwarfism of MPS I and II are quite similar; MPS II, however, occurs only in males, has X-linked inheritance, and patients are less retarded. MPS V is milder than either, with normal or near normal facies, stature, and intelligence. Two, MPS I and MPS V, share the same enzyme defect, and with MPS II, share the same abnormal products. MPS III, IV, and VI, on the other hand, share some clinical features but differ from each other in enzyme defects and/or corrective factors and excretory products.

The biochemical abnormalities of metachromasia and MPS excretion relate to the excessive storage of mucopolysaccharide polymer in cells, the degradation of which is normally catalyzed by hydrolases specific for the polymer's characteristic glycosaminoglycan component. Most, but not all, the involved hydrolases have been identified (Table VIII).

All share the abnormalities of metachromasia and excessive excretion of the acid mucopolysaccharides secondary to the effects of the enzyme deficiency (Table VIII). Although neither property is definitive, in many instances they are characteristic. The metachromasias of MPS III, IV, VI, and VII, for example, are especially characteristic. The MPS excretory patterns are also distinctive in several: Both heparan and dermatan sulfates are excessive in MPS I, II, and V, for example; heparan and keratan sulfates are excessive in MPS III and IV, respectively, and dermatan sulfate is excessive in MPS VI and VII.

131

Table VIII

CLINICAL SIGNS AND BIOCHEMICAL ABNORMALITIES IN THE MUCOPOLYSACCHARIDOSES

Signs	I_H Hurler	I_S or V Scheie	II Hunter	III San Filippo	IV Morquio	VI Maroteaux-Lamy	VII β-Glucuronidase Deficiency
Typical facies	+	+	+	+	+	±	+
Dwarfing	+	-	+	±	+	+	±
Skeletal malformations	+	+	+	±	+	+	+
Lumbar gibbus	+	-	-	-	+	-	+
Corneal clouding	+	+	-	-	+	+	±
Deafness	+	-	+	+	-	±	?
Retardation	+	-	±	+	±	-	+
Hepatosplenomegaly	+	+	+	-	+	?	+
Cardiovascular	+	+	+	-	+	+	?
Stiff joints	+	+	+	+	-	-	-
Early death	+	-	±	-	-	-	+
Inheritance[1]	R	R	X/R	R	R	R	R
Lymphocyte metachromasia	+	±	+	+	-	Coarse	Coarse
MPS excretion[2]	DS HS	DS HS	DS HS	HS	KS	DS	HS
Enzyme deficiency[3]	Id	Id	SIdS	HsS AcG	-	AS-B	β-G

[1] R, XR: Recessive, X-linked recessive, respectively.
[2] DS, HS, KS: Dermatan, heparan and keratan sulfates, respectively.
[3] Enzyme deficiencies are; iduronidase (Id), sulfoiduronate sulfatase (SIdS), heparan sulfate sulfatase (HsS), N-acetyl-α-D-glucosaminidase (AcG), aryl sulfatase B (AS-B), β-glucuronidase (β-G).

The inheritance patterns of all are recessive; MPS II differs in being X-linked, rather than autosomal. Carriers of all forms are clinically normal; they may, in some instances, be identified through cellular metachromasia and intracellular uronic acid levels of cultured fibroblasts and leukocytes.

Cellular metachromasia is usually demonstrated by staining fresh smears of peripheral leukocytes or cultured cells with toluidine blue or other mucopolysaccharide-specific dye (p. 138).

The gross excretory excesses of the acid mucopolysaccharides are detected by precipitation with acid albumin (p. 135), cetyl pyridinium compounds (p. 136), or metachromatic reaction on paper with toluidine blue (p. 133).

The pattern of excess is readily discerned in thin layer chromatographs (p. 140), and is a most helpful means of discriminating among the various types. The nitrous acid reaction reveals the extent of specific mucopolysaccharide excess in MPS III (p. 147), heparan sulfate. Total excretion rates of the acid mucopolysaccharides are estimated from quantitative assays (p. 136).

Assay for the enzyme defect of MPS VII, β-glucuronidase deficiency, is easily performed (p. 158). Assays for other enzyme deficiencies, for which substrate is readily available, are those for distinguishing Sanfilippo Type B by serum α-N-acetyl-glucosaminidase deficiency (p. 150), and Maroteaux-Lamy disease by urinary and leukocyte sulfatase B deficiency, pages 152 and 155, respectively.

SCREENING TESTS OF GENERAL APPLICABILITY

TOLUIDINE BLUE SPOT TEST (URINE)

Principle

Urine containing excessive acid mucopolysaccharides when dried on filter paper, stains purple with toluidine blue against a blue background. The color change, or metachromasia, occurs as the acidic groups on the polymer react with basic groups of the dye. The dye solution is buffered to prevent staining by compounds which ionize at weaker hydrogen ion concentrations (above pH 2.0).

Procedure

1. Spot 27λ aliquots of lyophilized and reconstituted urine sample (containing 40 μg creatinine) (p. 25) on prelined filter paper sheet in aliquots of about 10λ. Dry spot thoroughly (5 minutes) before applying next aliquot. Dry after last aliquot at least five minutes at room temperature.
2. Spot sheet with 27λ aliquots of standards and dry.
3. Dip sheet in toluidine blue solution in a half-filled 150 mm Petri dish, swirling dish gently until well covered. Swirl dish occasionally and remove sheet from dye after one minute. Let sheet drain momentarily and transfer to fresh Petri dish, half-filled with ethanol, swirling to wash thoroughly (one minute). Discard wash, add fresh ethanol, and swirl occasionally for thirty seconds. Remove sheet and hang to dry at room temperature.
4. Match purple color of test sample with those of standards.

Interpretation

Normal urine samples do not stain purple or only faintly so (less than that of the 0.1 mg/ml standard). Urine from normal infants under a year, however, may contain MPS in concentrations up to 0.1 mg/ml.

Purple staining darker than that of the 0.1 mg/ml standard indicates an abnormal MPS concentration. (See Color Illustration 7.)

Reagents

1. *Chondroitin Sulfate Standards, 0.1, 0.2, 0.3, 0.4, 0.5 mg/ml:* Dissolve 10 mg chondroitin sulfate C in 10 ml normal urine (1 mg/ml). Dilute the stock solution with various amounts of normal urine to give a series of standards (1 ml volumes) containing from 0.1 to 0.5 mg/ml. Can be stored at -20°C for up to six months.
2. *Toluidine Blue O Stain, 0.04%:* Dissolve 40 mg dye in 100 ml

demineralized water and adjust to pH 2.0 with concentrated hydrochloric ac'd (several drops). Store at 4° C. Make fresh every two months.

REFERENCE

Berry, K., and Spinanger, J.: A paper spot test useful in the study of Hurler's syndrome. *J Lab Clin Med.* 55:136, 1960.

ALBUMIN TURBIDITY SCREENING TEST (URINE)

Principle

Acid mucopolysaccharides in urine precipitate as insoluble complexes in the presence of buffered bovine albumin. The degree of turbidity is a measure of the excess.

Procedure

1. When samples, controls, and reagents have been brought to room temperature, acidify 1 ml clear urine sample and controls with 2 drops 5 N HCl. (Centrifuge urine sample to clarify, if necessary.) Mix.
2. Add 2 ml bovine albumin solution; mix.
3. Observe turbidity against a dark background twenty minutes later.

Interpretation

Urine containing few or no acid mucopolysaccharides remains clear. Urine containing mucopolysaccharides equivalent to 5 mg chondroitin sulfate or more per 100 ml becomes turbid.

Reagents

1. *Hydrochloric Acid, 5 N:* Add slowly, with mixing, 43.3 ml concentrated HCl to 40 ml demineralized water. Dilute to 100 ml in volumetric flask with demineralized water.

2. *Sodium Acetate Solution*: Dissolve 6.8 g sodium acetate trihydrate in 400 ml demineralized water; add 2.85 ml glacial acetic acid.
3. *Acid Bovine Albumin Solution, 0.1%*: Suspend 0.50 g bovine albumin, fraction V, in approximately 400 ml sodium acetate solution. Adjust to pH 3.75 with 10 N HCl, dilute to 500 ml and store at 4°C.
4. *Control Chondroitin Sulfate Solution, 10 mg%*: Dissolve 5 mg chondroitin sulfate in 50 ml normal urine. Store in 1.5 ml amounts in small, cork-stoppered test tubes at -20°C.

REFERENCE

Carter, C. H., Wan, A. T., and Carpenter, D. G.: Commonly used tests in the detection of Hurler's syndrome. *J Pediatr 73*:217, 1968.

CETYLPYRIDINIUM CHLORIDE TURBIDITY ASSAY (URINE)

Principle

Urinary mucopolysaccharides and mucoproteins are precipitated by cetylpyridinium chloride (CPC) in sodium citrate buffer. The turbidity is compared with that of chondroitin sulfate standards.

Procedure

1. Add 1.0 ml CPC reagent to 11 × 75 mm test tubes or Coleman cuvettes containing 1.0 ml aliquots of standard solutions, test urine, or demineralized water as CPC blank.
2. Add 1.0 ml aliquot citrate to 1.0 ml test urine as urine blank.
3. Mix contents of all tubes and let stand fifteen minutes.
4. Mix contents again and read turbidity promptly with 680 mμ filter. Read test urine samples against urine blank and standard solutions against CPC blank.
5. Express results in CPC units/g of creatinine. One CPC unit equals optical density of solutions containing 1 mg chondroitin

sulfate per 100 ml urine.

Interpretation

Urinary mucopolysaccharide concentrations are age-related; they vary from 375 CPC units/g or less in infants one year old or younger to 175 CPC units/g Cr or less in children up to nine years old. Urine from older children and adults contains 85 CPC units/g Cr or less.

Reagents

1. *Sodium Citrate Buffer, pH 4.8*: Dissolve 9.68 g citric acid and 15.88 g trisodium citrate and make to volume with demineralized water in 1 liter volumetric flask. Adjust to pH 4.8 with concentrated HC1.
2. *CPC Reagent*: Dissolve 250 mg cetylpyridinium chloride in 250 ml sodium citrate buffer.
3. *Standard Solutions*: Dissolve 1, 5, and 10 mg quantities chondroitin sulfate in 100 ml portions demineralized water.
4. *Negative Control*: Normal urine, filtered.

REFERENCE

Pennock, C. A.: A modified test for glycosaminoglycan excretion. *J Clin Pathol*, 22:379, 1969.

METACHROMATIC GRANULES (URINE)

Principle

Granular deposits in fresh urine from patients with lysosomal storage diseases often stain metachromatically. The glycolipid-protein complexes accumulate in the tubules and are excreted in various shapes, ranging from scattered sand to well-formed casts.

Procedure

1. Disperse sediment evenly in a fresh catch sample of urine, free

of bacteria and debris, by mixing. If turbid from urates, warm gently to dissolve crystals. Centrifuge 100 ml or more at 2500 R.P.M. for ten minutes.
2. Decant and discard supernatant urine.
3. Add 1 to 2 drops of 2% aqueous toluidine blue O solution to sediment, mix, and pipette two large drops on a glass slide.
4. Add cover slips and examine at 400X magnification.

Interpretation

Urinary metachromasia of the lipid storage diseases appears as golden-brown granular bodies not found in normal urine. In the mucopolysaccharidoses it forms reddish-purple flocculent casts.

Reagent

1. *Toluidine Blue 0, 2%:* Dissolve 2 g in 100 ml demineralized water and store at room temperature.

REFERENCE

Austin, J. A.: Metachromatic form of diffuse cerebral sclerosis diagnosis during life by urine sediment examination. *Neurology, 7*:415, 1957.

WHITE CELL METACHROMASIA

Principle

The white cells of patients with mucopolysaccharidoses and other lysosomal storage diseases contain cytoplasmic granules which stain metachromatically with basic dyes. The color, size, and location of the granules, as well as kinds of peripheral leukocytes affected, are often characteristic of the disease. The granules first described by Alder and Riley, for example, are now considered similar to the granulation of MPS VI and MPS VII.

Procedure

1. Prepare fresh blood smears on cover slips or slides and air

dry for thirty to sixty minutes. Fix ten minutes in cold, absolute methanol.
2. Stain by standing in 0.1% toluidine blue in 30% methanol for five minutes without agitating. Dehydrate by rinsing quickly through two changes each of acetone, acetone:xylol, 1:1, and xylol.
3. Seal in Fisher Permount® and observe granulation in cytoplasm when dry.

Interpretation

The granules of normal white cells are usually not metachromatic. True metachromasia, on the other hand, must be distinguished from toxic granulation.

Metachromasia is variable according to the disease and appears as cytoplasmic granules in shades of pink, lilac, or dark blue. Vacuoles may be common. The following table describes the kinds of metachromasia found in several lysosomal storage diseases (see Table IX). (See Color Illustrations 8 and 9.)

Reagents

1. *Methanol, 30%:* Dilute 30 ml absolute methanol to volume with demineralized water in 100 ml volumetric flask.
2. *Toluidine Blue 0 in 30% Methanol, 0.1%:* Dissolve 0.1 gm toluidine blue powder in 100 ml 30% methanol. Filter.

REFERENCES

Mittwoch, U.: Abnormal lymphocytes in gargoylism. *Br J Haematol,* 5:365, 1959.

Hansen, Hans G.: Hematologic studies in mucopolysaccharidoses and mucolipidoses. In Bergsma, Daniel (Ed): *Fourth Conference on the Clinical Delineation of Birth Defects, Part XIV Blood,* Baltimore, Williams and Wilkins, 1972, pp. 115-128.

Table IX

METACHROMASIA BY CELL TYPE AND GRANULATION

Disease	Cells	Granules
MPS I-V, II	Lymphocytes; neutrophiles	Blue-purple, evenly diffused in cytoplasm
MPS III	Lymphocytes	Red, distribution restricted to localized areas; occasional halo
MPS IV	Neutrophiles	1-3 plaque-like inclusions and fine, blue granules
MPS VI	Neutrophiles; eosinophiles	Coarse, closely packed; black-grey
MPS VII	Neutrophiles; lymphocytes	Like MPS VI
GM$_1$ gangliosidosis and fucosidosis	Lymphocytes	Most cells vacuolar; 20% cells granular
Metachromatic leukodystrophy	Like MPS VI	Like MPS VI
Mucolipidosis I	Lymphocytes	Granules & vacuoles
Mucolipidosis II (I-cell disease)	Lymphocytes	"Bulging" inclusions
Mucolipidosis III	Lymphocytes; neutrophiles	Vacuoles; granules in 10% of cells

DISCRIMINATORY TESTS

IDENTIFICATION OF MUCOPOLYSACCHARIDOSIS BY THIN-LAYER CHROMATOGRAPHY PATTERN

Principle

The urinary acid mucopolysaccharides in excess are concentrated by precipitation with cetyl pyridinium chloride and identified by thin-layer chromatography of the chloride salt solution on cellulose.

Procedure

1. Bring 15 ml aliquot of twenty-four-hour collection of thymol-preserved urine (fresh or frozen) to pH 5.5 with 1 N NaOH or 1 N HCl and clarify by centrifuging at 2000 R.P.M. for ten minutes.
2. Add 0.2 ml 5% cetylpyridinium chloride to 10 ml clarified urine sample in 12 ml Sorvall tube. Mix by inversion and stand in ice water bath for four hours.
3. Centrifuge at 3000 R.P.M. at 4°C for fifteen to twenty minutes, decant, and drain one minute.
4. Disperse precipitate in 10 ml absolute ethanol saturated with sodium chloride, centrifuge, decant, and drain as before. Repeat.
5. Disperse in ether, centrifuge, decant, and drain. Dry for about one minute by holding tube in palm of hand.
6. Dissolve precipitate in 2.0 ml 0.6 M sodium chloride and centrifuge at 2500 R.P.M. at 4°C for fifteen minutes to remove contaminants.
7. Tranfer supernatant fluid to clean 12 ml Sorvall tube and add 8 ml absolute ethanol. Mix by inversion and store overnight at 4°C.
8. Centrifuge precipitate at 3000 R.P.M. at 4°C for fifteen minutes; disperse in absolute ethanol, centrifuge, decant, and drain.
9. Disperse in ether, centrifuge, decant, drain, and dry as before.
10. Dissolve precipitate in 100 μl 0.6 M sodium chloride for chromatography or store at -20°C.
11. Apply 10 μl aliquot of dissolved precipitate and those of standards to precoated TLC sheet of cellulose (Merck 5502) at points on guide lines lightly drawn 2 cm long and 1 cm apart, 2 cm from and parallel to the bottom edge of sheet. Dry in stream of warm air.
12. Place sheet between clean glass plates and chromatograph in solvent system No. 1, until front moves 2 cm from application

points.
13. Remove glass plates from trough, blot bottom edges, remove sheet immediately, blot excess solvent from bottom edge of sheet, and place between another pair of clean glass plates.
14. Chromatograph in solvent system No. 2 until new front proceeds 2 cm.
15. Repeat procedures with solvent systems 3, 4, 5, and 6.
16. After chromatography in sixth solvent, air dry chromatogram for twenty minutes.
17. Stain by immersing sheet in 1% toluidine blue in glass dish for three minutes; drain.
18. Remove excess stain by immersing in successive rinses of 10% acetic acid in glass dishes until background is light blue; air dry. Compare pattern of urine sample with those of standards.

Interpretation

Urinary mucopolysaccharides from patients with known mucopolysaccharidoses form the patterns depicted in Figure 7. In MPS I, II, and V (Hurler, Hunter, and Scheie), for example, an intense band of dermatan sulfate appears at the origin, diffusing upward; two other bands appear half and three-fourths of the way to the front, consisting, respectively, of a slow-moving form of heparan sulfate and one or more of the chondroitin sulfates. In MPS III (Sanfilippo) the pattern consists of a single diffuse band of heparan sulfate with an Rf greater than that of the heparan sulfate of MPS I, II, and V and slightly less than that of chondroitin sulfates 4 and 6. In MPS IV (Morquio) an intense, discrete band of keratan sulfate forms at the final solvent front ahead of a lighter, more diffuse band of the chondroitin sulfates. MPS VI (Maroteaux-Lamy): The pattern resembles that of MPS I, II, and V in the appearance of an intense band of dermatan sulfate at the origin, diffusing upward. It lacks a band of slow-moving heparan sulfate, however, and contains a diffuse band of the chondroitin sulfates. (See Color Illustration 10.)

Reagents

1. *NaOH, 1 N*: Dissolve 4.0 g NaOH pellets in 50 ml demineral-

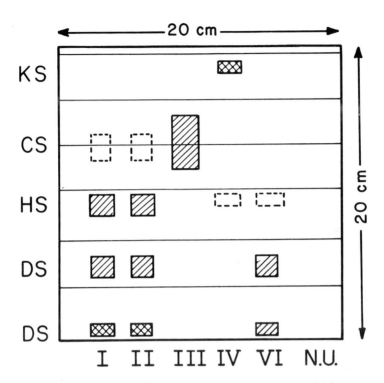

Figure 7. One-dimensional thin-layer cellulose chromatographic patterns of urinary mucopolysaccharides in the mucopolysaccharidoses. Cross-hatching indicates density. Patterns in MPS I and II are similar. Mucopolysaccharide excess of MPS III is heparan sulfate (HS) of greater mobility than HS of MPS I and II.

ized water in 100 ml Pyrex beaker. Dilute to volume in 100 ml volumetric flask with demineralized water.

2. *HCl, 1 N*: Dilute 8.6 ml concentrated hydrochloric acid to 100 ml in volumetric flask with demineralized water.

3. *Cetyl Pyridinium Chloride, 5%*: Dissolve 0.5 g CPC in 10 ml demineralized water.

4. *Acid Mucopolysaccharide (AMPS) Urine Standards*: Precipitate and apply AMPS from patients with known mucopolysaccharidoses, as described above.

5. *Absolute Alcohol Saturated with Sodium Chloride*: Add 0.5 g NaCl to 250 ml absolute ethanol in 500 ml Erlenmeyer flask

and stir for thirty minutes.

6. *NaCl, 0.6 M*: Dissolve 3.5 g NaCl in demineralized water and dilute to volume in 100 ml volumetric flask.

7. *Ethanol-Calcium Acetate - 0.5 N Acetic Acid Solvent Systems*: Combine the following volumes of absolute ethanol and calcium acetate solutions on the day of test:

System	%Ethanol (ml)	% Calcium Acetate (g)
1	60	2.5
2	50	5.0
3	40	5.0
4	30	5.0
5	20	5.0
6	10	5.0

Dissolve calcium acetate in from 10 to 60 ml portions of demineralized water in 300 ml Erlenmeyer flasks in inverse proportions to the amount of ethanol required, add 2.9 ml glacial acetic acid to each, and add the volumes of ethanol indicated. Bring to volume in 100 ml volumetric flasks with demineralized water.

8. *Toluidine Blue O, 1% in 70% Ethanol-Acetic Acid (95/5 v/v)*: Dilute 73.4 ml 95% ethanol to volume in 100 ml volumetric flask with demineralized water. Acidify 95 ml 70% ethanol with 5 ml glacial acetic acid in 250 ml Pyrex beaker and dissolve 1 g toluidine blue 0.

9. *Acetic Acid, 10%*: Dilute 200 ml glacial acetic acid to volume in 2 liter volumetric flask with demineralized water.

10. *Acid Mucopolysaccharide Standard Solutions*: Dissolve 2 mg amounts of heparan sulfate, keratan sulfate, dermatan sulfate, and a mixture of chondroitin sulfates in 10 ml aliquots of centrifuged normal urine and purify by CPC precipitation, washing, and extraction, as described in the procedure. (The heparan, keratan, and dermatan sulfates were obtained from J. A. Cifonelli (Chicago) as products from beef lung, human costal cartilage, and hog mucosal tissues, respectively. The chondroitin sulfates 4 and 6 were in a mixture of chondroitin sulfate isomers from whale and shark cartilage produced by Sigma Chemical Company.)

REFERENCES

Humbel, R.: Identification and quantitation of keratan sulfate in urine. *Clin Chim Acta, 52*:173, 1974.

Humbel, R., and Chamoles, N. A.: Sequential thin layer chromatography of urinary acidic glycosaminglycans. *Clin Chim Acta, 50*:290, 1972.

Lippiello, L., and Mankin, H. J.: Thin-layer chromatographic separation of the isomeric chondroitin sulfates, dermatan sulfate and keratan sulfate. *Anal Biochem, 39*:54, 1971.

IDENTIFICATION OF KERATAN SULFATE BY THIN-LAYER CHROMATOGRAPHY

Principle

The preparation of urine samples is the same as that for the identification of the mucopolysaccharidoses by thin-layer chromatography pattern (p. 141). Only four solvent systems, however, are needed for the separation and identification of the mucopolysaccharide keratan sulfate.

Procedure

1. - 14. As described on p. 141.
15. Repeat with solvent systems No. 3 and 4.
16. After chromatography in the fourth solvent system, air-dry chromatogram for twenty minutes.
17. Stain by immersing sheet in 1% toluidine blue in a glass dish for three minutes; drain.
18. Remove excess stain by immersing in successive rinses of 10% acetic acid in glass dishes until background is light blue; air dry. Compare unknown with standard.

Interpretation

Keratan sulfate, the chief urinary abnormality in Morquio's disease, is excreted by normal persons in trace amounts only. Excessive excretion also occurs in the mucolipidoses, generalized G_{M1}-gangliosidosis, and fucosidosis.

Reagents

1. *NaOH, 1N*: Dissolve 4.0 g NaOH pellets in 50 ml demineral-

ized water in 100 ml Pyrex beaker. Dilute to volume in 100 ml volumetric flask with demineralized water.

2. *HCl, 1 N*: Dilute 8.6 ml concentrated hydrochloric acid to 100 ml in volumetric flask with demineralized water.

3. *Cetylpyridinium Chloride, 5%*: Dissolve 0.5 g CPC in 10 ml demineralized water.

4. *Keratan Sulfate Standard, 1 mg/ml*: Dissolve 1 mg keratan sulfate in 1 ml 0.05 N NaOH (2 g/l).

5. *Absolute Alcohol Saturated with Sodium Chloride*: Add 0.5 g NaCl to 250 ml absolute alcohol in 500 ml Erlenmeyer flask and stir for thirty minutes.

6. *NaCl, 0.6 M*: Dissolve 3.5 g NaCl in demineralized water and dilute to volume in 100 ml volumetric flask.

7. *Ethanol-Calcium Acetate-0.5 N Acetic Acid Solvent Systems:* Combine the following volumes of absolute ethanol and calcium acetate solutions on the day of test:

Solvent System	% Ethanol (ml)	% Calcium Acetate (g)
1	60	2.5
2	50	5.0
3	40	5.0
4	30	5.0

Dissolve calcium acetate in from 30 to 60 ml portions of demineralized water in 300 ml Erlenmeyer flasks, in inverse proportions to the amount of ethanol required, add 2.9 ml of glacial acetic acid to each as well as the volumes of ethanol indicated. Bring to volume in 100 ml volumetric flasks with demineralized water.

8. *Toluidine Blue O, 1%, in 70% Ethanol-Acetic Acid (95/5 v/v)*: Dilute 73.4 ml 95% ethanol to volume in 100 ml volumetric flask with demineralized water. Acidify 95 ml 70% ethanol with 5 ml glacial acetic acid in 250 ml Pyrex beaker and dissolve 1 g toluidine blue 0.

9. *Acetic Acid, 10%*: Dilute 200 ml glacial acetic acid to volume in 2 liter volumetric flask with demineralized water.

REFERENCES

Humbel, R.: Identification and quantitation of keratan sulfate in urine. *Clin Chim Acta, 52*:173, 1974.

Lippiello, L., and Mankin, H. J.: Thin-layer chromatographic separation of the isomeric chondroitin sulfates, dermatan sulfate and keratan sulfate. *Anal Biochem, 39*:54, 1971.

HEPARAN SULFATE AS N-SULFATE GLYCOSAMINOGLYCAN

Principle

Heparan sulfate, a glycosaminoglycan excreted in several of the mucopolysaccharidoses, is measured colorimetrically by reaction with indole. Preparatory steps include isolation by cetylpyridinium chloride, and precipitation and deamination of the N-sulfated-D-glucosamine groups.

Procedure

1. Adjust 15 ml catch urine sample, containing at least 0.1 mg/ml creatinine, or toluene-preserved twenty-four-hour collection, to pH 5 with 1 N HCl or 1 N NaOH in 50 ml Nalgene® Sorvall tube. Add 0.5 ml 5% cetylpyridinium chloride and let precipitate form overnight at 4°C. If smaller volumes of urine are used, adjust volumes of reactants accordingly.
2. Centrifuge at 3000 R.P.M. at 4°C for fifteen to twenty minutes.
3. Decant supernatant fluid carefully and discard. Wash precipitate three times with 15 ml sodium chloride-saturated ethanol and centrifuge at 4°C, dissociating CPC from the acid mucopolysaccharides.
4. Dissolve the final acid mucopolysaccharide-containing sediment in 5 ml 0.05 N sodium hydroxide. Clarify turbid supernatant fluid by centrifuging at 2500 R.P.M. for fifteen to twenty minutes at 4°C.
5. Remove and save supernatant fluid (AMPS).
6. Add 0.2 ml aliquots of supernatant fluid (AMPS) and heparan working standards, in duplicate, into respective 10 ml tubes.
7. Add 0.2 ml 5% sodium nitrite and 0.2 ml 33% acetic acid, mix by shaking, and let stand at room temperature for eighty minutes for deamination.
8. Add 0.1 ml 12.5% ammonium sulfamate, shake vigorously,

and let stand fifteen minutes. Repeat step with another 0.1 ml aliquot of the sulfamate.
9. Add 1 ml 5% HCl and 0.1 ml 1% indole, mix, and let stand at room temperature for ten minutes.
10. Place tubes in boiling water bath for five minutes. Remove and cool to room temperature.
11. Add 1 ml absolute ethanol, mix, and read absorbance at 492 $m\mu$ and 520 $m\mu$.

Calculations

1. Subtract O.D.$_{520}$ from O.D.$_{492}$ of samples and standards for O.D. of N-sulfate hexosamine.
2. Plot standard curve of O.D. versus concentration of N-sulfate hexosamine.
3. Obtain μg N-sulfate hexosamine per ml AMPS from standard curve. Divide by 3 to correct for three fold concentration by precipitation with CPS and express as μg N-sulfate hexosamine per ml urine.
4. Divide μg N-sulfate hexosamine per ml urine by concentration of urinary creatinine in mg/ml and express as μg N-sulfate hexosamine per mg creatinine.

Interpretation

The excretion of glycosaminoglycan N-sulfate hexosamines by normal children falls gradually from a peak of up to 11 μg/mg Cr during infancy to less than 3 μg/mg Cr by age sixteen years. Excessive concentrations in the mucopolysaccharidoses range from 300-500 μg/mg Cr in severe forms, like MPS I (Hurler) and lesser amounts in MPS II (Hunter), to 20-40 μg/mg Cr in the milder MPS I (Scheie) form.

Reagents

1. *Cetylpyridinium Chloride, 5%*: Dissolve 0.5 g cetylpyridinium chloride in 10 ml demineralized water.
2. *Ethanol Saturated with Sodium Chloride*: Add 0.5 g sodium

chloride to 250 ml 95% ethanol in 500 ml Erlenmeyer flask and mix with magnetic stirrer for one-half hour. Decant and save the saturated alcohol.

3. *Sodium Hydroxide, 0.05N:* Dissolve 1 g sodium hydroxide in 500 ml demineralized water.
4. *Sodium Nitrite, 5%:* Dissolve 2.5 g sodium nitrite in 50 ml demineralized water. Store in brown bottle for up to one week at 4°C.
5. *Acetic Acid, 33%:* Mix 33 ml glacial acetic acid and 77 ml demineralized water.
6. *Ammonium Sulfamate, 12.5%:* Dissolve 12.5 g ammonium sulfamate in 100 ml demineralized water.
7. *Hydrochloric Acid, 5%:* Add 13.7 ml concentrated HCl to 86.3 ml demineralized water.
8. *Indole, 1%:* Just before use, dissolve 0.1 g indole in 10 ml absolute ethanol.
9. *Heparin Standard Stock Solution, 2 mg/ml:* Dissolve 10 mg heparin (sodium salt) (170 units/mg) in 5 ml demineralized water.
10. *Working Heparin Standards:* Dilute the heparin standard stock solution, as follows:

Hep/ml (μg)	Stock Standard (ml)	NaOH (ml)
50	0.25	9.75
100	0.5	9.5
200	1.0	9.0
400	2.0	8.0

REFERENCES

Lagunoff, D., Pritzl, P., and Scott, C. R.: Urinary N-sulfate glycosaminoglycan excretion in children: Normal and abnormal values. *Proc Soc Exp Biol Med, 126:*34, 1967.

Teller, W. M., Burke, E. C., Rosevear, J. W., and McKenzie, B. F.: Urinary excretion of acid mucopolysaccharides in normal children and patients with gargoylism. *J Lab Clin Med, 59:*95, 1962.

Lagunoff, D. and Warren, G.: Determination of 2-deoxy-2-sulfoamino-hexose content of mucopolysaccharides. *Arch Biochem Biophys, 99:*396, 1962.

SERUM α-N-ACETYLGLUCOSAMINIDASE DEFICIENCY

Principle

The enzyme defect of the Sanfilippo B form of mucopolysaccharidosis, absence of α-N-acetylglucosaminidase, is detectable in serum. The enzyme of normal serum hydrolyzes the artificial substrate, p-nitrophenyl-N-acetyl-α-D-glycopyranoside. The freed p-nitrophenol, a red solution when alkaline, is released stoichiometrically.

Procedure

1. Combine 0.2 ml fresh or frozen serum or plasma, 0.1 ml demineralized water, 0.1 ml sodium azide solution, 0.1 ml p-nitrophenyl-N-acetyl-α-D-glucopyranoside in 16×100-mm test tube and mix by swirling. Substitute 0.1 ml citrate buffer for substrate in blank tube (one for each sample).
2. Incubate at 37°C in water bath four hours.
3. Remove from bath, add 0.2 ml 0.825 M perchloric acid solution, and mix.
4. Centrifuge ten minutes at 1500 R.P.M.
5. Prepare p-nitrophenol standards.
6. Remove 0.5 ml supernatant fluid from pellet with a 1 ml Schwartz/Mann Biotip-Biopipette® and add to 1.0 ml glycine-NaOH buffer in 10×75 mm round cuvettes; mix.
7. Measure optical density of sample and standards at 430 nm, using glycine/NaOH buffer as instrument blank.

Calculations

1. Plot standard curve of absorbance versus concentration of nitrophenol.
2. Obtain nmoles nitrophenol released from standard curve, divide by 1.5 (ml) for nmoles/ml.
3. Multiply by 9.5, to correct for dilution of 0.143 ml sample in 1.5 ml reaction mixture.

4. Divide by 240 (minutes) and express activity in nmoles p-nitrophenol released/min/ml at 37°C.

Interpretation

Normal serum, according to Figura, et al. (1973) contains from 0.30 to 0.60 units enzyme activity (nmoles/min/ml at 37°C); serum from homozygous persons has practically no activity; serum from heterozygous persons displays partial activity. Since the assay components produce high "blank" absorbance, the interpretation is best based on values obtained in one's own laboratory.

Reagents

1. *Sodium Citrate Buffer 0.1875 M, pH 3.8:* Dissolve 2.43 g citric acid (M.W. 192) and 1.79 g sodium citrate (M.W. 294) in demineralized water; dilute to the mark in 100 ml volumetric flask.
2. *p-Nitrophenyl-N-Acetyl-α-D-Glucopyranoside Substrate, 0.1 M:* Dissolve 4.0 mg (M.W. 342) in 1 ml citrate buffer (per sample). Heat at 37°C and mix vigorously.
3. *Sodium Azide Solution, 0.1%:* Dissolve 0.1 g in 100 ml demineralized water.
4. *Perchloric Acid, 0.825 M:* Add 0.629 ml $HClO_4$ (70%) to 50 ml demineralized water, mix, and dilute to volume in 100 ml volumetric flask.
5. *Glycine/Sodium Hydroxide Buffer, 0.4 M, pH 10.4:* Dissolve 3.0 g glycine in 50 ml demineralized water. Mix to dissolve; adjust to pH 9 with 10 N NaOH (40 g/100 ml). Adjust to pH 10.4 with 1 N NaOH (4 g/100 ml). Bring to volume in 100 ml volumetric flask with demineralized water.
6. *p-Nitrophenol Standard Stock Solution, 1 μmole/ml:* Dilute 0.1 ml Sigma p-nitrophenol standard solution (10 μmoles/ml) with 0.9 ml glycine/NaOH buffer.
7. *p-Nitrophenol Working Standards:* Dilute p-nitrophenol standard stock solution as follows:

Conc. p-Nitrophenol (nmoles/ml)	Stock Solution (ml)	Glycine Buffer (ml)
9	0.0	5.0
10	0.1	9.9
20	0.1	4.9
30	0.1	3.2
50	0.2	3.8

Mix thoroughly.

REFERENCES

von Figura, K., Lögering, M., Kresse, H.: Serum α-N-acetylglucosaminidase: Determination, characterization, and corrective activity in *Sanfilippo B* fibroblasts. *Z Klin Chem Klin Biochem, 13*:285, 1975.

von Figura, K., Lögering, M., Mersmann, G., and Kresse, H.: Sanfilippo B disease: Serum assays for detection of homozygous and heterozygous individuals in three families. *J Pediatr, 83*:607, 1973.

URINARY SULFATASE B DEFICIENCY

Principle

Urinary deficiency of arylsulfatase B in the patient with Maroteaux-Lamy syndrome is demonstrable in the presence of A by inhibiting the latter with high substrate concentration, neutral pH, and barium ions. The activity of B is measured colorimetrically as the amount of 4-nitrocatechol released from conjugated substrate.

Procedure

1. Adjust 5 ml fresh or frozen catch sample of urine to pH 6.0 to 6.3 and centrifuge in clinical centrifuge for ten minutes.
2. Place clear supernatant fluid in 10-inch length of cylindrical 1/4-inch dialysis tubing (retention porosity of molecular weight [M. W.] 12,000) and dialyze for eighteen hours against two changes of tap water at 1°C with stirring.
3. Adjust volume of dialyzed urine to 6 ml with tap water (if second method of calculation is used).

4. Add 1.2 ml dialyzed urine to 1.2 ml buffered substrate in 16 × 125 mm screw-cap tubes (in duplicate). Add 1.2 ml dialyzed urine to tubes without substrate as blanks (in duplicate).
5. Incubate tubes at 37°C. Remove 1 ml aliquots from sample tubes at thirty minutes and add to 16 × 100 mm tubes containing 1.5 ml 1 N NaOH to stop reaction. Also at thirty minutes, add 1.2 ml substrate mixture to one of the blanks per sample; mix, remove 1 ml aliquot and add to 1.5 ml 1 N NaOH.
6. Continue incubation with remaining sample and blank tubes for a total of ninety minutes. Stop reaction as described in step 5.
7. Centrifuge suspensions at 4000 R.P.M. for five minutes, if not clear. Collect supernatant fluids and measure optical density of samples and 4-nitrocatechol standards at 515 nm.

Calculations

1. Subtract blank from test sample O.D.
2. Subtract contribution of arylsulfatase A to the total activity of urinary enzyme by subtracting O.D. at thirty minutes from O.D. at ninety minutes and the intercept value/5 when $O.D._{30 min}$ and $O.D._{90 min}$ are extrapolated to zero time (A).
3. When using standard curve, estimate microgram 4-nitrocatechol released per ml per hour from standard curve.
4. When using molecular extinction coefficient, estimate microgram 4-nitrocatechol released per ml per hour by multiplying A by 94, a factor obtained by multiplying molecular weight of 4-nitrocatechol (M.W. 155) expressed in μg (10^6), the reciprocal of the extinction coefficient of 4-nitrocatechol ($\frac{1}{12,400}$), the reciprocal of the volume of sample in ml ($\frac{1}{10^3}$), and the dilution factor of the urine sample as a result of the dialysis (6/4) and assay procedure ($\frac{2.5}{0.5}$).

Interpretation

Arylsulfatase B activity in urine samples from ten healthy adult males ranged from 0.3 to 3.0 μg per ml per hour when tested by Baum et al. (1959). In our hands, the method revealed a complete deficiency in a patient with Maroteaux-Lamy syndrome.

Reagents

1. *Sodium Acetate Buffer 0.5 M pH 6.0, containing barium acetate, 10^{-2} M*: Dissolve 6.8 g sodium acetate · 3 H_2O and 0.26 g barium acetate in 80 ml demineralized water. Adjust to pH 6.0 with glacial acetic acid and bring to volume in 100 ml volumetric flask.
2. *Potassium 2-Hydroxy-5-Nitrophenyl Sulfate (Nitrocatechol sulfate) Buffered Substrate, 0.05 M*: On the day of test dissolve 160 mg p-nitrocatechol sulfate (disodium salt) in 10 ml 0.5 M sodium acetate buffer containing 10^{-2} M barium acetate.
3. *Sodium Hydroxide, 0.5 N*: Dissolve 4 g NaOH and bring to 200 ml in volumetric flask with demineralized water.
4. *Sodium Hydroxide, 1 N*: Dissolve 4.0 g NaOH and bring to 100 ml in volumetric flask with demineralized water.
5. *4-Nitrocatechol Stock Standard Solution for Standard Curve (10 µg/ml)*: Dissolve 10 mg 4-nitrocatechol in 10 ml 0.5 N NaOH solution. Add 100 µl to 9.9 ml 0.5 N NaOH solution.
6. *Nitrocatechol Working Standard Solutions for Standard Curve*: Combine the following volumes of nitrocatechol stock standard solution and 0.5 N NaOH:

µg Nitrocatechol (per 5.0 ml NaOH)	Volume Stock Standard (µl)	Volume NaOH (ml)
0.5	50	4.95
1.0	100	4.9
2.0	200	4.8
3.0	300	4.7
4.0	400	4.6
5.0	500	4.5
7.0	700	4.3
10	1000	4.0

REFERENCES

Shapira, E., DeGregorio, R. R., Matalon, R., and Nadler, H. L.: Reduced arylsulfatase B activity of the mutant enzyme protein in Maroteaux-Lamy syndrome. *Biochem Biophys Res Commun, 62*:448, 1975.

Baum, H., Dodgson, K. S., and Spencer, B.: The assay of arylsulphatases A and B in human urine. *Clin Chim Acta,* 4:453, 1959.

MICROMETHOD FOR LEUKOCYTE SULFATASE B

Principle

Arylsulfatase B, the enzyme defect of Maroteaux-Lamy disease (MPS VI), is measured in leukocytes isolated from 50 μl blood and incubated with synthetic substrate, 4-methylumbelliferyl sulfate. The method employs Peters' procedures for separating leukocytes and increasing sensitivity of the assay with taurocholate, Baum and coworkers' conditions for optimum activity, and Harinath and Robins' selection of substrate.

Procedure

1. Collect approximately 0.5 ml capillary blood in heparinized hematocrit tubes or venous blood in EDTA (not heparinized) tubes. If heparinized, transfer samples to 10 $\times$ 75 mm tube.
2. To 50 μl aliquots of sample in seven 10 ml (15 $\times$ 100 mm) tubes add 5 ml 0.2% NaCl and mix by inversion several times. Note time. Exactly two minutes later, add 1.5 ml 3.6% NaCl to restore isotonicity; mix by inversion.
3. Centrifuge at maximum speed in a clinical centrifuge five to seven minutes.
4. Remove supernatant fluid containing hemoglobin and red cell ghosts with a fine Pasteur pipette, as follows: Hold tube at an angle of about 30° from the vertical and slide pipette tip along the side opposite the leukocyte pellet; aspirate last ml of fluid slowly, completely removing red cell ghosts from top of pellet.
5. Add 100 μl substrate solution to four of the tubes containing leukocyte pellets and mix on Vortex until suspension is uniform. Cool fifth tube at 4°C until ready for protein estimation (step 8).
6. Add 3.0 ml glycine-NaOH buffer to the two remaining tubes (blanks) and mix on Vortex.
7. Incubate sample and blank tubes at 37°C. Remove and stop

reactions in two sample tubes and one blank tube at thirty minutes by adding 3.0 ml glycine-NaOH buffer. Mix.

8. During preceding wait, suspend leukocyte pellet of fifth tube (step 5) in 0.1 ml demineralized water and measure protein as described in section on leukocyte branching enzyme (p. 238, Steps 17-19).

9. Continue incubation of remaining sample tubes and blank for ninety minutes. Stop reactions with glycine-NaOH buffer, as above.

10. Centrifuge suspensions in clinical centrifuge at maximum speed five to seven minutes, if not clear. Save supernatant fluids and measure fluorescence of standards, blanks, and samples on Turner fluorometer, Model 110, using primary filter 7-60 and secondary filters 2A and 48, overlaid with 10% neutral density filter.

Calculation

1. Plot standard curve of fluorescence against concentration of 4-methylumbelliferone.

2. Subtract blank from sample fluorescence values.

3. Correct total fluorescence for that contributed by activity of arylsulfatase A by subtracting fluorescence value at thirty minutes' incubation from that at ninety minutes. Also subtract one-fifth the intercept value when fluorescence values at thirty and ninety minutes are extrapolated to zero time for fluorescence due to activity of arylsulfatase B per hour.

4. Plot standard curve of absorbance at 750 nm versus mg protein.

5. Estimate mg protein per 0.1 ml leukocyte suspension from protein standard curve.

6. Obtain nanomoles 4-methylumbelliferone released per 0.1 ml leukocyte suspension from standard curve, and express activity of arylsulfatase B activity per mg protein per hour.

Interpretation

Leukocytes from healthy adults (four) contained from 5 to 10 units of activity (nmoles 4-methylumbelliferome released/hr/mg protein), when tested by this method. Humbel found little or no activity in leukocytes from a patient with Maroteaux-Lamy disease when tested by a macromethod. Until found otherwise, it can be presumed that carriers have half-normal levels of enzyme.

Reagents

1. *NaCl, 0.2%*: Dissolve 0.5 g NaCl in 250 ml demineralized water.
2. *NaCl, 3.6%*: Dissolve 3.6 g NaCl in 100 ml demineralized water.
3. *Sodium Acetate Buffer, 0.2 M, pH 6.0, Containing Barium Acetate, 5 mM*: Dissolve 0.49 g sodium acetate $\cdot$ 3 H_2O and 128 mg barium acetate in 80 ml demineralized water. Adjust to pH 6.0 with glacial acetic acid and bring to volume in 100 ml volumetric flask.
4. *4-Methylumbelliferyl Sulfate Buffered Substrate, 10 mM*: On the day of test, dissolve 60 mg taurocholic acid, sodium salt, in 10 ml freshly prepared, warm 0.2 M sodium acetate buffer, pH 6, (on heater-stirrer for approximately fifteen minutes), cool to 37°C, add 30 mg 4-methylumbelliferyl sulfate, and dissolve by stirring.
5. *Glycine-NaOH Buffer, 1.0 M, pH 10.5*: Dissolve 18.7 g glycine in 200 ml demineralized water. Adjust to pH 10.5 with 10 N sodium hydroxide and bring to volume in 250 ml volumetric flask.
6. *4-Methylumbelliferone Stock Standard Solution, (10 nmoles/3.1 ml)*: Dissolve 14.2 mg 4-methylumbelliferome in 10 ml glycine-NaOH buffer and bring to 250 ml in volumetric flask with demineralized water. Dilute 1 ml to 100 ml with glycine-NaOH buffer.
7. *4-Methylumbelliferone Working Standards*: Combine the following volumes of stock standard and glycine buffer:

Concentration (nanomoles/3.1ml)	Volume of Stock Standard (ml)	Volume of Buffer (ml)
0	0	5
0.1	0.05	4.95
0.2	0.1	4.9

Concentration (nanomoles/3.1ml)	Volume of Stock Standard (ml)	Volume of Buffer (ml)
0.4	0.2	4.8
0.6	0.3	4.7
0.8	0.4	4.6
1.0	0.5	4.5
1.2	0.6	4.4
1.4	0.7	4.3
2.0	1.0	4.0

REFERENCES

Baum, H., Dodgson, K. S., and Spencer, B.: The assay of arylsulfatases A and B in human urine. *Clin Chim Acta, 4*:453, 1959.

Harinath, B. C., and Robins, E.: Arylsulfatases in human brain: Assay, some properties and distribution. *J Neurochemistry, 18*:237, 1971.

Humbel, R.: Rapid method for measuring arylsulfatase A and B in leucocytes as a diagnosis for sulfatidosis, mucosulfatidosis and mucopolysaccharidosis VI. *Clin Chim Acta, 68*:339, 1976.

Peters, S. P., Lee, R. E., and Glen, R. H.: A microassay for Gaucher's disease. *Clin Chim Acta, 60*:391, 1975.

Bakhru-Kishore, R. and S. Kelly: A microfluorometric assay of the lysosomal arylsufatases in leukocytes. *Clin Chim Acta*, In press.

SERUM β-GLUCURONIDASE DEFICIENCY

Principle

Deficiency of β-glucuronidase is detectable in the serum of patients with Type VII mucopolysaccharidosis by a fluorometric method in which 4-methylumbelliferone is released from conjugated substrate by the hydrolase.

Procedure

1. Add 50λ aliquots of fresh or frozen sample and control sera in triplicate to 25 × 75 mm rubber-stoppered tubes. Add 200λ 4-methylumbelliferyl-β-D-glucuronide to two per set; the third tubes are blanks.
2. Incubate all tubes at 37°C for one hour. Stop reaction by cooling tubes in ice water bath and quickly adding 7.5 ml

glycine-carbonate buffer.
3. Add 200λ 4-methylumbelliferyl-β-D-glucuronide to blanks.
4. Measure fluorescence in standards, samples, and control in Turner Fluorometer, using primary Filter 760 and secondary filters, 2A and 48, overlaid with 10% neutral density filter. Zero instrument with zero nanomole standard.

Calculations

1. Plot standard curve of fluorescence against nm methylumbelliferone.
2. Subtract blank from sample fluorescence.
3. Obtain nanomoles 4-methylumbelliferone/7.75 ml diluted reaction mixture or per 0.05 ml serum from standard curve.
4. Multiply by 20 and express activity in units or nanomoles 4-methylumbelliferone released/ml serum/hour at 37°C.

Interpretation

Normal serum contains from 75 to 377 units/ml of activity; levels in plasma are slightly lower. Carriers are not distinguished from the normal state by the method.

Reagents

1. *Acetic Acid, 0.1 M*: Dilute 0.57 ml glacial acetic acid to 100 ml in volumetric flask.
2. *Acetate Buffer, 0.1 M, pH 4.8*: Dissolve 1.36 g sodium acetate trihydrate in 100 ml demineralized water. Adjust to pH 4.8 with approximately 60 ml 0.1 M acetic acid.
3. *4-Methylumbelliferyl-β-D-Glucuronide, 10 mM*: Dissolve 11.6 mg 4-methylumbelliferyl-β-D-glucuronide · 2 H_2O in 3.0 ml 0.1 M acetate buffer, pH 4.8.
4. *Glycine-Carbonate Buffer, 320 mM Glycine; 200 mM Carbonate, pH 10*: Dissolve 24.0 g glycine and 21.2 g Na_2CO_3 in 800 ml demineralized water. Adjust to pH 10 with 10 N NaOH and bring to volume in 1 liter volumetric flask.
5. *4-Methylumbelliferone Stock Standard, 1μmole/7.75 ml*: Dis-

solve 4.55 mg 4-methylumbelliferone in 200 ml glycine · carbonate buffer.

6. *4-Methylumbelliferone   Working   Standards:* Dilute stock standard as follows:

4-Methylumbelliferone (nmoles/7.75 ml)	Stock Standard (ml)	Glycine-CO_3 Buffer (ml)
0	0	5
1.0	0.010	9.99
2.5	0.025	9.975
5	0.05	9.95
7.5	0.075	9.925
10	0.1	9.9

REFERENCE

Glaser, J. H., and Sly, W. S.: β-Glucuronidase deficiency mucopolysaccharidosis: methods for enzymatic diagnosis, *J Lab Clin Med,* *82*:969, 1973.

MUCOLIPIDOSES

THE mucolipidoses are a transitional group of diseases with characteristics of both the mucopolysaccharidoses and the sphingolipidoses. Patients have various degrees of Hurler-like features, usually without mucopolysacchariduria; biochemical abnormalities, on the other hand, refer to lysosomal storage, chiefly lipid, sometimes in combination with some degree of mucopolysaccharide excess (see Table X).

Specific enzyme defects have been demonstrated in only two: In fucosidosis and G_{MI}-gangliosidosis, deficiencies of the hydrolases, fucosidase, and β-galactosidase, respectively. All the mucolipidoses are characterized biochemically, however, by the hyperactivity of other lysosomal enzymes in the tissues and body fluids, suggesting that the permeability of lysosomal membranes is involved. The ultrastructure of lysosomal membranes, furthermore, is typically altered. As in other lysosomal storage diseases, the cells often contain abnormal cytoplasmic granules or inclusions, and urine contains breakdown products of the stored glycolipids.

The diseases are probably autosomal recessive. Where specific enzyme defects are known, carriers, in some instances, may be identified by partial deficiencies. Alternately, they may or may not be recognized by typical cytologic inclusions or vacuoles.

The enzyme defect of fucosidosis is detected in serum (p. 169) and that of G_{MI}-gangliosidosis in urine or leukocytes (p. 172 and 174).

Urinary oligosaccharide patterns of the various mucolipidoses are interpreted from thin-layer chromatograms (p. 164). Excesses of serum β-glucuronidase are measured by a modification of the method used for demonstrating the deficiency (p. 166). Excessive serum sulfatase A is measured by the method described on p. 168.

Metachromasia in white cells and urine is demonstrated by methods described on pp. 138 and 137, respectively.

Table X

THE MUCOLIPIDOSES

	Storage product	*Enzyme defect*
Mucolipidosis Type I		
Mucolipidosis Type II (I-Cell Disease)		
Mucolipidosis Type III		
G$_{M1}$-Gangliosidosis	G$_{M1}$/Ganglioside; Desulfated keratan sulfate	Generalized deficiency of acid β-galactosidase
Fucosidosis	Fucosides: glycolipid and polysaccharide	Generalized deficiency of α-fucosidase
Mannosidosis	Mannose-rich oligosaccharides	Acid α-mannosidase deficiency
Mucosulfatidosis		Generalized deficiency of arylsulfatase A and partial deficiencies of B & C

Table X

THE MUCOLIPIDOSES

Clinical signs	*Laboratory Findings*
Hurler-like, but variable; Peripheral neuropathy; Cherry-red macular spot;	Alterations in lysosomal ultrastructure Acid hydrolases in urine (β-galactosidase and others); Vacuolated lymphocytes; bone marrow storage cells; Liver acid-hydrolases hyperactive;
Hurler-like; Growth slows by age two;	Granular inclusions in cultured fibroblasts (I-cells); Polyenzyme deficiency in I-cells; Vacuolated lymphocytes; Acid hydrolases in serum (β-glucuronidase and others); Moderate alterations in lysosomal ultrastructure; Liver acid-hydrolases normal;
Hurler-like;	Bone marrow storage cells; Lymphocytes not vacuolated; Slight alterations in lysosomal ultrastructure;
Hurler-like; Progressive psychomotor disturbances; Hypotonia, spasticity, convulsions; Macular cherry red spot Respiratory infections;	Vacuolated white cells Bone marrow storage cells; Occasional keratan sulfaturia; Hurler-like changes in lysosomal ultrastructure; Liver acid-hydrolase hyperactivity (other than β-galactosidase);
Hurler-like Angiokeratoma corporis diffusion; psychomotor retardation; Spasticity; Frequent respiratory infections;	Vacuolated white cells Liver acid-hydrolase hyperactivity (other than fucosidase); Altered ultrastructure of liver lysosomes;
Hurler-like; Progressive psychomotor retardation Frequent infections;	Vacuolated white cells and bone marrow; Mannose-rich oligosacchariduria; Altered ultrastructure of liver lysosomes (Hurler-like);

Hurler-like
Progressive neurologic
degeneration.
	Mucopolysacchariduria;
	Golden-brown urinary metachromatic granules
	   (leukodystrophic-like);
	Vacuolated white cells and bone marrow;
	Altered ultrastructure of liver lysosomes (Hurler-like);
	Altered ultrastructure of nerve cells (leukodystrophic-like);
	Liver acid-hydrolase hyperactivity
	   (other than sulfatases and β-galactosidase).

SCREENING

THIN-LAYER CHROMATOGRAPHY
OF OLIGOSACCHARIDES

Principle

The oligosaccharides excreted in certain lysosomal storage diseases, especially the mucolipidoses, form characteristic patterns discernible in thin-layer chromatograms stained with orcinol. Mannosidosis, fucosidosis, G_{M1}-gangliosidosis Type I, and aspartylglucosaminuria are among those with distinctive patterns.

Procedure

1. Lightly draw guide lines, 5 cm long and 1 cm apart, 2 cm from and parallel to the bottom edge of a precoated TLC sheet of silica gel 60 (Merck 5506).
2. Streak 20 μl aliquots of lactose standard and catch urine samples along respective guidelines. Dry streaks thoroughly with a heat gun (90°C for about one minute).
3. Develop overnight in butanol-acetic acid-water solvent (sixteen hours).
4. Dry sheet at room temperature for an hour and at 70°C for five minutes.
5. Spray sheet with orcinol solution and dry at 100°C for ten minutes.

Interpretation

The chromatograms of urine from patients with glycoprotein storage diseases contain substances with R_f values less than that of lactose, as indicated in Figure 8. The mannosidosis pattern includes an intense red-brown band; the fucosidosis pattern includes a yellow-brown band; the G_{M1}-gangliosidosis Type I patterns contain intense bands near the origin and slightly below that of lactose, and an abnormal band remains near the origin in aspartylglucosaminuria. Keratan sulfate of fucosidosis, G_{M1}-

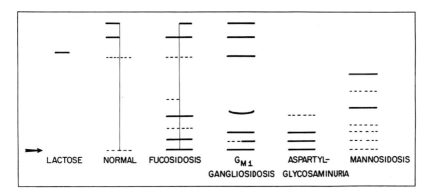

Figure 8. One-dimensional thin-layer silica gel chromatographic patterns of urinary oligosaccharides in the mucolipidoses. Patterns on lower half are definitive.

gangliosidosis and Morquio disease remains at the origin.

Reagents

1. *TLC Sheet of Silica Gel 60 (Merck 5506)*
2. *n-Butanol:Acetic Acid:Water Solvent, 10:5:5:* On the day of test, mix thoroughly 50 ml n-butanol, 25 ml glacial acetic acid, and 25 ml demineralized water in 300 ml Erlenmeyer flask.
3. *Sulfuric Acid, 20% By Weight:* Estimate volume of concentrated sulfuric acid required to obtain weight of 20 g from formula:

$$V = \frac{20}{D \times \dfrac{C}{100}}$$

where D is density and C is concentration of acid in percent (as given on the bottle label). Add this volume carefully to 80 ml demineralized water in 250 ml Pyrex beaker and dilute to volume in 100 ml volumetric flask.
4. *Orcinol Reagent, 0.2%:* On the day of test, dissolve 0.1 g orcinol in 50 ml 20% sulfuric acid.
5. *Lactose Standard, 10 μg/20 μl:* Dissolve 1 mg lactose in 2 ml demineralized water (10 μg in 20 μl).

REFERENCE

Humbel, R., and Collart, M.: Oligosaccharides in urine of patients with glycoprotein storage diseases. I. Rapid detection by thin-layer chromatography. *Clin Chim Acta, 60*:143, 1975.

TYPE II (I-CELL DISEASE)

*EXCESSIVE SERUM β-*GLUCURONIDASE

Principle

DenTandt's observation of a striking increase in hydrolases in patients with I-cell disease is a clue to the diagnosis of patients with the mucolipidoses. Of four especially active hydrolases, β-D-glucuronidase was the most active, the level being twenty-five or more times that in normal serum. The method described for demonstrating β-D-glucuronidase excess is modified from the fluorimetric assay for demonstrating a deficiency of the enzyme in mucopolysaccharidosis Type VII.

Procedure

1. Dilute serum sample 0, 1:10, 1:25, and 1:50 times with saline. Also dilute rabbit serum 1:2 for diluted control.
2. Pipette triplicate 50λ aliquots of the undiluted and diluted serum samples, and undiluted and diluted rabbit serum controls into 10 ml screw-capped tubes.
3. Add 200λ 4-methyl umbelliferyl-β-D-glucuronide substrate, 10 mM, to two tubes of each set, leaving third tubes as blanks.
4. Incubate all tubes at 37°C for one hour.
5. Stop reaction by placing tubes in ice water bath and quickly add 7.5 ml glycine-carbonate buffer.
6. Add 200λ substrate (4-methylumbelliferyl-β-D-glucuronide) to blanks.
7. Measure fluorescence of methylumbelliferone standard solutions and samples in Turner fluorometer with Turner primary

filter 7-60 and secondary filters, 2A and 48, overlaid with 10% neutral density filter. Zero the instrument with the zero standard.

Calculations

1. Plot concentration of methylumbelliferone standards against fluorescence.
2. Subtract blank from test readings.
3. Obtain 4-methylumbelliferone in nanomoles per 7.75 ml diluted reaction mixture from standard curve.
4. Multiply by dilution factor for nanomoles 4-methylumbelliferone per 0.05 ml serum per hour, then by 20, and express activity as nanomoles 4-methylumbelliferone per ml serum per minute.

Interpretation

Excesses of the serum hydrolases, especially β-glucuronidase, N-acetyl-β-D-glucosaminidase, and β-D-mannosidase, support the diagnosis of I-cell disease.

Reagents

1. *Saline*: Weight 0.85 grams sodium chloride. Dilute to 100 ml with demineralized water.
2. *Sodium Acetate Buffer, 0.1 M, pH 4.8*: Dissolve 1.36 g Na Acetate · 3 H_2O in 100 ml demineralized water. Adjust to pH 4.8 with 0.1 M acetic acid (0.57 ml glacial acetic acid diluted to 100 ml).
3. *4-Methylumbelliferyl-β-D*-Glucuronide Substate, 10 mM: Dissolve 116 mg 4-methylumbelliferyl-β-D-glucuronide · 2 H_2O in 3.0 ml 0.1 M acetate buffer, pH 4.8.
4. *Glycine-Carbonate Buffer, pH 10, 320 mM Glycine; 200 mM Carbonate*: Dissolve 24.0 g glycine and 21.2 g Na_2CO_3 in 800 ml demineralized water. Adjust to pH 10 with 10 NaOH and bring to volume with water in a liter volumetric flask.
5. *4-Methylumbelliferone Stock Standard, 1 μmole/7.75 ml*:

Dissolve 4.55 mg 4-methylumbelliferone in 200 ml glycine-carbonate buffer.

6. *4-Methylumbelliferone Working Standards*: Dilute stock standard, as follows:

Working Standard Concentration (nanomoles/7.75 ml)	Volume Stoek Standard (ml)	Volume Glycine-CO₃ Buffer (ml)
0	—	5
1.0	0.01	9.99
2.5	0.025	9.975
5	0.05	9.95
7.5	0.075	9.925
10	0.01	9.9

REFERENCES

DenTandt, W. R., Lassila, E., and Philippart, M.: Leroy's I-cell disease: markedly increased activity of plasma acid hydrolases. *J Lab Clin Med,* *83*:403. 1974.

Glaser, J. H., and Sly, W. S.: β-Glucuronidase deficiency mucopolysaccharidosis: methods for enzymatic diagnosis. *J Lab Clin Med,* *82*:969, 1973.

TYPE III

EXCESSIVE SERUM ARYLSULFATASE A

Principle

The excessive levels of serum arylsulfatase A in mucolipidosis Types II and III are detectable by a colorimetric method for nitrocatechol. When released from nitrocatechol sulfate by hydrolysis, nitrocatechol is red in strong alkaline solution.

Procedure

1. Combine 0.2 ml aliquots of sample and control sera with 0.5 ml nitrocatechol sulfate substrate in respective 10 × 75 ml screw-capped test tubes. Mix.
2. Incubate tubes for one hour in 37°C water bath.
3. Add 1.5 ml aliquots of 10% NaOH and observe color.

Interpretation

Reaction mixtures remaining pale yellow indicate normal levels of enzyme; deep orange or red solutions indicate excessive sulfatase.

Reagents

1. *Acetic Acid-Sodium Acetate Buffer, 0.5 M, pH 5.0*: Dissolve 13.6 g $NaC_2H_3O_2 \cdot 3 H_2O$ in 175 ml demineralized water. Adjust to pH 5.0 with glacial acetic acid. Bring to volume in 200 ml volumetric flask with demineralized water.
2. *Nitrocatechol Sulfate Reagent*: Dissolve 156 mg p-nitrocatechol sulfate, 11.2 mg sodium pyrophosphate ($NaP_2O_7 \cdot 10 H_2O$) and 5.0 g sodium chloride in 50 ml 0.5 M acetate buffer. Store at 4°C in brown bottle.
3. *Sodium Hydroxide, 10%*: Dissolve 10 g sodium hydroxide in final volume of 100 ml demineralized water.
4. *Positive Controls*: Guinea pig serum, undiluted; guinea pig serum diluted 1 to 10 with acetate buffer.
5. *Negative Control*: Rabbit serum, undiluted.

REFERENCE

Kelly, T. E., Thomas, H., and Taylor, H. A., Jr.: Screening for mucolipidosis. *Lancet, 2*:1089, 1973.

FUCOSIDOSIS

α-L-FUCOSIDASE IN SERUM

Principle

Serum from patients with fucosidosis lacks the enzyme fucosidase. The enzyme is demonstrable in a colorimetric assay for the nitrophenol released from conjugated substrate, when incubated with enzyme-containing serum from healthy persons. The lysosomal enzyme also splits the fluorigenic substrate, 4-methylumbelliferyl-fucoside; neither assay, however, discriminates heterozygote levels from normal with certainty.

Procedure

1. Add 0.2 ml serum sample to 1.0 ml 2.0 mM p-nitrophenol-α-L-fucoside substrate in two 8.5 × 75 mm Nalgene Sorvall tubes and 0.2 ml sample only in a third tube (blank).
2. Stopper tubes and incubate in shaking water bath at 37°C for thirty minutes; stop reaction by quickly adding 0.4 ml 10% trichloroacetic acid.
3. Add 1.0 ml substrate to blank tube.
4. Centrifuge tubes at 5000 R.P.M. at 4°C for ten minutes. Add 0.5 ml clear supernatant fluid to 0.5 ml 0.25 M glycine-carbonate buffer.
5. Measure absorbance of sample and standards at 420 nm.

Calculations

1. Plot curve of concentration of nitrophenol standards against $O.C._{420}$.
2. Subtract O.D. of blank from that of test sample for ΔO.D. nitrophenol formed.
3. Convert O.D. to mmoles nitrophenol/1000 ml final mixture from standard curve.
4. Divide by 1000 for mmoles per ml; multiply by 10_6 for nanomoles/ml final mixture. Correct for sixteen fold dilution of serum sample in final mixture, i.e. multiply by 16.
5. Mulitiply result by 2 for one hour reaction figures and express activity (E) as

$$E = \text{Nanomoles/ml/hr @ 37°C.}$$

Interpretation

Serum from patients with fucosidosis contains little or no activity, while that from normal persons contains from 282 to 659 units of activity (nanomoles per ml per hour). Levels in the serum of obligate carriers may be in the normal range.

Normal serum occasionally lacks enzyme, the significance of which must be verified by measuring activity of leukocyte enzyme. The level of leukocyte enzyme is also necessary to distinguish carriers from normal.

Reagents

1. *Citrate-Phosphate Buffer, 0.1 M, pH 5.0*: Dissolve 2.84 g $Na_2H\ PO_4$ and 2.04 g citric acid in 180 ml demineralized water. Adjust to pH 5.0, if necessary, with 0.1 M citric acid solution and bring to volume in 200 ml volumetric flask.
2. *p-Nitrophenyl-α-L-Fucoside, 2.0 mM*: Dissolve 14.25 mg p-nitrophenyl-α-L-fucoside in 25 ml citrate-phosphate buffer.
3. *Glycine-Carbonate Buffer, 0.25 M, pH 10.5*: Dissolve 2.65 g sodium carbonate and 1.88 g glycine in 80 ml demineralized water. Adjust to pH 10.5 with 10 N NaOH and bring to volume in 100 ml volumetric flask.
4. *p-Nitrophenol Stock Standard Solution, 1 mM*: Dilute 0.1 ml p-nitrophenol commercial standard solution (10 μmoles/ml) with 0.9 ml glycine-carbonate buffer.
5. *p-Nitrophenol Working Standards*:

p-Nitrophenol (mM)	Stock Standard (ml)	Glycine-Co₃ Buffer (ml)
0.00	0.0	5.0
0.01	0.1	9.9
0.02	0.1	4.9
0.03	0.1	3.2
0.05	0.2	3.8

REFERENCES

Zielke, K., Okada, S., and O'Brien, J. S.: Fucosidosis: Diagnosis by serum assay of α-L-fucosidase. *J Lab Clin Med, 79*:164, 1972.

Levvy, G. A., and McAllan, A.: Mammalian fucosidase.2 α-L-fucosidase. *Biochem J, 80*:435, 1961.

Ng, W. G. Donnell, G. N., and Koch, R.: Serum α-L-fucosidase activity in the diagnosis of fucosidosis. *Pediatr Res, 7*:391, 1973.

GENERALIZED G$_{MI}$-GANGLIOSIDOSIS

URINARY β-GALACTOSIDASE DEFICIENCY

Principle

The urine of patients with generalized G$_{MI}$ gangliosidosis contains little or no β-galactosidase, as measured by the amount of nitrophenol released from conjugated substrate. The activity is compared to that of a reference enzyme subject to the same variables to compensate for artifactual changes, and the relative activity of the two is expressed as a ratio.

Procedure

1. Filter fresh sample of catch urine through Whatman #1 filter paper. Collect in chilled beaker (ice water bath).
2. Dialyze 10.0 ml filtered urine in 5/8-inch diameter casing, six inches long, of retention porosity, M. W. 12,000 and above, against 3 one-liter changes of demineralized water at 4° C, over a period of at least fifteen hours.
3. Remove dialyzed urine without spilling, record volume, and process as below, storing at -20° C for up to a week, if necessary.
4. Distribute the dialyzed urine in six tubes in aliquots of 0.8 ml; add 0.2 ml aliquots of galactoside substrate to two, glucosaminide substrate to two, and acetate buffer to the two remaining (blank) tubes. Cool blank tubes immediately in an ice water bath.
5. Incubate all but blank tubes at 37° C for exactly sixty minutes.
6. Stop reaction in all tubes, including blanks, with 0.4 ml 0.25 M glycine buffer.
7. Measure optical density at 400 nm against a water blank.
8. Combine 0.8 ml aliquots of the nitrophenol working standards with 0.2 ml acetate buffer; quickly add 0.4 ml glycine buffer and measure O.D. at 400 nm.

Calculations

1. Plot curve of concentration of nitrophenol standards versus O.D.
2. Subtract blank O.D. from O.D. of test samples.
3. Obtain mμ moles p-nitrophenol cleaved by 0.8 ml dialyzed sample per hour at 37°C from standard curve and multiply by 1.25 for activity per ml dialyzed sample.
4. Correct for dilution during dialysis and express as activity in ml urine sample.
5. Divide β-D-glucosaminidase activity by β-galactosidase activity for ratio.

Interpretation

The ratio of β-D-glucosaminidase/β-galactosidase is strikingly elevated in urine from patients with G_{MI} gangliosidosis, ranging from 100 to 1400. Ratios in normal urine range from 0.4 to 20.

Reagents

1. *Acetic Acid, 0.5 M*: Dilute 2.86 ml glacial acetic acid with demineralized water in 100 ml volumetric flask.
2. *Acetate Buffer, 0.5 M, pH 5.0*: Dissolve 4.8 g $C_2H_3O_2$ Na · 3 H_2O (sodium acetate) in 60 ml demineralized water and 29.6 ml 0.5 M acetic acid. Adjust to pH 5.0 and bring to volume with water in 100 ml volumetric flask.
3. *p-Nitrophenyl-β-D-Galactoside, 0.005 M*: Dissolve 6.02 mg p-nitrophenyl-β-D-galactoside · 1 H_2O in 4.0 ml acetate buffer.
4. *p-Nitrophenyl-N-acetyl-β-D-Glucosaminide, 0.00375 M*: Dissolve 5.12 mg p-nitrophenyl-N-acetyl-β-D-glucosaminide in 4.0 ml acetate buffer.
5. *Glycine Buffer, 0.25 M, pH 10.0*: Dissolve 1.88 g glycine and 2.65 g sodium carbonate in 80 ml demineralized water. Adjust to pH 10.0 and bring to volume in 100 ml volumetric flask.
6. *p-Nitrophenol Stock Standard Solution (1000 mμ moles/ml)*: Dilute 1 ml Sigma standard p-nitrophenol solution (10

μmoles/ml) with 9 ml demineralized water.

7. *Working p-nitrophenol Standards:* Dilute the stock standard solution as follows:

mμ moles/ 0.8 ml	Stock Standard (ml)	H$_2$0 (ml)
0	0	3
8	0.1	9.9
20	0.05	1.95
40	0.1	1.9
80	0.2	1.8
120	0.3	1.7
160	0.4	1.6

REFERENCE

Thomas G. H.: β-D-Galactosidase in human urine: Deficiency in generalized gangliosidosis. *J Lab Clin Med, 74*:725, 1969.

LEUKOCYTE β-GALACTOSIDASE DEFICIENCY

Principle

Patients with G$_{MI}$-gangliosidosis are distinguished from those with other lysosomal storage diseases by demonstrating a deficiency of leukocyte β-galactosidase. The enzyme is measured colorimetrically as the amount of nitrophenol hydrolyzed from conjugated specific substrate, p-nitrophenyl-β-D-galactopyranoside, by cell-free homogenate.

Procedure

1. Separate white cells from 5 to 10 ml fresh heparinized blood in 50 ml Nalgene Sorvall tube, as follows: Add two volumes 3% dextran, mix thoroughly for five minutes, and let cells settle for one hour at 4°C. Remove leukocyte-rich supernatant fluid with Pasteur pipette and centrifuge in clean 50 ml Nalgene Sorvall tube for ten to fifteen minutes at 3000 R.P.M. at 4°C. Decant and discard platelet-rich supernatant fluid.

2. Suspend white blood cell pellet in 2 ml 0.85% NaCl, add 6 ml

demineralized water, and immediately shake gently for exactly one minute to lyse contaminating red cells; restore isotonicity immediately by adding 2 ml 0.6 M NaCl. Mix.

3. Centrifuge at 3000 R.P.M. for ten to fifteen minutes and discard supernatant fluid. Repeat steps 2 and 3 to remove remaining red cells.

4. Wash cells twice with 10 ml 0.85% NaCl to remove red cell ghosts.

5. Suspend leukocytes in sucrose-detergent solution, using one-fifth the volume of the initial heparinized blood sample. Transfer to glass homogenizing tube and homogenize manually.

6. Centrifuge homogenate at 34,000 × g (16,800 R.P.M.) at 4°C for twenty minutes. Save supernatant fluid for enzyme assay and protein determination.

7. Add 0.1 ml aliquots of supernatant fluid to 0.1 ml volumes of 0.1 M acetate buffer, pH 3.6, in three 15 ml conical centrifuge tubes. Add substrate to two. The third tube is blank.

8. Mix, incubate at 37°C for ninety minutes, and stop reactions by adding 0.1 ml 1 M trichloroacetic acid.

9. Add 0.1 ml substrate to blank, add 2 ml cold absolute ethanol to all tubes and shake.

10. Centrifuge at 1500 R.P.M. for ten minutes, decant and collect clear, supernatant fluid (ethanol layer) in 10 ml tube.

11. Add 1.5 ml glycine·carbonate buffer to the alcoholic solution, mix, and measure O.D. at 410 nm. Color is stable for at least an hour.

12. Measure O.D. of nitrophenol standards at 410 nm.

13. Estimate protein concentration in supernatant fluid of high-speed white cell homogenate as follows: add 50λ supernatant fluid and 50λ working standards to 2.0 ml aliquots of working alkaline copper reagent in respective tubes. Let stand at room temperature for fifteen minutes; add 0.2 ml dilute phenol reagent to all tubes quickly, mix, and let stand at room temperature at least thirty minutes. Measure optical density at 750 nm.

Calculations

1. Plot O.D.$_{410}$ versus concentration of p-nitrophenol standards.

2. Subtract O.D.$_{410}$ of blank from O.D. of substrate-containing tubes.
3. Read nanomoles substrate hydrolyzed in 3.9 ml reaction mixture (0.1 ml leukocyte homogenate) per ninety minutes at 37°C from standard nitrophenol curve. Divide by 90 and multiply by 1000 for nanomoles substrate hydrolyzed by 100 ml leukocyte homogenate per minute at 37°C.
4. Plot O.D.$_{750}$ versus protein concentration.
5. Estimate mg protein in 100 ml leukocyte homogenate from standard protein curve.
6. Express activity as nanomoles substrate hydrolyzed per minute per mg protein.

Interpretation

Leukocytes from patients with G$_{M1}$ gangliosidosis contain no more than 1 unit (nmoles substrate hydrolyzed/min/mg protein) β-galactosidase activity; obligate heterozygote levels range from 2 to 4 units and leukocytes from normal persons (and patients with the mucopolysaccharidoses) contain from 6 to 10 units of activity.

Reagents

1. *Dextran, 3%*: On the day of test, dissolve 1.5 g dextran (average mol. wt: 139,000 to 230,000) in 50 ml 0.85% NaCl.
2. *NaCl, 3.5%*: Dissolve 3.5 g sodium chloride in 100 ml demineralized water.
3. *Sucrose, 0.25 M, Containing 2.5% Detergent:* Dissolve 8.56 g sucrose in 2.5 ml Cutscum® detergent (Fisher) and 97.5 ml demineralized water.
4. *Acetate Buffer, 0.1 M, pH 3.6*: Dissolve 0.102 g sodium acetate · 3 H$_2$O in 60 ml demineralized water; add 18.5 ml 0.5 M acetic acid (2.86 ml glacial acetic acid/100 ml). Adjust to pH 3.6. Bring to volume in 100 ml volumetric flask with demineralized water.
5. *Substrate, p-Nitrophenyl-β-D-Galactopyranoside, (20 mM):*

Dissolve 19.7 mg p-nitrophenyl-β-D-galactopyranoside · H₂O in 3 ml demineralized water.

6. *Trichloroacetic Acid, 1 M*: Dissolve 16.3 g trichloroacetic acid in demineralized water and bring to volume in 100 ml volumetric flask.

7. *Glycine · Carbonate Buffer, 0.2 M, pH 10.7*: Dissolve 1.52 g glycine in 2.12 g sodium carbonate in 80 ml demineralized water. Adjust to pH 10.7 and bring to volume in 100 ml volumetric flask.

8. *p-Nitrophenol Stock Standard (500 nanomoles/3.9 ml)*: Combine 0.1 ml p-nitrophenol Sigma reagent (10 µmole/ml) with 7.7 ml glycine·carbonate buffer.

9. *p-Nitrophenol Working Standards*: Combine the following volumes of stock standard and glycine · carbonate buffer:

Nanomoles (in 3.9 ml)	Stock Standard (ml)	Buffer (ml)
0	0	5
25	0.25	4.75
50	0.5	4.5
100	1.0	4.0
150	1.5	3.5
200	2.0	3.0

10. *Dilute Phenol Reagent*: Dilute 2.0 ml Fisher phenol reagent with 2.0 ml demineralized water.

11. *Alkaline Tartrate Reagent*: Dissolve 2.0 g Na₂CO₃ and 50 mg Na or K tartrate in 100 ml 0.1 N NaOH (0.4 g/100 ml).

12. *Copper Sulfate, 0.1%*: Dissolve 100 mg CuSO₄ · 5 H₂O in 100 ml demineralized water.

13. *Working Alkaline Copper Reagent*: On the day of test combine 27 ml alkaline tartrate reagent and 3 ml 0.1% CuSO₄.

14. *Stock Protein Standard, 600 mg%*: Dissolve 1.0 mg 30% bovine albumin in 49.0 ml demineralized water.

15. *Working Protein Standards*: Combine the following volumes of stock protein standard and demineralized water:

Protein (mg%)	Stock Standard (ml)	Water (ml)
0	0	2
50	0.25	2.75

Protein (mg%)	Stock Standard (ml)	Water (ml)
100	0.50	2.5
200	1.0	2.0
300	1.0	1.0
400	2.0	1.0

REFERENCES

Lowry, O. H., Rosebrough, N. J., Farr, A. L., and Randall, R. J.: Protein measurement with the Folin phenol reagent. *J Biol Chem, 193*:265, 1951.

Singer, H. S., Nankervis, G. A., and Schafer, I. A.: Leukocyte beta-galactosidase activity in the diagnosis of generalized GM$_1$ gangliosidosis. *Pediatrics, 49*:352, 1972.

Singer, H. S., and Schafer, I. A.: White-cell β-galactosidase activity. *New England J Med, 282*:571, 1970.

Skoog, W. A., and Beck, W. S.: Studies on the fibrinogen, dextran, and phytohemagglutinin methods of isolating leukocytes. *Blood, 11*:436, 1956.

WOLMAN DISEASE

LEUKOCYTE ACID LIPASE

Principle

Tissues from patients with Wolman disease and cholesterol ester storage disease are deficient in acid lipase. One of the many lysosomal enzymes active on both natural and artificial substrates, the leukocyte enzyme, hydrolyzes the artificial substrate p-nitrophenyl-palmitate in the assay described here. The p-nitrophenol freed is measured colorimetrically.

Procedure

1. Centrifuge 10 ml heparinized blood at 1000 g at 4°C for five minutes.
2. Remove carefully and discard supernatant plasma, leaving white cell plaque and red cells undisturbed. Resuspend plaque and red cells in one volume 0.9% saline; recentrifuge. Collect leukocyte plaque at interface with Pasteur pipette.
3. Wash leukocytes twice with 1 ml portions 0.9% NaCl, centri-

fuging at 2900 R.P.M. after each wash.

4. Suspend cells in 1 ml cold demineralized water and centrifuge immediately at 2900 R.P.M. five minutes at 4°C.

5. Repeat cold water wash and centrifugation.

6. Suspend cells in 0.5 ml 1% aqueous Triton ® X-100.

7. Homogenize cells with Teflon pestle one to two minutes. Centrifuge at 1500 g five minutes at 4°C.

8. Collect supernatant fluid for determination of enzyme activity and protein concentration. Store supernatant fluid at 4°C until ready for protein determination. Measure enzyme activity immediately, as described below.

9. Add 0.05 ml homogenate supernatant fluid and 0.5 ml glycine-HCl buffer to three 3 ml Sorvall tubes. Add 0.2 ml plamitate-Triton X-100 dispersion substrate to two, leaving third tube as blank.

10. Incubate all tubes at 37°C for thirty minutes; stop reactions with 0.25 ml 20% perchloric acid, including blank.

11. Add 0.2 ml palmitate-Triton X-100 dispersion substrate to blank. Let all tubes stand at room temperature five minutes.

12. Centrifuge at 5000 R.P.M. five minutes.

13. Add 0.5 ml supernatant fluids to 3.0 ml bicarbonate-carbonate buffer, mix by shaking, and determine O.D. at 400 nm immediately (one-half to one minute).

14. Prepare p-nitrophenol working standards and determine O.D. at 400 nm.

15. To 2.0 ml of working alkaline copper reagent in respective tubes add 50λ aliquots working protein standards and supernatant fluid portion of white cells homogenate.

16. Let stand at room temperature fifteen minutes.

17. Quickly add 0.2 ml dilute phenol reagent, mix by shaking, and let stand at room temperature one-half hour.

18. Centrifuge test samples at 1000 R.P.M., save clear supernatant fluids; measure O.D. of sample and working protein standards at 750 nm.

Calculations

1. Plot standard curve of p-nitrophenol concentration versus O.D. at 400 nm.

2. Subtract O.D. of blank from test samples.
3. Obtain concentration p-nitrophenol in mM of final solution of test samples from standard curve.
4. Multiply by 3.5×10^{-3}. Express activity as nmoles p-nitrophenol per thirty minutes in 3.5 ml final solution, 0.5 ml reaction mixture or 25λ cell homogenate.
5. Multiply by 4000 for activity in 100 ml homogenate; divide by 30 for activity per 100 ml homogenate per minute; multiply by 10^6, expressing activity in nmoles.
6. Plot standard curve of protein concentration versus O.D. at 750 nm.
7. Obtain concentration protein in mg per 100 ml of homogenate from standard curve.
8. Divide nmoles p-nitrophenol per 100 ml homogenate per minute by mg protein per 100 ml homogenate; express activity as nmoles p-nitrophenol per mg protein per minutes at 37°C.

Interpretation

Acid esterase activity increases gradually with age, ranging from a low of from 6.5 to 17 nmoles/mg protein/min at 37°C in normal cord blood to activities of from 30 to 84 units in adult samples.

Reagents

1. *Triton X-100, 1%*: Dilute 0.5 ml stock Triton X-100 (Sigma) with 49.5 ml demineralized H_2O.
2. *Glycine ·HCl Buffer, 50 μmoles/0.5 ml, pH 4.0*: Dissolve 375 mg glycine in 40 ml demineralized H_2O. Adjust to pH 4.0 with 0.1 M HCl and bring to volume in 50 ml volumetric flask.
3. *Palmitate · Triton X-100 Dispersion, 3 μmoles/0.2 ml*: Combine 56.6 mg p-nitrophenyl palmitate (Koch-Light) with 0.5 ml Triton X-100. Add 1-2 ml petroleum ether and warm in 50°C water bath with constant shaking for about ten minutes. When the dispersion is complete, the two layers are clear. Remove the ether layer by vacuum aspiration and discard. Agitate and warm the lower layer, while adding, in drops, 5 ml demineral-

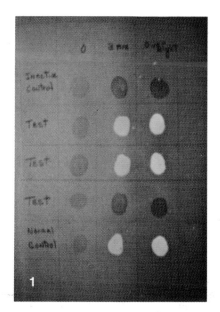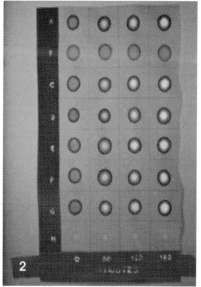

Illustration 1. Photograph of fluorescent spot test for deficiency of red cell galactose-1-phosphate uridyl transferase, the enzyme defect of galactosemia. Nonfluorescent sample (row 4) indicates deficiency. Row 1 is control sample of heat-inactivated enzyme.

Illustration 2. Photograph of fluorescent spot test for red cell galactokinase deficiency. Nonfluorescent sample (row B) indicates deficiency. Row H is control sample of heat-inactivated enzyme.

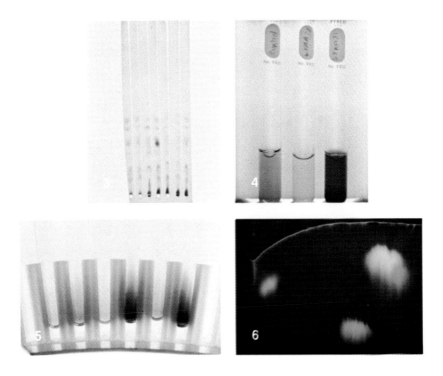

Illustration 3. Paper chromatogram of amino acids in dried blood spot samples, ninhydrin-stained. Middle channel contains sample from patient with citrullinemia.

Illustration 4. Nitroprusside test for urinary cystine. Tube on right contains sample from patient with cystinuria.

Illustration 5. Nitroaniline test for urinary methylmalonic acid. Fourth tube contains urine from patient with untreated methylmalonic aciduria. Sixth tube displays artifact from brown chromogen.

Illustration 6. Paper chromatogram of urinary tryptophane metabolites in ultraviolet. In hydroxykynureninuria, hydroxykynurenine is present (upper right, dull spot) and anthranilic acid is absent (extreme left spot).

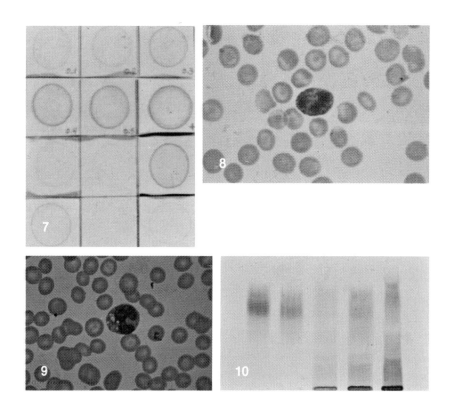

Illustration 7. Toluidine blue spot test of mucopolysaccharides in urine. Two upper rows are chondroitin sulfate standards. Last spot in third row is sample from patient with Hurler disease (MPS I).

Illustration 8. Coarse metachromatic granules in leukocyte from girl with Maroteaux-Lamy disease (MPS VI). Giemsa-stained.

Illustration 9. Vacuoles in granulocyte of patient with lipofuscinosis storage disease. Compare with granules in Illustration 8. Toluidine blue-stained.

Illustration 10. Toluidine blue-stained chromatographic patterns of urinary mucopolysaccharides on thin-layer cellulose. Samples from patients with MPS diseases, from left to right: Maroteaux-Lamy (VI), Hunter (II), Hurler/Scheie genetic compound (I/V), and Sanfilippo (III) (two samples).

Erratum: Color illustration 10 has been reversed.

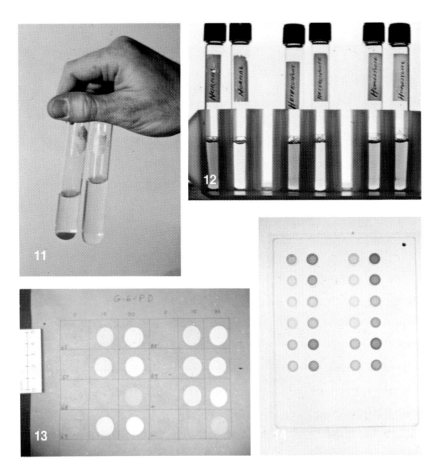

Illustration 11. Nitrocatechol test for urinary sulfatase. Nitrocatechol, released by sulfatase action in normal urine, forms red solution. Nitrocatechol is not released by reaction with sulfatase-deficient urine, as from patient with metachromatic leukodystrophy, and solution is colorless or yellow.

Illustration 12. Paired solutions reveal phenotypes for the pseudocholinesterase variant gene. From left to right: normal, carrier and homozygous phenotypes. α-Naphthol, released by hydrolytic action of pseudocholinesterase or pseudocholinesterase variant, forms pink solutions. Second tubes of pairs contain inhibitor. Normal pseudocholinesterase enzyme, in the presence of inhibitor (second tube of first pair) does not hydrolyze substrate and solution is colorless.

Illustration 13. Fluorescent spot test for deficiency of red cell glucose-6-phosphate dehydrogenase (G-6-PD). Nonfluorescing spots in third horizontal row (left) contain sample from patient with G-6-PD deficiency. Spots in fourth horizontal row (right) contain heat-inactivated enzyme control.

Illustration 14. Solubility spot test for hemoglobins SS and AS. Horizontal pairs consist of hemolysates from dried blood spots, without and with urea, respectively. Hemolysates contain, from top to bottom: hemoglobins AA, AS, SS, SC, AC, and F. Pairs on left are made with Ortho Diagnostic's Sickledex reagents; those on right are made with phosphate and phosphate-urea solutions.

ized water. Add 0.75 ml Triton X-100, and bring to volume in 10 ml volumetric flask with demineralized water. Use within an hour.

4. *Perchloric Acid, 20%*: Dilute 10 ml perchloric acid (70%) with 25 ml demineralized water.

5. *Bicarbonate · Carbonate Buffer, 1 M, pH 9.0*: Dissolve 16.8 g $NaHCO_3$ in 200 ml demineralized H_2O. Adjust to pH 9.0 with 1 M Na_2CO_3 (21.2 g/200 ml).

6. *p-Nitrophenol Stock Standard, 1 mM*: Dilute 0.5 ml Sigma standard p-nitrophenol solution (10 μmoles/ml) in 4.5 ml demineralized H_2O.

7. *p-Nitrophenol Working Standards*: Immediately before use dilute the p-nitrophenol stock solution as follows:

Concentration of p-nitrophenol	Volume Stock Standard	Volume Carbonate· Bicarbonate Buffer
(mM)	(ml)	(ml)
0.0	—	5
0.01	0.1	9.9
0.02	0.1	4.9
0.03	0.1	3.2
0.05	0.2	3.8
0.075	0.3	3.7
0.1	0.5	4.5

Reagents for Protein Determination

1. *Dilute Phenol Reagent (Fresh)*: Dilute 2.0 ml Fisher phenol reagent with 2.0 ml demineralized water.

2. *Alkaline Tartrate Reagent*: Dissolve 2.0 g Na_2CO_3 and 50 mg Na or K tartrate in 100 ml 0.1 N NaOH (0.4 g/100 ml).

3. *Copper Sulfate, 0.1%*: Dissolve 100 mg $CuSO_4 \cdot 5\ H_2O$ in 100 ml demineralized H_2O.

4. *Working Alkaline Copper Reagent (Fresh)*: Dilute 27 ml alkaline tartrate reagent with 3 ml 0.1% $CuSO_4$.

5. *Stock Protein Standard, 600 mg%*: Dilute 1.0 ml 30% bovine albumin with 49.0 ml demineralized H_2O.

6. *Working Protein Standards*: Dilute stock protein standard as follows:

Protein (mg%)	Volume of Stock (ml)	Volume H_2O (ml)
0	0	2
50	0.25	2.75
100	0.5	2.5
200	1.0	2.0
300	1.0	1.0
400	2.0	1.0

REFERENCES

Young, E. P., Patrick, A. D.: Deficiency of acid esterase activity in Wolman's disease. *Arch Dis Child, 45*:664, 1970.

Mahadevan, S., Tappel, A. L.: Hydrolysis of higher fatty acid esters of p-nitrophenol by rat liver and kidney lysosomes. *Arch Biochem Biophys, 126*:945, 1968.

ASPARTYLGLYCOSAMINURIA

ASPARTYLGLYCOSAMINE IN URINE

Principle

Aspartylglycosamine is separated from amino acids and other ninhydrin-positive compounds in urine by thin-layer chromatography on cellulose and is distinguished by the development of a blue-green color when overstained with a mixture of acetic and hydrochloric acids. The test is used as a screening method for aspartylglycosaminuria and to verify an abnormal oligosaccharide pattern (p. 164).

Procedure

1. Apply 2 µl aliquots of test and control catch urine samples in duplicate on Eastman Chromagram Sheet of 13255 cellulose (No. 6064) in streaks, 1.5 cm long, 1 cm apart, 1.5 cm from side, and 2 cm from bottom edges of sheet. Overstreak one of each pair with 5 µl aspartylglycosamine standard.
2. Develop in acetone-n-butanol-acetic acid-water solvent system until front rises 10 cm (about one hour). Dry sheet at 80°C five

minutes in explosion-proof oven and redevelop in same system. Dry ten minutes.

3. Spray with 0.2% solution ninhydrin in propanol. Heat sheet at 60°C ten minutes or until ninhydrin-positive (blue) spots appear.
4. Remove sheet from oven and lightly spray with acid counterstain until amino acid spots begin to fade. Excessive counterstain masks the development of color by aspartylglycosamine.
5. Heat at 60°C until aspartylglycosamine standard appears blue (about five minutes). Examine immediately, as color fades.

Interpretation

Aspartylglycosamine appears as a blue streak about 1.5 cm from the origin.

Reagents

1. *Aspartylglycosamine Standard*: Dissolve 2 mg aspartylglycosamine in 1 ml demineralized water.
2. *Acetone-n-Butanol-Acetic Acid-Water Chromatographic Solvent, 35:35:10:20*: Mix the following thoroughly in 300 ml Erlenmeyer flask: 35 ml acetone, 35 ml n-butanol, 10 ml glacial acetic acid, and 20 ml demineralized water.
3. *Ninhydrin Stain, 0.2% in n-Propanol*: Dissolve 100 mg ninhydrin in 50 ml n-propanol.
4. *Acid Counterstain*: Add 10 ml concentrated hydrochloric acid to 40 ml glacial acetic acid in 125 ml Erlenmeyer flask. Mix well.

REFERENCE

Humbel, R. and Marchal, C.: Screening test for aspartylglycosaminuria. *J Pediatr, 84*:456, 1974.

CHAPTER 7

SPHINGOLIPIDOSES

Excessive storage of the sphingolipids causes a variable group of diseases involving the erythropoietic organs of destruction and disposal. Defects in specific hydrolases of reticuloendothelial cells are at fault and lead to the accumulation of sphingolipids. The liver, spleen, kidneys, and bone marrow become engorged; the central nervous system degenerates in infantile and some juvenile forms. The chief clinical signs and laboratory findings of the sphingolipidoses are listed in Table XI. Although treatment is nonspecific at present, the clinical signs may be alleviated in the future by organ transplants or enzyme replacement.

Clinical impressions are confirmed by demonstrating deficiencies of specific hydrolases in urine, fresh leukocytes, cultured fibroblasts, or appropriate excised tissues. Metachromasia in leukocytes and fresh urine sediments accompanies the enzyme defects.

GAUCHER

β-GLUCOSIDASE IN LEUKOCYTES

Principle

A deficiency of the leukocyte β-glucosidase normally active at pH 4.0 is demonstrable in patients with Gaucher disease. The lysosomal enzyme is measured by a fluorometric method in which conjugated substrate is hydrolyzed to fluorescent methylumbelliferone. Another form of the enzyme, normally active at pH 5.3, is not measured, as it is only slightly less active than normal in Gaucher disease.

Procedure

1. Sediment red cells in 10 ml fresh venous blood (with or

Table XI

THE SPHINGOLIPIDOSES

Disease	Ceramide	Enzyme defect	Clinical signs	Laboratory findings
Gaucher	Glucocerebroside	β-glucosidase	H, S, B, R* Anemia	Marrow: Gaucher's cells Serum: > acid phosphatase Tissues: > cerebroside RE organs and leukocytes: >β-glucosidase
Metachromatic leukocystrophy	Sulfatide	Arylsulfatase A	Dementia; Weakness	Urine: Metachromasia and <sulfatase Leukocytes: < sulfatase
Niemann-Pick	Sphingomyelin	Sphingomyelinase	H, S, B, R* Olive skin; Cherry red spot	Marrow: foam cells Liver: >sphingomyelin RE organs and leukocytes: <sphingomyelinase
Fabry	Trihexoside (GL-3)	β-galactosidase Trihexosidase	X-linked; Renal failure; Joint pain; Pigmented Papules; Opacities	Small intestine mucosa and plasma:<β-galactosidase
Tay-Sachs	Ganglioside GM$_2$	Hexosaminidase A	H, S, B, R* Cherry red spot; Blindness; Early death	Muscle, cell cultures and leukocytes: <hexosaminidase A
Generalized gangliosidosis	Ganglioside GM$_1$	β-galactosidase	H, R* Early death; Milder forms	Leukocytes Liver Urine } <β-galactosidase

*Key: H = hepatomegaly
    S = splenomegaly
    B = bone erosion
    R = mental retardation in infancy

without heparin) with 3.3 ml 3% sodium citrate · PVP. Mix by inverting and let settle at 37°C for thirty to forty-five minutes.

2. Aspirate and save supernatant layer containing leukocytes; centrifuge at 1000 R.P.M. at 4°C for ten minutes.

3. Discard supernatant fluid, suspend cells in 0.7 ml ice cold demineralized water for fifty seconds and quickly add 0.7 ml 2% NaCl to restore isotonicity.

4. Dilute a 1 ml aliquot with 4 ml saline.

5. Count white cells per cmm on one portion and sediment the remainder at 2700 R.P.M. at 4°C for ten minutes.

6. Discard supernatant fluid, resuspend cells in 0.5 ml saline, and proceed immediately with assay for enzyme activity.

7. Combine 0.020 ml 0.2 M acetate buffer and 0.050 ml substrate in four test tubes per sample, adding 0.020 ml cell suspension to three (triplicate sample tubes) and 0.020 ml saline to the fourth (blank).

8. Incubate all tubes at 37°C for sixty minutes; stop reaction by partially submerging tubes in an ice bath and quickly adding 3 ml 0.2 M glycine buffer, pH 10.7.

9. Measure fluorescence of working standards and test solutions with Turner 110 fluorometer, using primary filter 7-60 and secondary filters 2-A and 48, overlaid with a 10% neutral density filter. Zero the instrument with the 0 nmole methylumbelliferone standard.

Calculations

1. Correct for the concentrated leukocyte suspension by multiplying cell count by 10; express as cells per mm^3 in 0.5 ml concentrated cell suspension. Multiply figure by 20 for cells in 20λ original cell suspension.

2. Plot fluorescence versus concentration of standard 4-methylumbelliferone solutions.

3. Subtract fluorescence of blank from that of test sample.

4. Read nanomoles 4-methylumbelliferone cleaved per 3.09 ml final dilution from standard curve, or per 20λ cell suspension per sixty minutes. Divide by the number of cells in 20λ cell suspension and multiply by 10^7 for nanomoles methylumbelli-

ferone/10^7 cells/60 minutes.

5. Divide by 60, multiply by 1000 and express as enzyme units or picomoles 4-methylumbelliferone formed/10^7 cells/minute at 37°C.

Interpretation

Normal white cells contain from 17 to 44 μU β glucosidase/10^7 cells, while those from patients with Gaucher disease have only 0-4 μU. Obligate heterozygotes have about half normal levels; the upper ones (up to 25 μU) overlap with those in the lower portion of the normal range. Levels of lymphocyte β-glucosidase (p. 190) are more discriminatory of the carrier state than leukocyte enzyme.

Reagents

1. *Sodium Citrate, 3%, Containing PVP, 5%*: Dissolve 0.75 g sodium citrate and 1.25 g polyvinylpyrrolidone (PVP) in demineralized water in 25 ml volumetric flask. Bring to volume.
2. *Acetate Buffer, 0.2 M, pH 4.0*: Dissolve 2.72 g Na · Acetate · 3 H_2O in 100 ml demineralized water. Adjust to pH 4.0 with 0.2 M acetic acid.
3. *4-Methylumbelliferyl-β-D-Glucopyranoside Substrate 1 mM*: Dissolve 16.9 mg 4-methylumbelliferyl-β-D-glucopyranoside from Koch-Light in 50 ml H_2O. If Sigma substrate is used, extract first with 4 volumes ether to remove fluorescent contaminant.
4. *Glycine Buffer, 0.2 M, pH 10.7*: Dissolve 15.01 g glycine in 700 ml demineralized H_2O. Adjust to pH 10.7.
5. *Stock 4-Methylumbelliferone Standard, 300 Nanomoles per 3.09 ml*: Dissolve 4.3 g 4-methylumbelliferone in 250 ml glycine buffer.
6. *Working 4-Methylumbelliferone Standards*: Combine the following volumes of stock standard and glycine buffer:

Nanomoles (3.09)	Stock Standard (ml)	Glycine Buffer (ml)
0	0	10

Nanomoles (3.09)	Stock Standard (ml)	Glycine Buffer (ml)
0.25	0.005	6
0.50	0.010	6
1.0	0.020	6
1.5	0.025	5
2.0	0.020	3
2.5	0.050	6

MICROMETHOD FOR LEUKOCYTE β-GLUCOSIDASE

Principle

β-glucosidase activity in leukocytes, isolated from 50 μl blood, is measured on synthetic substrate 4-methylumbelliferyl-β-D-glucopyranoside, at the hydrogen ion concentration optimum for authentic enzyme in the presence of sodium taurocholate.

Procedure

1. Collect approximately 0.40 ml capillary blood in heparinized hematocrit tubes or venous blood in EDTA (not heparinized) tubes. If heparinized, transfer sample to 10 × 75 mm tube.
2. Have a second person count white cells in aliquots of samples.
3. Add 5 ml aliquots of 0.2% NaCl to 0.050 ml sample in a 10 ml (15 × 100 mm) tube and mix by inversion several times. (Cover tube with Parafilm® .) Note time. Exactly two minutes later, add 1.5 ml of 3.6% NaCl to restore isotonicity; mix by inversion. Repeat with three more aliquots of NaCl and sample (three replicates and a blank).
4. Centrifuge all tubes at maximum speed in a clinical centrifuge for five to seven minutes.
5. Remove supernatant fluid containing hemoglobin and red cell ghosts with a fine Pasteur pipette, as follows: Hold tube at an angle of about 30° from the vertical and slide pipette tip along the side opposite the leukocyte pellet; aspirate last ml of fluid slowly, completely removing red cell ghosts from top of leukocyte pellet.
6. Add 100 μl substrate solution to tubes containing pellets and mix (Vortex).
7. Add 3.0 ml glycine · NH₄OH buffer to blank tubes; mix and

incubate all tubes at 37°C for one hour.
8. Add 3.0 ml glycine · NH_4OH buffer to sample tubes (omit blanks) and mix.
9. Measure fluorescence of standard, blank, and sample tubes on Turner fluorometer, Model 110, using primary filter 7-60 and secondary filters 2-A and 48 overlaid with 10% neutral density filter.

Calculations

1. Multiply cell count (cells/mm^3) by 50 for cell count in 50λ blood or 3.1 ml final solution; express as number $\times 10^7$ cells.
2. Plot standard curve of fluorescence (F) against concentration of 4-methylumbelliferone.
3. Estimate nanomoles substrate cleaved per 3.1 ml final solution from standard curve.
4. Subtract blank values, divide by cell count/3.1 ml final solution and express activity as nanomoles substrate cleaved per 10^7 cells per hour at 37°C.

Interpretation

β-glucosidase activities in normal leukocytes range from 3.40 to 7.20 nanomoles/10^7 cells/hour; those in patients with Gaucher disease (homozygotes) range from 0.71 to 1.32 nanomoles/10^7 cells/hour. Leukocytes in one of six heterozygotes tested by Peters, et al. (1975), contained low normal levels of β-glucosidase (3.89); cells from most heterozygotes contain from 1.74 to 2.27 units of activity.

Reagents

1. *NaCl, 0.2%*: Dissolve 0.5 g NaCl in 250 ml demineralized water.
2. *NaCl, 3.6%*: Dissolve 3.6 g NaCl in 100 ml demineralized water.
3. *Sodium Acetate, 0.2 M, pH 5.5*: On the day of test, dissolve 2.41 g sodium acetate · 3 H_2O in 70 ml demineralized H_2O. Adjust to pH 5.5 with 0.2 M acetic acid (1.15 ml glacial acetic

acid to 100 ml) and bring to volume in 100 ml volumetric flask.
4. *Substrate Solution*: Add 120 mg taurocholic acid, sodium salt, to 20 ml of hot 0.2 M sodium acetate buffer, pH 5.5, while stirring. Stir until dissolved ($\approx$15 minutes). Cool and add 23.7 mg 4-methylumbelliferyl-β-D-glucopyranoside (4-MUB Glu) (Koch-Light); stir with magnetic stirrer until dissolved and added to pellet.

β-GLUCOSIDASE IN LYMPHOCYTES
IN ADULT-TYPE DISEASE

Principle

Peripheral leukocytes reflect the enzyme defect of Gaucher disease, lack of β-glucosidase. Enzyme levels in the lymphocyte fraction, however, are a more sensitive index of the carrier state than those of the total white cell component. Assay for the lymphocyte enzyme is similar to that for β-glucosidase in leukocytes, described on p. 184, once the lymphocytes have been isolated.

Procedure

A. *Separation of lymphocytes*
  1. Combine 3 ml 3% sodium citrate solution (containing 5% PVP) and 10 ml fresh heparinized blood sample in 50 ml Sorvall tube.
  2. Mix by inversion, and let red cells settle for thirty to forty-five minutes at 37°C. Decant and save supernatant suspension.
  3. Centrifuge supernatant suspension containing leukocytes and platelets at 4°C for ten minutes at 100 g (950 R.P.M).
  4. Discard the platelet-rich supernatant layer and suspend leukocyte pellet in 1 ml 0.85% NaCl.
  5. Gently layer leukocyte suspension over 10 ml layering solution, and centrifuge at 20°C for twenty to twenty-five minutes at 400 g (1475 R.P.M).
  6. Collect lymphocyte plaque at interface of two upper layers by aspirating top layer and a small portion (1 ml) of second

layer. Centrifuge aspirated suspension at 2000 R.P.M. at 4° C for ten minutes.

7. Discard supernatant layer and suspend lymphocyte pellet in 1 ml saline. Centrifuge at 2000 R.P.M., wash again in saline and centrifuge.

8. Resuspend pellet in 0.5 ml saline, remove small aliquot, dilute 1 to 20, and count cells. Estimate number of cells in 0.02 ml saline suspension (approximately 1-5 $\times$ 10^6 lymphocytes/20λ).

B. *β-Glucosidase Assay*

1. Combine 0.020 ml acetate buffer and 0.05 ml substrate in four tubes. Add 0.020 ml cell suspension to three and 0.020 ml saline to the fourth (blank).

2. Incubate tubes at 37° C for sixty minutes; stop reaction by submerging tubes in ice water bath, and quickly adding 3 ml 0.2 M glycine buffer, pH 10.7.

3. Obtain fluorescence of working standard solutions in Turner 110 fluorometer with primary filter 7-60 and secondary filters 2-A and 48 overlaid with 10% neutral density filter.

4. Obtain fluorescence in blank and test solutions, zeroing fluorometer with 0 nanomole methylumbelliferone standard.

5. *Glycine · NH₄OH buffer, 0.2 M, pH 10.5*: Dissolve 3.75 g glycine in 200 ml demineralized water, adjust to pH 10.5 with concentrated NH₄OH (18 to 20 ml) and bring to volume in 250 ml volumetric flask.

6. *4-Methylumbelliferone Stock Standard, 1000 nmoles/3.1 ml*: Dissolve 14.2 mg 4-methylumbelliferone in 200 ml water in 300 ml Erlenmeyer flask; bring to volume in 250 ml volumetric flask.

7. *4-Methylumbelliferone Working Standards*: Dilute 1 ml stock standard to 100 ml (10 nmole/3.1 ml) and combine with glycine · NH₄OH buffer as follows:

Nanomoles (3.1 ml)	Volume Standard (ml)	Volume Buffer (ml)
0	—	5
0.05	0.05	9.95

Nanomoles (3.1 ml)	Volume Standard (ml)	Volume Buffer (ml)
0.1	0.05	4.95
0.2	0.1	4.9
0.3	0.15	4.85
0.4	0.2	4.8
0.5	0.25	4.75

Interpretation

β-glucosidase activity in normal lymphocytes ranged from 37 to 76 $\mu U/10^7$ cells. Activity in lymphocytes from patients with Gaucher disease ranged from 2 to 5 μU and from 17 to 40 μU in those of obligate carriers.

Calculations

1. Plot fluoresce versus concentration of 4-methylumbelliferone.
2. Subtract fluorescence of blank from that in test samples.
3. Obtain nanomoles of 4-methylumbelliferone cleaved per 3.09 ml of final dilution per sixty minutes (or 20λ of cell suspension) from standard curve.
4. Divide by number of cells in 20λ cell suspension and multiply by 10^7 for nanomoles/10^7 cells/60 minutes.
5. Divide by 60 and multiply by 1000 for picomoles of 4-methylumbelliferone per 10^7 cells per minute at 37°C.

$$1 \ \mu\text{Unit} = \frac{1 \ \text{picomole 4-methylumbelliferone}}{10^7 \ \text{cells} \cdot \text{minute}}$$

Reagents

1. *Sodium Citrate, 3%, PVP, 5%*: Dissolve 0.75 g sodium citrate and 1.25 g polyvinylpyrrolidone in demineralized water in 25 ml volumetric flask. Bring to volume.
2. *Sodium Diatrizoate, 34%*: Just before use, dissolve 8.5 g sodium diatrizoate in demineralized water in 25 ml volumetric flask. Bring to volume.
3. *Ficoll, 9%*: Just before use, dissolve 2.25 g Pharmacia Ficoll in demineralized water in 25 ml volumetric flask. Bring to volume.

4. *Layering Solution*: Combine 10 ml of the sodium diatrizoate and 24 ml of the Ficoll solutions.
5. *Acetate Buffer, 0.2 M, pH 4.0*: Dissolve 2.72 g Na · Acetate · 3 H_2O in 100 ml demineralized water. Adjust to pH 4.0 with 0.2 M acetic acid.
6. *4-Methylumbelliferyl-β-D-Glucopyranoside Substrate, 1 mM*: Dissolve 16.9 mg 4-methylumbelliferyl-β-D-glucopyranoside from Koch-Light in 50 ml H_2O. If Sigma substrate is used, extract first with four volumes ether to remove fluorescent contaminant.
7. *Glycine Buffer, 0.2M, pH 10.7*: Dissolve 15.01 g glycine in 700 ml demineralized H_2O. Adjust to pH 10.7.
8. *Stock 4-Methylumbelliferone Standard, 300 Nanomoles Per 3.09 ml*: Dissolve 4.3 g 4-methylumbelliferone in 250 ml glycine buffer.
9. *Working 4-Methylumbelliferone Standards*: Combine the following volumes of stock standard and glycine buffer:

Nanomoles (3.09)	Stock Standard (ml)	Glycine Buffer (ml)
0	0	10
0.25	0.005	6
0.50	0.010	6
1.0	0.020	6
1.5	0.025	5
2.0	0.020	3
2.5	0.050	6

REFERENCES

Beutler, E., Kuhl, W.: The diagnosis of the adult type of Gaucher's disease and its carrier state by demonstration of deficiency of β-glucosidase activity in peripheral blood leukocytes. *J Lab Clin Med, 76*:747, 1970.

Beutler, E., and Kuhl, W.: Detection of the defect of Gaucher's disease and its carrier state in peripheral-blood leukocytes. *Lancet, 1*:612, 1970.

Perper, R. J., Zee, T. W., and Mickelson, M. M.: Purification of lymphocytes and platelets by gradient centrifugation. *J Lab Clin Med, 72*:842, 1968.

NIEMANN-PICK

PHOSPHODIESTERASE IV DEFICIENCY IN LIVER

Principle

Tissues and cultured fibroblasts of patients with Niemann-Pick disease are deficient in acid phosphodiesterase IV, an enzyme active in vivo on lyso-bisphosphatidic acid. Enzyme activity can be measured in vitro by incubating with the synthetic substrate, bis (p-nitrophenyl) phosphate (Bis pNPP), and measuring the nitrophenol liberated colorimetrically.

Procedure

1. Mince 1 g fresh or frozen (-20°C) liver tissue with scissors and homogenize in Tenbroeck glass tube with 9 volumes ice cold 0.25 M sucrose solution. Centrifuge suspension at 4°C at 9500 R.P.M. thirty minutes. Store supernatant fluid at -20°C, if necessary. (Enzyme is stable for several weeks at -20°C.)
2. Combine 0.2 ml 100 mM sodium acetate buffer, pH 5.0, and 0.5 ml 1 mM Bis pNPP in three Sorvall tubes per sample and preincubate thirty minutes at 37°C.
3. Add 0.2 ml homogenate to two tubes, leaving third tube as blank. Mix (Vortex).
4. Stopper all tubes and incubate in shaking water bath at 37°C for two hours.
5. End reaction quickly by adding 0.1 ml 10% trichloroacetic acid to all tubes.
6. Add 0.2 ml homogenate to blank.
7. Centrifuge tubes at 5000 R.P.M. at 4°C fifteen minutes, remove, and add 0.5 ml clear supernatant fluid to 4.5 ml 0.25 M glycine-carbonate buffer, pH 10.5. Mix.
8. Measure absorbance of sample and nitrophenol standards at 410 nm.

Calculations

1. Plot standard curve of optical density versus concentration of p-nitrophenol standards.
2. Subtract blank from sample O.D. for O.D. difference of enzyme reaction.
3. Obtain nanomoles nitrophenol released per ml glycine-carbonate buffer from standard curve; multiply by 10 for activity per ml homogenate.

4. Divide by 2 (hours) and express activity of homogenate enzyme in nanomoles p-nitrophenol released/ml/hour at 37°C.

Interpretation

Normal human liver contains from 76 to 192 units of acid phosphodiesterase IV activity (nanomoles p-nitrophenol released/ml/hr), whereas liver from patients with Niemann-Pick disease, Types A or C, contains half-normal activity. The liver enzyme from persons with other types of Niemann-Pick disease has not been measured by this method.

Reagents

1. *Sodium Acetate Buffer, 100 mM, pH 5.0*: Dissolve 1.36 gm sodium acetate · $3H_2O$ in 100 ml demineralized water. Adjust to pH 5.0 with glacial acetic acid.
2. *Bis (p-nitrophenol) Phosphate, Sodium Salt, 1 mM*: Dissolve 3.62 mg Bis (p-NPP) in 10 ml 100 mM sodium acetate buffer, pH 5.0.
3. *Sucrose Solution, 0.25 M*: Dissolve 8.56 gm in 100 ml demineralized water.
4. *Glycine-Carbonate Buffer, 0.25 M, pH 10.5*: Dissolve 2.65 g $NaCO_3$ and 1.88 g glycine in 80 ml demineralized water. Adjust to pH 10.5 with 10 N NaOH and bring to volume in 100 ml volumetric flask.
5. *p-Nitrophenol Stock Standard Solution, 100 micromoles/ml*: Add 0.1 ml Sigma p-nitrophenol stock standard solution (10 μmole/ml) to 9.9 ml glycine-carbonate buffer.
6. *p-Nitrophenol Working Standards*: Combine the following volumes of the diluted p-nitrophenol stock standard solution (100 μmoles/ml) and glycine-carbonate buffer:

Concentration p-Nitrophenol (nmoles)	Stock Standard (ml)	Buffer (ml)
0	0.0	5.0
10	0.1	4.9
20	0.2	4.8

Concentration p-Nitrophenol (nmoles)	Stock Standard (ml)	Buffer (ml)
50	0.5	4.5
70	0.7	4.3
100	1.0	4.0

REFERENCE

Callahan, J. W.: Phosphodiesterases in human tissues: Decreased hydrolysis of synthetic substrate by tissues from patients with the Niemann-Pick syndrome. *Biochem Med, 11*:262, 1974.

METACHROMATIC LEUKODYSTROPHY

SULFATASE A IN SERUM

Principle

The sulfatases are lysosomal enzymes which catalyze hydrolytic desulfations. The following method for sulfatase A, the enzyme deficiency of metachromatic leukodystrophy, utilizes the artificial substrate, p-nitrocatechol sulfate. Free nitrocatechol is released during the incubation, forms a red complex in alkaline solution, and is measured colorimetrically.

Procedure

1. Measure optical density at 515 nm ($O.D._{515}$) of standard 4-nitrocatechol solutions in the Coleman, Jr. spectrophotometer and calculate extinction coefficient (E) for use in the following assay. Repeat whenever the assay conditions change, e.g. photocells replaced, light path length, etc.
2. Add 0.5 ml of fresh or fresh-frozen fasting serum to two 12 × 75-mm test tubes.
3. Add 0.5 ml of p-nitrocatechol sulfate substrate to one tube.
4. Incubate both tubes for four hours in a carefully controlled 37°C water bath.

5. Remove tubes from bath; add substrate to second tube (zero time blank).
6. Immediately add 0.2 ml of 2.5 N sodium hydroxide to both tubes and mix. Centrifuge, if turbid. (10 g NaOH/100 ml sol)
7. Measure $O.D._{515}$ of both tubes in Coleman Jr. spectrophotometer. Subtract O.D. of zero time blank from O.D. of first tube and express as O.D. difference.
8. Compare O.D. of control nitrocatechol solution with standard curve.
9. Calculate amount of nitrocatechol released in nanomoles/ml/4 hr, as described below.

Calculations

1. Estimate extinction coefficient from the average of several standard p-nitrocatechol solutions, ranging from 15 to 60 nanomoles/ml, from the formula:

$$E \text{ (nanomoles/ml)} = \frac{O.D._{515}}{\text{conc. (nanomoles/ml)}}$$

2. Calculate the amount of nitrocatechol released as nanomoles/ml/4 hr from the relation:

$$\text{conc. (nanomoles/ml)} = \frac{O.D._{515} \times 2.4}{E \text{ (nanomoles/ml)}}$$

where O.D. is the O.D. difference and 2.4 is the dilution factor of the sample from 0.5 to 1.2 ml.

Interpretation

Sulfatase A activity in normal blood is greater than 27 nanomoles/ml/4 hrs. Blood from homozygous persons contains little or no activity. The test does not reliably distinguish heterozygotes from normal.

Reagents

1. *Sodium Acetate-Acetic Acid, 1 M, Tetrasodium Pyrophosphate, 5×10^{-4} M, and Sodium Chloride, 1.7 M, Substrate*

Buffer pH 4.9: Dissolve 13.6 g sodium acetate trihydrate, dissolve 22.3 mg tetrasodium pyrophosphate and 9.8 g sodium chloride in 80 ml demineralized water. Adjust to pH 4.9 with 1 M acetic acid (approximately 8.7 ml) and bring to final volume of 100 ml with demineralized water. Store at 4°C for up to three months. (60 ml glacial acetic acid/100 ml sol).

2. *Nitrocatechol Sulfate Substrate, 0.02 M*: Dissolve 31.2 mg p-nitrocatechol sulfate in 5.0 ml substrate buffer (6.23 mg/ml).

3. *Nitrocatechol Standards for Estimation of Extinction Coefficient*: Dissolve 9.3 mg 4-nitrocatechol in 1.0 ml of 0.5 N sodium hydroxide (60 micromoles/ml). Dilute the stock solution with 0.5 N sodium hydroxide to give a series of solutions of from 15 to 60 nanomoles/ml, with O.D. of from 0.150 to 0.590 at 515 mμ. (2.0 g NaOH/100 ml sol)

4. *Control Nitrocatechol Solution, 30 nanomoles/ml*: Dilute 10 μl of the stock 4-nitrocatechol solution (60 micromoles/ml) to 20 ml with 0.5 N sodium hydroxide.

REFERENCE

Beratis, N., Aron, A., and Hirschhorn, K.,: Metachromatic leukodystrophy: Detection in serum. *J Pediatr, 83*:824, 1973.

SULFATASE A IN URINE

Principle

The lysosomal enzyme, arylsulfatase A, in normal urine is partially purified and concentrated. The concentrate catalyzes the hydrolysis of nitrocatechol sulfate, the reaction product of which, nitrocatechol, is red in alkaline solution.

Procedure

1. Collect catch sample of urine after morning meal. If necessary, continue collecting after meals until sample volume is at least 100 ml.
2. Dialyze 100 ml sample overnight against cold running tap

water to remove inhibitory phosphates.

3. Warm dialyzed urine in 37°C water bath, and filter through coarse, fluted filter paper. Measure volume after filtration.

4. Add 47.3 g ammonium sulfate to 100 ml of urine, stirring with magnetic bar.

5. Centrifuge suspension at 7500 R.P.M. for twenty minutes in 250 ml centrifuge bottle at 4°C.

6. Decant supernatant fluid and resuspend pellet in 1.7 ml 0.1 M acetate buffer.

7. Adjust to pH 5.0 with 1 N HCl or 1 N NaOH, using narrow-range pH paper.

8. Add 1.5 ml sulfatase reagent to three 20 ml screw capped tubes; add 1.5 ml pellet suspension to two (sample and standard) and 1.5 ml acetate buffer to the third tube (control).

9. Incubate tubes at 75°C±3 for ten minutes; stop reaction with 10 ml 0.01 N HCl, mix by inverting five times, and let stand five minutes. Temperatures over 80°C inactivate the enzyme.

10. Add 5 ml acidified ether, mix by inverting five times, and let stand ten minutes. If foam forms, separate layers by centrifuging at 2000 R.P.M.

11. Remove and save ether layers in clean 20 ml screw-capped tubes.

12. Repeat extractions twice with 5 ml portions of fresh acidified ether; pool extracts.

13. Add 2 drops 6 N NaOH to extracts, and mix by tapping tube firmly with the fingers, creating a vortex. Do not invert.

14. Observe and record color of bottom aqueous layer after five minutes.

15. If bottom layer is not red, check its hydrogen ion concentration with wide-range paper. If not strongly alkaline, add NaOH in drops. Wait five minutes for color to form.

Interpretation

If sulfatase is present, as in normal urines, the bottom layer will be red. If absent, the layer will be colorless or yellow. (See Color Illustration 11.)

Reagents

1. *Sodium Acetate Buffer, 0.1 M, pH 5.0*: Add 13 g sodium acetate to 500 ml demineralized water and stir until dissolved. Adjust to pH 5.0 with glacial acetic acid. Transfer to 1-liter volumetric flask and dilute to mark. Store at room temperature.
2. *Sodium Acetate Buffer, 0.5 M, pH 5.0*: Add 13.6 g sodium acetate to 150 ml demineralized water and stir until dissolved. Adjust to pH 5.0 with glacial acetic acid. Transfer to 200 ml volumetric flask and dilute to mark. Store at room temperature.
3. *Sulfatase Reagent*: Dissolve in 50 ml 0.5 M pH 5.0 acetate buffer: 165 mg p-nitrocatechol sulfate, 11.2 mg sodium pyrophosphate $(Na_4P_2O_7 \cdot 10\ H_2O)$, and 5.0 g sodium chloride.
4. *Hydrochloric Acid Solution, 1.0 N*: Add 8.6 ml concentrated HCl to 75 ml demineralized water and dilute to mark in 100 ml volumetric flask.
5. *Hydrochloric Acid Solution, 0.05 N HCl*: Dilute 5.0 ml 1.0 N HCl with demineralized water to mark in 100 ml volumetric flask.
6. *Hydrochloric Acid Solution, 0.01 N HCl*: Dilute 1.0 ml 1.0 N HCl with demineralized water to mark in 100 ml volumetric flask.
7. *Acidified Ether Solution*: For three tubes, shake 50 ml diethyl ether with 10 ml 0.05 N HCl in separatory funnel immediately before use. Allow phases to separate. Draw off lower acid layer and discard. Save ether layer in Erlenmeyer flask.
8. *Sodium Hydroxide, 6 N*: Dissolve 60 g NaOH in 150 ml demineralized water. Cool, transfer to 250 ml volumetric flask, and dilute to mark. Store in plastic bottle.

REFERENCE

Austin, J., Armstrong, D., Shearer, L., McFee, D.: Metachromatic form of diffuse cerebral sclerosis. *Arch Neur, 14*:259, 1966.

SULFATASE A IN LEUKOCYTES

Principle

Leukocyte aryl sulfatase A is measured in the presence of arylsulfatase B as the amount of p-nitrocatechol released when B is inhibited with low substrate concentrations and sodium pyrophosphate.

Procedure

1. Separate leukocytes from 10 ml heparinized blood as follows: Add 2 ml Sigma dextran-NaCl solution, mix by gentle inversion, and let settle forty-five minutes at room temperature.
2. Collect supernatant fluid containing plasma and leukocytes with a Pasteur pipette, place in 13 ml Sorvall tube, and centrifuge at 2250 R.P.M. (600 × g), ten minutes at 4°C.
3. Wash cells three times with 5 ml saline, centrifuging as above.
4. Suspend cells in 1 ml demineralized water; shell-freeze and thaw quickly seven times for lysis.
5. Centrifuge at 4000 R.P.M. (1800 × g) for five minutes at 4°C.
6. Collect supernatant fluid (leukocyte lysate) for enzyme assay and protein determination. (May be stored at -20°C for at least twenty-four hours).
7. Measure activity of enzyme by adding triplicate 0.1 ml portions of leukocyte lysate (or 0.05 ml lysate and 0.05 ml water) to 0.5 ml buffered substrate in 3 ml Sorvall tubes. 0.1 ml leukocyte lysate without substrate is blank A and 3 ml buffered substrate without lysate is blank B.
8. Incubate all tubes at 37°C for thirty minutes.
9. Bring another water bath to boiling.
10. Add 0.5 ml buffered substrate to blank A and place all tubes immediately in boiling water bath for ninety seconds.
11. Add 0.5 ml 1 N NaOH to all tubes, mix, and centrifuge at 4000 R.P.M. (1800 × g) for five minutes.
12. Collect supernatant fluid and measure optical density at 515 nm against zero standard.
13. Measure O.D.$_{515}$ of 4-nitrocatechol standard solutions.
14. Measure protein in duplicate 25λ aliquots of leukocyte lysate and working protein standard by adding to 2 ml alkaline copper reagent. Mix and let stand at room temperature fif-

teen minutes. Add rapidly 0.2 ml dilute phenol reagent, mix immediately, and let stand at least thirty minutes. Read optical density of all solutions at 750 nm.

15. Estimate hemoglobin concentration in 0.025 ml leukocyte lysate by adding 0.975 ml demineralized water in 1.0 ml microcuvette. Mix by inversion and read optical density at 410 nm on Beckman DU-2 spectrophotometer, using water blank.

16. Obtain correction factor, 528, as mg protein per 100 ml lysate required to give O.D.$_{410}$ of 1.000, calculated from slope of curve, when protein concentrations of a series of hemolysate dilutions in water (from 1:100 to 1:50,000) are plotted against O.D.$_{410}$

Calculations

1. Plot p-nitrocatechol concentration against optical density at 515 nm on linear scale.

2. Measure nanomoles p-nitrocatechol released in 1.1 ml final solution for all blank and test samples directly from standard curve (0.1 ml leukocyte lysate).

3. Subtract blank from test values for net nanomoles p-nitrocatechol per 0.1 ml lysate.

4. Plot protein concentration against optical density at 750 nm on linear scale.

5. Measure mg protein per 100 ml leukocyte lysate directly from standard curve.

6. Correct for residual hemoglobin in leukocyte lysate by multiplying optical density at 410 nm of dilute lysate by 528 (correction factor when measured with Beckman DU-2 spectrophotometer) for mg erythrocyte protein per 100 ml lysate; subtract from (5) for mg leukocyte protein per 100 ml lysate.

7. Divide by 1000 mg protein per 0.1 ml leukocyte lysate.

8. Divide net nanomoles p-nitrocatechol per 0.1 ml lysate (step 3) by mg leukocyte protein per 0.1 ml lysate for nanomoles nitrocatechol per mg protein per thirty minutes; multiply by 2

and express activity as nanomoles nitrocatechol/mg protein/hour.

Interpretation

Normal leukocytes contain from 110 to 275 units of activity (nanomoles p-nitrocatechol/mg protein/hr); those from obligate heterozygotes contain from 36 to 74 units and those from homozygous patients have little or no activity.

Reagents

1. *Dextran-NaCl Solution*: On the day of test, dissolve 0.5 g Sigma dextran-500 and 70 mg sodium chloride in 10 ml demineralized water.
2. *Acetate Buffer, 0.5 M, pH 5.0 (Containing 5×10^{-4} M $Na_4P_2O_7$ and 10% NaCl)*: Dissolve 4.77 g Na acetate. 3 H_2O, 22.3 mg $Na_4P_2O_7 \cdot 10$ H_2O and 10 g NaCl in 50 ml demineralized water. Add 30 ml 0.5 M acetic acid (2.88 ml glacial acetic acid per 100 ml solution). Adjust to pH 5.0, if necessary, and dilute to volume in 100 ml volumetric flask.
3. *p-Nitrocatechol Sulfate Buffered Substrate 0.01 M*: On the day of test, dissolve 31.1 mg p-nitrocatechol-sulfate, dipotassium salt, in 10 ml 0.5 M acetate buffer, containing 5×10^{-4}M $Na_4P_2O_7$ and 10% NaCl.
4. *NaOH, 1 N*: Dissolve 4.0 g NaOH in 100 ml demineralized water.
5. *NaOH, 0.5N*: Dissolve 4.0 g NaOH in 200 ml demineralized water.
6. *4-Nitrocatechol Stock Standard, 1µ mole per 1.1 ml*: Dissolve 14.1 mg p-nitrocatechol in 100 ml 0.5 N NaOH.
7. *4-Nitrocatechol Working Standards*: Combine the following:

Nanomoles/1.1 ml	Volume Stock Standard (ml)	Volume 0.5 N NaOH (ml)
0	0	
10	0.05	4.95
20	0.1	4.9
40	0.2	4.8
60	0.3	4.7
80	0.4	4.6

8. *Dilute Phenol Reagent*: Combine 2 ml Fisher phenol reagent with 2 ml demineralized water.
9. *Alkaline Tartrate Reagent*: Dissolve 2.0 g sodium carbonate (Na_2CO_3) and 50 mg Na or K tartrate in 100 ml 0.1 N NaOH.
10. *Copper Sulfate, 0.1%*: Dissolve 100 mg $CuSO_4 \cdot 5 H_2O$ in 100 ml demineralized water.
11. *Working Alkaline Copper Reagent*: Combine 27 ml alkaline tartrate reagent and 3 ml 0.1% copper sulfate.
12. *Stock Protein Solution, 1200 mg%*: Dilute 2 ml 30% bovine albumin with 48 ml demineralized water.
13. *Working Protein Solutions*: Combine the following:

mg/100 ml	*Volume Stock Standard* (ml)	*Volume H_2O* (ml)
0	0	3
200	0.50	2.50
400	1.00	2.00
600	1.50	1.50
800	2.0	1.0
1000	2.50	0.50

REFERENCES

Beratis, N. G., Danesino, C., and Hirschhorn, K.: Detection of homozygotes and heterozygotes for metachromatic leukodystrophy in lymphoid cell lines and peripheral leukocytes. *Ann Hum Genet, 38*:485, 1975.

Percy, A. K., and Brady, R. O.: Metachromatic leukodystrophy: Diagnosis with samples of venous blood. *Science, 161*:594, 1968.

Kampine, J. P., Brady, R. O., Kanfer, J. N., Feld, M., and Shapiro, D.: Diagnosis of Gaucher's disease and Niemann-Pick disease with small samples of venous blood. *Science, 155*:86, 1967.

Baum, H., Dodgson, K. S., and Spencer, B.: The assay of arylsulphatases A and B in human urine. *Clin Chim Acta, 4*:453, 1959.

FABRY

α-GALACTOSIDASE IN BODY FLUIDS

Principle

The body fluids and cells of boys with Fabry's disease, an X-linked recessive disease, lack the hydrolase α-galactosidase. The defect is detectable in serum, plasma, or urine by a fluorometric assay in which the enzyme frees fluorescent 4-methyumbelliferone by hydrolysis from methylumbelliferyl-conjugated substrate. An assay for β-galactosidase is also performed to include the variables which might affect hydrolase levels in vitro.

Procedure

1. Combine duplicate 50λ aliquots of serum, plasma, or centrifuged urine and 300λ portions of the appropriately-buffered α- and β-pyranoside substrates in respective 10 ml screw-capped tubes. Duplicate 50λ aliquots of sample alone serve as blanks for the two substrates.
2. Incubate the six tubes in 37°C water bath for two hours; stop reactions with 4.65 ml 0.1 M ethylenediamine.
3. Add 300λ appropriate buffer-substrate to blanks.
4. Measure fluorescence in Turner fluorometer with filters 7-60, 48, and 2A, overlaid with 10% neutral density filter, if serum or plasma; overlay with 1% neutral density filter, if urine. Zero instrument with 0 mg% standard.

Calculations

1. Plot standard curve of fluorescence versus nanomoles 4-methylumbelliferone. Use 1% neutral density filter for concentrations of 8 and 16 nmoles/5.0 ml.
2. Read nanomoles substrate cleaved per 120 min per 5.0 ml reaction mixture (RM) from standard curve (nmoles$_{RM}$).
3. Convert to nanomoles cleaved per ml sample by multiplying by 20, since volume of sample is 50λ in 5.0 ml reaction mixture; convert to nanomoles cleaved per hour by dividing by 2. The conversions can also be made by substituting in the formula:

$$\text{nmoles/ml/hr} = \text{nmoles}_{RM} \times 10$$

Interpretation

α-Galactosidase levels in normal serum and plasma range from

8 to 15 nanomoles/ml/hr, from 3 to 6 nanomoles in the heterozygous state and from 0.3 to 0.9 nanomoles in the hemizygous, affected boy.

Urinary α-galactosidase ranges from 15 to 56, 9 to 19, and 1 to 4 nanomoles/ml/hr in the three groups, respectively.

Serum β-galactosidase levels range from 1.3 to 4 nanomoles/ml/hr in the three groups; plasma levels range up to 6.8 nanomoles. Urinary β-galactosidase levels range from 49 to 530 nanomoles, and in hemizygous boys from 100 to 520 nanomoles/ml/hr.

Reagents

1. *Citrate-Phosphate Buffer, 0.10 M, pH 4.5 (30 μmole/300λ for urine)*: Dissolve 2.10 g citric acid · H_2O in 50 ml demineralized water. Adjust to pH 4.5 with $\simeq$20 ml 1.0 M Na_2HPO_4 · 2 H_2O (14.2 g/100 ml) and bring to volume in 100 ml volumetric flask with demineralized water.

2. *Citrate-Phosphate Buffer, 0.05 M, pH 4.6 (15 μmole/300λ for plasma)*: Adjust 25 ml 0.10 M citrate-phosphate buffer, pH 4.5, to pH 4.6 with 1.0 M Na_2HPO_4 · 2 H_2O and bring to volume in 50 ml volumetric flask.

3. *Citrate-Phosphate Buffer, 0.05 M, pH 4.8 (15 μmole/300λ for serum)*: Adjust 25 ml 0.10 M citrate-phosphate buffer, pH 4.5, to pH 4.8 with 1 M Na_2HPO_4 · 2 H_2O, and bring to volume in 50 ml volumetric flask.

4. *4-Methylumbelliferyl-α-D-Galactopyranoside*, 30 mM (1.5 μmole/300λ): Dissolve 8.53 mg α-pyranoside substrate in 5 ml appropriate citrate-PO_4 buffer.

5. *4-Methylumbelliferyl-β-D-Galactopyranoside, 4.0 mM (0.2 μmole/300λ)*: Dissolve 5.63 mg β-pyranoside substrate in 25 ml appropriate citrate-PO_4 buffer.

6. *Ethylenediamine, 0.1 M, pH 11.4*: Dissolve 6.65 g ethylenediamine dihydrochloride in 400 ml demineralized water. Adjust to pH 11.4 with 10 N NaOH and bring to volume in 500 ml volumetric flask.

7. *4-Methylumbelliferone Stock Standard, 80 μM (0.4 μmole/5.0*

ml): Dissolve 2.8 mg 4-methylumbelliferone in 200 ml demineralized water.

8. *Working Standards*: Dilute 4-methylumbelliferone stock standard as follows:

Standard (nmoles/5.0)	Volume Stock Standard (λ)	Volume Ethylenediamine (ml)
0	0	5.0
0.4	10	10.0
1.0	25	10.0
2.0	50	9.95
4.0	100	9.9
8.0	200	9.8
16.0	400	9.6

REFERENCE

Desnick, R. J., Allen, K. Y., Desnick, S. J., Mohanreddy, K., et al: Fabry's disease: Enzymatic diagnosis of hemizygotes and heterozygotes. *J Lab Clin Med, 81*:157, 1973.

TAY-SACHS AND VARIANTS

SERUM HEXOSAMINIDASE A

Principle

The enzyme defect of Tay-Sachs disease, deficiency of the heat-labile, isozyme A fraction of hexosaminidase, can be demonstrated in serum by comparing the proportions of isozyme A and the heat-stable, isozyme B fraction. Normal serum contains the two hydrolases, both of which split methylumbelliferyl-conjugated substrate and free fluorescent methylumbelliferone.

Procedure

1. Dilute 0.1 ml serum sample with 0.9 ml citrate-phosphate buffer and cool in ice bath ten minutes.
2. Distribute 50 µl aliquots of the diluted serum in eight 10-ml

screw-cap tubes; freeze four immediately in CO_2-alcohol bath and incubate the remaining four tubes in shaking water bath at 50°C (must *not* be 52°C). Remove two tubes after three hours' incubation and the other two after four hours; freeze both sets of tubes immediately and keep frozen until continuation of assay, described below.

3. Thaw contents of all tubes, add 100 μl substrate to all but one (blank), and incubate sixty minutes in shaking water bath at 37°C.
4. Stop reaction by partially submerging tubes in ice bath; quickly add 5 ml 0.17 M glycine-carbonate buffer to all, including blank.
5. Add 100 μl substrate to blank.
6. Read fluorescence of samples and standards in Turner fluorometer, using primary filter 7-60 and secondary filters 2A and No. 48, overlaid with 10% neutral density filter.

Calculations

1. Plot standard curve of fluorescence versus concentration of 4-methylumbelliferone working standards.
2. Subtract fluorescence of blanks from those of the unheated and heated serum samples.
3. Convert fluorescence of all test samples into 4-methylumbelliferone cleaved per 5.15 ml final reaction mixture or per 0.005 ml serum from the standard curve.
4. Multiply by 200 for nmoles 4-methylumbelliferone cleaved per 1 ml serum at 37°C in one hour.
5. Estimate hexosaminidase A content by subtracting activity in heated serum (hexosaminidase B) from that in unheated serum (total hexosaminidase) and express as percent of total hexosaminidase.

Interpretation

The hexosaminidase A content of normal serum ranges from 49 to 68%, in Tay-Sachs patients is 4% or less, and in carriers, from 26 to 45%.

Reagents

1. *Sample*: Centrifuge serum or plasma from clot or red cells at 3000 R.P.M. for fifteen minutes. Stable for up to six months at -20°C.
2. *Citrate-Phosphate Buffer, 0.04 M, pH 4.4*: Dissolve 1.7 g citric acid in demineralized water and dilute to mark in 100 ml volumetric flask. Dissolve 4.8 g Na_2HPO_4 in demineralized water and dilute to mark in 100 ml volumetric flask. Adjust 50 ml of the citric acid solution to pH 4.4 with the phosphate solution and bring volume to 100 ml with demineralized water.
3. *4-Methylumbelliferyl-N-Acetyl-β-D-Glucosaminide Substrate, 1.0 mM*: Dissolve 9.5 mg 4-methylumbelliferyl-N-acetyl-β-D-glucosaminide in 25 ml citrate-phosphate buffer. Heat in running tap water to dissolve. Make fresh on day of test.
4. *Glycine-Carbonate Buffer, 0.17 M, pH 9.9*: Dissolve 12.7 g glycine in 500 ml demineralized water. Dissolve 26.5 g Na_2CO_3 in 500 ml demineralized water. Adjust 500 ml of the glycine solution to pH 9.9 with the sodium carbonate solution and bring to volume in 1000 ml volumetric flask.
5. *4-Methylumbelliferone Stock Standard Solution, 10 nmoles/5.15 ml*: Dissolve 8.55 mg 4-methylumbelliferone in 250 ml glycine-carbonate buffer. Dilute 2.5 ml to volume with glycine-carbonate buffer in 250 ml volumetric flask.
6. *4-Methylumbelliferone Working Standards*: Dilute the 4-methylumbelliferone stock standard solution as follows:

nMoles (per 5.15 ml)	Stock Solution (ml)	Buffer (ml)
10	5.0	0
6.0	6.0	4.0
5.0	5.0	5.0
2.5	2.5	7.5
0	0	5

REFERENCE

O'Brien, J. S., Okada, S., Chen, A., and Fillerup, D. L.: Tay-Sachs disease. Detection of heterozygotes and homozygotes by serum hexosaminidase assay. *N Engl J Med, 283*:15, 1970.

HEXOSAMINIDASE A IN AMNIOTIC FLUID

Principle

As described in the section on serum hexosaminidase A, (p. 207).

Procedure

1. Centrifuge freshly-drawn amniocentesis fluid and cells at 2000 R.P.M. at 4°C for ten minutes. Decant and save clear fluid for test or store at -60°C.
2. Dilute 0.1 ml of clear amniotic fluid with 0.9 ml citrate-phosphate buffer and cool in ice bath ten minutes. Remainder of procedure is similar to that for serum hexosaminidase, steps 2 through 6 (p. 207).

Calculations

Calculations as described in the section on serum hexosaminidase A, (p. 208).

Interpretation

Normal amniotic fluid contains 283 to 592 units of total hexosaminidase activity, of which 11 to 26% is hexosaminidase A. Fluid from the Tay-Sachs fetus contains 383 to 726 units total activity, of which 4 to 8% is hexosaminidase A.

The interpretation should be verified by assays of enzyme in uncultured and cultured cells.

Reagents

Reagents as described in section on Serum Hexosaminidase A, Reagents 2-6, p. 209.

REFERENCES

O'Brien, J. S., Okada, S., Fillerup, D., et al: Tay-Sachs disease: Prenatal diagnosis, *Science, 172*:61, 1971.

O'Brien, J. S., Okada, S., Chen, A., and Fillerup, D. L.: Tay-Sachs disease: Detection of heterozygotes and homozygotes by serum hexosaminidase assay. *N Engl J Med, 283*:15, 1970.

HEXOSAMINIDASE A IN CULTURED AMNIOTIC CELLS

Principle

Hexosaminidase A deficiency of Tay-Sachs disease can be demonstrated prenatally in cultured amnion cells by methodology similar to that for measuring hexosaminidase A activity in serum (p. 207). The assay verifies the test results of enzyme activity in freshly drawn amniotic fluid and uncultured cells.

Procedure

1. Sediment cells from 20 ml of freshly drawn amniotic fluid by centrifuging in sterile tube at 1200 R.P.M. for five minutes.
2. Discard supernatant fluid. Suspend packed cells in 4 ml growth medium.
3. Transfer aseptically to four plastic tissue culture flasks (25 cm²), flush with filtered air containing 5% carbon dioxide, and incubate at 37°C. Change media weekly.
4. Harvest cells of two flasks three weeks later (or subculture until confluent cell layer is obtained), as follows: Decant growth medium, rinse cell layers quickly with two 1 ml portions 0.25% trypsin-EDTA solution, and save rinses; add approximately 2 ml trypsin solution to cell layers, agitate gently, and let stand at room temperature for about ten minutes or until cells are evenly suspended, as determined microscopically.
5. Combine rinses and trypsinized cell suspensions from both flasks. Centrifuge in 10 ml Sorvall tube at 4°C at 1000 R.P.M. for five minutes.

6. Decant supernatant fluid, suspend cell pellet in 5 ml saline, and centrifuge. Repeat saline rinse.
7. Suspend packed cells in 2.0 ml 0.05 M citrate buffer, pH 5.0, and count cells in an aliquot diluted twenty-fold with 0.1 N HCl.
8. Freeze and thaw remaining cell suspension four times.
9. Centrifuge at 9300 R.P.M. at 4° C for thirty minutes; draw off and save supernatant fluid (enzyme extract). Store at -60° C until assayed.
10. Add 0.2 ml enzyme extract to seven 10 ml screw-cap tubes; freeze four immediately in CO_2-alcohol bath; incubate the remaining three tubes at 50° C in a shaking water bath. Remove tubes from water bath after three hours' incubation; freeze immediately and keep frozen until continuation of the assay, described below.
11. Thaw contents of all tubes, add 0.4 ml substrate to all but one (blank) and incubate thirty minutes in shaking water bath at 37° C.
12. Remove tubes from bath and stop reaction, including blank, by adding 1.6 ml 0.2 M glycine-NaOH buffer.
13. Add 0.4 ml substrate to blank.
14. Read fluorescence of samples and standards in Turner fluorometer, using primary filter 7-60 and secondary filters 2-A and 48, overlaid with a 1% neutral density filter.

Calculations

1. Plot standard curve of 4-methylumbelliferone concentration versus fluorescence (F units).
2. Subtract fluorescence of blank from those of heated and unheated samples.
3. Convert fluorescence into nanomoles 4-methylumbelliferone cleaved per 2.2 ml final reaction mixture or per 0.2 ml cell extract/30 minutes from standard curve.
4. Multiply cell count or number of cells per mm^3 or 0.001 ml cell culture suspension by 200 for number of cells represented in 0.2 ml cell extract.
5. Divide nanomoles 4-methylumbelliferone/0.2 ml cell ex-

tract/30 minutes by number of cells in 0.2 ml and multiply by 10^5 for nanomoles/10^5 cell/30 minutes.

6. Multiply by 2 for nanomoles of 4-methylumbelliferone cleaved by 10^5 cells in one hour at 37°C.

7. Estimate hexosaminidase A content by subtracting activity in heated extract (hexosaminidase B) from that in unheated extract (total hexosaminidase) and express as percent of total hexosaminidase.

Interpretation

Hexosaminidase A levels differ according to age of the fetus and, at the time of assay, should be compared with those in normal fetuses of similar gestational age. Levels in normal fetuses of an age when amniocentesis is usually performed, from sixteen to twenty-five weeks, range from 50 to 70 percent. Fetuses heterozygous for Tay-Sachs disease may have enzyme levels of from 27 to 45 percent at twenty to twenty-eight weeks' gestation, and fetuses homozygous for Tay–Sachs disease at eighteen weeks' gestation, as little as 1 per cent.

Reagents

1. *Trypsin-EDTA, 0.25%*: Store solution at -20°C until needed. Thaw and bring to 37°C before using.

2. *Citric Acid Solution, 0.05 M, Containing 0.1% Bovine Albumin*: Dissolve 10.5 g citric acid in 100 ml demineralized water; add and mix with 0.33 ml 30% bovine serum albumin.

3. *Sodium Citrate, 0.05 M, Containing 0.1% Bovine Albumin*: Dissolve 1.47 g sodium citrate·2 H_2O in 100 ml demineralized water; add and mix with 0.33 ml 30% bovine serum albumin.

4. *Citrate Buffer, 0.05 M, pH 5, with 0.1% Bovine Albumin*: Adjust 50 ml 0.05 M citric acid solution to pH 5.0 with 0.05 M sodium citrate.

5. *Citrate Buffer, 0.05 M, pH 4.5, with 0.1% Bovine Albumin*: Adjust 50 ml 0.05 M citric acid solution to pH 4.5 with 0.05 M sodium citrate.

6. *4-Methylumbelliferyl-N-Acetylglucosamine Substrate, 0.25*

mM: Dissolve 4.75 mg 4-methylumbelliferyl-N-acetyl-glucosamine in 50 ml 0.05 M citrate-albumin buffer, pH 4.5.

7. *Glycine-NaOH Buffer, 0.2 M, pH 10.6*: Dissolve 3.75 g glycine in 220 ml demineralized water. Adjust to pH 10.6 with 10 N NaOH and bring to volume in 250 ml volumetric flask.

8. *Stock 4-Methylumbelliferone Standard, 1000 nanomoles/2.2 ml*: Dissolve 8.0 mg 4-methylumbelliferone in 100 ml glycine-NaOH buffer.

9. *Working 4-Methylumbelliferone Standards*: Combine the stock 4-methylumbelliferone standard with glycine-NaOH buffer in the following volumes.

Nanomoles/2.2 ml	Volume Stock Standard (ml)	Volume Glycine · NaOH (ml)
0	0	10
1	0.01	10
5	0.05	9.95
10	0.1	9.9
20	0.2	9.8
30	0.3	9.7
40	0.4	9.6
50	0.5	9.5

REFERENCES

Navon, R., and Padeh, B.: Prenatal diagnosis of Tay-Sachs genotypes. *Br Med J, 4*:17, 1971.

Paul, B.: Unpublished method in use at the N. Y. State Department of Health, 1973.

HEXOSAMINIDASE A IN UNCULTURED AMNIOTIC CELLS

Principle

Hexosaminidase A deficiency of Tay-Sachs disease can be demonstrated prenatally in uncultured amnion cells by methodology similar to that for enzyme in cultured cells (p. 211).

Procedure -

1. Gently invert two 5 ml aliquots of freshly drawn amniotic

fluid to obtain a homogeneous suspension; centrifuge at 2000 R.P.M. at 4°C for five minutes.

2. Remove and store clear supernatant amniotic fluid at -60°C for assay of enzyme in amniotic fluid, as described on p. 210. Continue with assay for enzyme in uncultured cells by suspending cell pellet in 3 ml saline.

3. Centrifuge suspended cells at 2000 R.P.M. and repeat saline wash.

4. Suspend cell pellet in 1.5 ml 0.05 M citrate buffer, pH 5.0. Count cells on aliquot diluted twenty fold with 0.1 N HCl. (0.83 ml concentrated HCl/100 ml solution.)

5. Disrupt cell membranes by freezing and thawing four times in a CO_2-alcohol bath.

6. Centrifuge thirty minutes at 9500 R.P.M. at 4°C.

7. Remove and save supernatant fluid (enzyme extract) for immediate assay or store at -20°C.

8. Follow procedure as outlined in the assay for enzyme in cultured amniotic cells, steps 10 through 14 (p. 212). Measure fluorescence with 10%, rather than 1%, neutral density filter.

Calculations

As in method for cultured amniotic cells, (p. 212).

Interpretation

Hexosaminidase A levels in uncultured amniotic cells are informative when the three-week period required for culture is prohibitive. The values, however, are lower and less reliable than those of cultured cells from the same age fetus. Uncultured cells from normal fetuses of sixteen through twenty-five weeks gestational age have hexosaminidase A activity of from 23 to 40 percent; fetuses heterozygous for Tay-Sachs disease of 20 to 28 weeks gestational age have from 22 to 27 percent of hexosaminidase A activity; homozygous cells have up to 6 percent.

Reagents

Details are as given in method for cultured amniotic cells (p. 211), except where noted.

1. *Citric Acid Solution, 0.05 M, Containing 0.1% Bovine Albumin.*
2. *Sodium Citrate, 0.05 M, Containing 0.1% Bovine Albumin.*
3. *Citrate Buffer, 0.05 M, pH 5.0, with 0.1% Albumin.*
4. *Citrate Buffer, 0.05 M, pH 4.5 with 0.1% Albumin.*
5. *4-Methylumbelliferyl-N-Acetylglucosamine Substrate, 0.25 mM.*
6. *Glycine-NaOH Buffer, 0.2 M, pH 10.6.*
7. *Stock 4-Methylumbelliferone Standard (1000 nmoles/2.2 ml).*
8. *Working 4-Methylumbelliferone Standards*: Combine stock 4-methylumbelliferone standard with glycine-NaOH buffer in the following volumes:

Nanomoles/2.2 ml	*Volume Stock Standard* (ml)	*Volume Glycine-NaOH* (ml)
0	0	10
0.5	0.005	10
1.0	0.010	10
1.5	0.015	10
2.0	0.020	10

REFERENCE

Navon, R., and Padeh, B.: Prenatal diagnosis of Tay-Sachs genotypes. *Br Med J, 4*:17, 1971.

ELECTROPHORESIS OF N-ACETYL-HEXOSAMINIDASE ISOZYMES IN AMNIOTIC FLUID

Principle

Isozymes of amniotic fluid hexosaminidase separate electrophoretically on cellulose acetate and are visualized in ultraviolet after staining with specific fluorogenic reaction mixture.

Procedure

1. Mark strips of cellulose acetate (1 × 6 3/4-inches) (Sepraphore® III) 1 inch (A) and 1 1/2 inches (B) from the cathodal end. Soak in electrophoresis buffer one-half hour.
2. Place 100 ml electrophoresis buffer in chambers of Gelman Sepra Tek   cell.
3. Remove strips from buffer, blot, and lay in electrophoresis chamber so that Mark B is over cathodal baffle. Hold in place with magnets.
4. Apply test samples and control amniotic fluid three times with Gelman #51220 electrophoresis sample applicator at mark A on respective strips. Strips at either end of chamber are blanks.
5. Place cell at 4°C, fill both chambers with electrophoresis buffer, attach to power supply, cover, and adjust source to supply 250 V constant voltage for forty minutes and current of from 5 to 7 ma per strip.
6. Prepare staining agar gel during electrophoresis period.
7. When electrophoresis is complete, remove strips from chamber and lay face down on staining agar. Do not move strips, once laid. Remove air bubbles between strip and gel with gentle pressure.
8. Incubate at 37°C for thirty minutes.
9. Spray strips with 1 M sodium carbonate and examine under long-wave ultraviolet.

Interpretation

Hexosaminidase isozymes in normal amniotic fluid and that from the Tay-Sachs carrier fetus separate into two bands. Hexosaminidase B is the slower, major component. Hexosaminidase A stains less intensely and moves faster. Amniotic fluids from the fetus homozygous for the Tay-Sachs gene contain only the slower band of hexosaminidase B.

Reagents

1. *Sodium Phosphate Electrophoresis Buffer, 0.1 M, pH 6.85:*

Dissolve 7.1 g Na_2HPO_4 anhydrous and 6.9 g $NaH_2PO_4 \cdot H_2O$ in 900 ml demineralized water. Adjust to pH 6.85 and bring to volume in 1000 ml volumetric flask.

2. *Phosphate-Citrate Buffer, 0.1 M, pH 4.5*: Dissolve 2.84 g Na_2HPO_4 in 100 ml demineralized water. Adjust to pH 4.5 with 0.2 M citric acid (4.2 g/100 ml) and bring to 200 ml volume in volumetric flask.

3. *Staining Agar, 1%*: Dissolve 0.5 g Ionagar in 50 ml 0.1 M phosphate-citrate buffer. Heat to boiling until agar dissolves. Remove from heat promptly and add 25 mg 4-methylumbelliferyl-β-D-N-acetylglucosaminide; swirl until dissolved. Pour approximately 20 ml volumes into two Petri dishes and cool at room temperature.

4. *Sodium Carbonate, 1 M, pH 10*: Dissolve 10.6 g Na_2CO_3 in 80 ml demineralized water. Adjust to pH 10 with 4 N HCl (33.3 ml concentrated HCl/100 ml) and bring to volume in 100 ml volumetric flask.

REFERENCES

Singer, J. D., Cotlier, E., and Krimmer, R.: Hexosaminidase A in tears and saliva for rapid identification of Tay-Sachs disease and its carriers. *Lancet,* 2:1116, 1973.

Saifer, A., Schneck, L., Perle, G., et al.: Caveats of antenatal diagnosis of Tay-Sachs disease. *Am J Obstet Gynecol, 115*:553, 1973.

CHAPTER 8

GLYCOGEN STORAGE DISEASES (GSD)

PATIENTS with the glycogen storage diseases usually present with hepatomegaly or muscle weakness or both. Age at onset and physical appearance also are sometimes characteristic (Table XII).

The primary clinical signs arise from the deposition of excessive or unusual forms of glycogen in various organs. The target organ often determines the extent and severity of clinical signs. The biochemical defects involve blocks in the synthesis or degradation of glycogen by enzymes, the sites of which are specific for the particular glycogenosis. Identification of the specific enzyme defect has become part of the differential diagnosis of these diseases.

Most of the GSD diseases have autosomal recessive patterns of inheritance. The obligate carriers can be identified, in some instances, by demonstrating partial enzyme defects.

The enzyme defects are found in a variety of tissues. (Table XII). The sampling site chosen should reflect the enzyme defect itself or some form of its biochemical expression, and be free of interfering enzymes. Leukocytes and urine are satisfactory samples for demonstrating some defects, for example, while excised tissues are required for others. Assays utilizing the former are more convenient, of course, and, when more available, should improve the differential diagnosis of this large group of rare diseases.

Characterizing the liver glycogen is of special value for the diagnosis of one of the glycogenoses, GSD IV, in addition to demonstrating the specific enzyme defect.

TYPE I (VON GIERKE)

GLUCOSE-6-PHOSPHATASE IN LIVER

Principle

Glucose-6-phosphatase is measured as the difference between

Table XII

DIFFERENTIATION OF THE GLYCOGEN STORAGE DISEASES (GSD)

Type	Eponym	Clinical Features	Defect	Sampling Site
I	Von Gierke	Hypoglycemic seizures (neonates) Hepatomegaly Acidotic episodes "Doll face," small stature Respiratory infections, bleeding Gout	Glucose-6-phosphatase	Liver Kidney Intestinal mucosa
II a.	Pompe Generalized GSD Acid maltase deficiency	Cardiomegaly Muscle weakness and hypotonia Death in infancy	α-1,4-glucosidase (α glucosidase)	Muscle Leukocytes Urine
b.		Muscle weakness - survival	α-1,4-glucosidase	Muscle
III	Cori; Forbes Debrancher GSD Limit dextrinosis	Similar, but less severe than Type I Adult myopathy Normal life span	Amylo-1,6-glucosidase "Debrancher"	Liver Muscle

IV	Brancher deficiency	Cirrhosis in infancy	Amylo-(1,4 to 1,6) trans glucosidase "Brancher"	Liver
	Anderson Amylopectinosis	Muscle weakness and contractures Early death	Amylopectin-like glycogen	Leukocytes
V	Myophosphorylase deficiency	Muscle pain, weakness	Phosphorylase	Muscle
	McArdle	Exercise-induced cramping Occasional myoglobinuria		
VI	Hers	Cherubic, small stature Hepatomegaly Normal life span	Phosphorylase	Liver Leukocytes
VI a.		Hepatomegaly in childhood Mild muscle weakness Usually X-linked	Phosphorylase kinase	Liver Leukocytes
VII		Exercise-induced muscle cramps Myoglobinuria	Phosphofructokinase	Muscle Red cell

total phosphatase and β-glycerol phosphatase activity in liver homogenate. Total and β-glycerol phosphatases are measured as the amounts of inorganic phosphate liberated from glucose-6-phosphate and β-glycerol phosphate, respectively.

Procedure

1. Homogenize from 35 to 135 mg fresh or frozen liver in 1 ml demineralized water in ice water bath, using greater amounts of tissue when little activity is anticipated.
2. Centrifuge at 4°C at 3000 R.P.M. for fifteen minutes, draw off, and save supernatant fluid (cell-free homogenate) in ice water bath.
3. Add 0.3 ml buffer to four 15 ml conical centrifuge tubes, (A, B, C, and D) and 0.1 ml demineralized water to two (tubes A and B). Add 0.1 ml glucose-6-phosphate to tubes A and C, and 0.1 ml β-glycerolphosphate to tubes B and D. Add 0.1 ml cell-free homogenate to tubes C and D.
4. Mix solutions and incubate tubes in 37°C water bath for exactly fifteen minutes. Stop reaction with 1 ml 10% TCA.
5. Chill in ice water bath five minutes, centrifuge at 2000 R.P.M. for fifteen minutes, remove, and save supernatant fluids for phosphate determination.
6. Combine 0.5 ml aliquots of the supernatant fluids with 0.2 ml 5.0 M H_2SO_4, 0.4 ml 2.5% ammonium molybdate, 0.2 ml amino naphthol sulfonic acid (ANSA), and 4.5 ml demineralized water.
7. Mix, let stand ten minutes, and measure optical density at 730 nm.
8. Repeat steps 6 and 7 with 0.5 ml aliquots of the standard phosphate solutions.
9. Dilute 10λ cell-free homogenate (step 2) with 30λ demineralized water. Add 20λ diluted homogenate to 1.0 ml working alkaline copper reagent and let stand fifteen minutes.
10. Repeat step 9 with 20λ of the standard protein solutions.
11. Add 0.1 ml dilute phenol reagent rapidly to all tubes, mix

immediately, let stand one-half hour, and measure O.D. at 750 nm.

Calculations

1. Plot standard curves of phosphate and protein concentrations versus respective optical densities.
2. Obtain O.D. phosphate from glucose-6-phosphatase activity from O.D. phosphate from total and β-glycerol phosphatase activities as

$$O.D. = [O.D._C - (O.D._D - O.D._B + O.D._A)]$$

3. Convert O.D. to mmoles phosphate/100 ml from standard curve of phosphate concentrations. Obtain mg protein per 100 ml from standard curve of protein concentration.
4. Calculate activity of glucose-6-phosphatase in mg P/g liver protein (E) as:

$$E = \frac{\text{mmoles } PO_4^=/100 \text{ ml} \times 15 \times 31 \times 1000}{\text{mg protein}/100 \text{ ml} \times 4},$$

where 15 is the dilution factor in phosphate assay, 31 is atomic weight of phosphorus, 1000 is the number of mg protein in 1 gram protein, and 4 is dilution factor in protein assay.

Interpretation

Liver from normal persons contains approximately 27 units (mg P/g protein) activity. Little or no glucose-6-phosphatase activity is detected in liver from patients with GSD I (Von Gierke).

Reagents

1. *Maleic Acid Buffer, 0.1 M, pH 6.5*: Dissolve 1.16 g maleic acid in 80 ml demineralized water, adjust to pH 6.5 with 1 N NaOH (40 g/l), and bring to volume in 100 ml volumetric flask.
2. *Glucose-6-Phosphate, 0.1 M*: 36.4 mg/ml demineralized water.
3. *β-Glycerophosphate, 0.1 M*: 17.2 mg/1.0 ml.
4. *Trichloroacetic Acid, 10%*: Dissolve 10 g trichloroacetic acid

in 100 ml demineralized water.

5. *Ammonium Molybdate, 2.5%*: Dissolve 2.5 g in 100 ml demineralized water.

6. *Sulfuric Acid, 5 M*: Dilute 27.8 ml concentrated H_2SO_4 with 72.2 ml demineralized water by adding acid slowly to the water.

7. *Amino Naphthol Sulfonic Acid Reagent*: Dissolve the following, in the order given, in 10 ml demineralized water: 25 mg 1, 2, 4-aminonaphthol-sulfonic acid; 1.50 g $NaHSO_3$; 50 mg Na_2SO_3. Filter, if necessary.

8. *Phosphate Standard Stock Solution, 0.2 mmoles/100 ml:* Dissolve 27.6 mg $NaH_2PO_4 \cdot H_2O$ in 100 ml demineralized water.

9. *Phosphate Standards*: Dilute the phosphate standard stock solution with demineralized water as follows:

nmoles/100 ml	Stock (ml)	Water (ml)
0.15	3	1
0.10	2	2
0.075	1.5	2.5
0.05	1	3
0.025	0.5	3.5

10. *Dilute Phenol Reagent*: At the time of test, add one part phenol reagent 2 N solution (Fisher) to one part demineralized water.

11. *Alkaline Tartrate Reagent*: Dissolve 2.0 g Na_2CO_3 and 50 mg Na or K tartrate in 100 ml 0.1 N NaOH (4 g/1).

12. *Copper Sulfate, 0.1%*: Dissolve 100 mg $CuSO_4 \cdot 5 H_2O$ in 100 ml demineralized water.

13. *Working Alkaline Copper Reagent*: At the time of test, combine 9 volumes alkaline tartrate reagent with 1 volume 0.1% copper sulfate.

14. *Bovine Albumin Standard Protein Solutions*: Combine the following volumes of bovine albumin and demineralized water as follows:

Standard (mg%)	Bovine Albumin 30% (ml)	600 mg% (ml)	Water (ml)
600	1		49

Standard (mg%)	Bovine Albumin 30% (ml)	600 mg% (ml)	Water (ml)
500		2.5	0.5
400		2.0	1.0
300		1.0	1.0
200		1.0	2.0
100		0.5	2.5
50		0.25	2.75

REFERENCES

Field, J. B., Epstein, S., and Egan, T.: Studies in glycogen storage disease. I. Intestinal glucose-6-phosphatase activity in patients with Von Gierke's disease and their parents. *J Clin Invest, 44*:1240, 1965.

Lowry, O. H., Rosebrough, N. J., Farr, A. L., and Randall, R. J.: Protein measurement with the Folin phenol reagent. *J Biol Chem, 193*:265, 1951.

Fiske, C. H., and Subbarow, Y.: The colorimetric determination of phosphorous. *J Biol Chem, 66*:375, 1925.

TYPE II (POMPE)

URINARY α-GLUCOSIDASE

Principle

The urinary acid α-glucosidase (pH optimum of 4) of patients with GSD Type II (Pompe) is deficient, whereas the neutral form of the enzyme (pH optimum of 6) remains normally active.

Both α-glucosidases are determined by a fluorometric method for the amount of 4-methylumbelliferone formed by the hydrolysis of 4-methylumbelliferyl-α-D-glucoside at their respective pH optima.

Procedure

1. Pipette 100λ volumes sodium acetate buffer, pH 4.0, and sodium cacodylate buffer, pH 6.0, into respective 10 ml screw-capped tubes, three tubes per buffer. Add 200λ aliquots urine sample, clarified by centrifugation, to the six tubes.
2. Add 100λ 1.0 mM 4-methylumbelliferyl-α-D-glucoside to four tubes, leaving one tube of each buffer as blank.
3. Place tubes in 37°C water bath. Stop reactions in all tubes one

hour later with 5.6 ml 1.0 M glycine-NaOH buffer.
4. Add 100λ 1.0 mM 4-methylumbelliferyl-α-D-glucoside to both blanks.
5. Measure fluorescence in Turner 110 fluorometer, with primary filter 760, secondary filters 2A, 48, and 10% neutral density filter. Use glycine-NaOH buffer as blank.
6. Prepare and measure fluorescence of 4-methylumbelliferone standards from 4-methylumbelliferone stock solution during the incubation period, as follows:

Concentration Standard (nmoles/3 ml)	Volume Stock Solution (λ)	Volume Glycine-NaOH Buffer (ml)
0.0	-	3
0.25	5	10
0.5	10	10
1.0	20	10
2.5	50	10

Calculations

1. Plot standard curve of fluorescence versus concentration of 4-methylumbelliferone.
2. Obtain nmole 4-methylumbelliferone formed per 3 ml reaction mixture per hour at the two hydrogen ion concentrations from standard curve.
3. Multiply by 1000 for nmole/100 ml urine per hour, (since 3.0 ml of the reaction mixtures contain 100λ of urine); divide by creatinine concentration in mg/100 ml for nmole/mg creatinine per hour (units of activity).
4. Divide units at pH 4.0 by units at pH 6.0 for ratio.

Interpretation

The ratio of urinary enzyme activity at pH 4 and 6 in patients with Pompe's disease is less than 1, between 1 and 2 in normal infants less than two years old and from 2.5 to 7 in children and adults.

Reagents

1. *Acetic Acid, 0.2 M*: Dilute 1.15 ml glacial acetic acid with 100 ml demineralized water in volumetric flask.
2. *Sodium Acetate Buffer, 0.2 M, pH 4.0*: Dissolve 2.72 g sodium acetate (trihydrate) in 100 ml demineralized water. Adjust to pH 4.0 with approximately 200 ml 0.2 M acetic acid.
3. *Sodium Cacodylate Buffer, 0.2 M, pH 6.0*: Dissolve 8.56 g sodium cacodylate in 140 ml demineralized water. Adjust to pH 6.0 with 1N HCl and bring volume to 200 ml.
4. *4-Methylumbelliferyl-α-D*-Glucoside, *1.0 mM*: Dissolve 8.45 mg Sigma 4-methylumbelliferyl-α-D-glucoside in 25 ml demineralized water by shaking suspension in hot water bath three to four hours.
5. *Stock 4-Methylumbelliferone Standard*: Dissolve 7.35 mg 4-methylumbelliferone in 250 ml demineralized water by shaking suspension in hot water bath three to four hours.
6. *Glycine-NaOH Buffer, 1.0 M, pH 10.5*: Dissolve 15 g glycine in 130 ml demineralized water. Adjust to pH 10.5 with concentrated NaOH and bring to volume in 200 ml volumetric flask.

REFERENCE

Salafsky, I. S., and Nadler, H. L.: Deficiency of acid alpha glucosidase in the urine of patients with Pompe's disease. *J Pediatrics, 82*:294, 1973.

MICROMETHOD FOR LEUKOCYTE α-GLUCOSIDASE

Principle

Salafsky and Nadler's (1973) assay for cellular α-1, 4-glucosidase activity on the synthetic substrate, 4-methylumbelliferyl-α-D-glucopyranoside, is modified by isolating leukocytes and estimating activity by methods described by Peters et al. (1975) for β-glucosidase, i.e. in the presence of taurocholate.

Procedure

1. Steps 1-8 as described in "Procedure" for leukocyte β-

glucosidase, (p. 184), with the exception of different substrate and buffer, as listed in "Reagents" in this section.

9. Centrifuge all tubes at maximum speed in clinical centrifuge for five minutes. Decant clear supernatant fluids and measure fluorescence on Turner fluorometer model 110, using primary filter #7-60 and secondary filters 48 and 2-A, overlaid with 25% neutral density filter.

10. Calculate and express activity as described in "Calculations" for leukocyte β-glucosidase (p. 186).

Interpretation

Leukocytes from five normal adult controls contained from 12.1 to 19.8 units of α-glucosidase activity (nanomoles 4-methylumbelliferyl-α-glucopyranoside cleaved per 10^7 cells per hour at 37° C). Patients with Pompe's disease are expected to have little or no detectable activity, and heterozygotes have 50% of normal activity.

Reagents

1. *NaCl, 0.2%*: Dissolve 0.5 g NaCl in 250 ml demineralized water.

2. *NaCl, 3.6%*: Dissolve 3.6 g NaCl in 100 ml demineralized water.

3. *Sodium Acetate, 0.2 M, pH 4.0*: Dissolve 0.49 g Na · Acetate · 3 H_2O in 80 ml demineralized water. Adjust to pH 4.0 with glacial acetic acid and bring to volume in 100 ml volumetric flask.

4. *Substrate Solution*: Dissolve 600 mg taurocholic acid·Na salt in 100 ml warm acetate buffer (on heater-stirrer for approximately one-quarter hour). Cool to 37° C, add 16.9 mg 4-methylumbelliferyl-α-glucopyranoside and dissolve by stirring.

5. *Glycine · NaOH, Buffer, 1.0 M, pH 10.5*: Dissolve 18.7 g glycine in 200 ml demineralized water. Adjust to pH 10.5 with 10 N NaOH and bring to volume in 250 ml volumetric flask.

6. *4-Methylumbelliferone Stock Standard, (10 nmoles/3.1 ml)*:

Dissolve 14.2 mg 4-methylumbelliferone in 200 ml demineralized water in 300 ml Erlenmeyer flask; bring to volume in 250 ml volumetric flask. Dilute 1 ml to 100 ml with glycine buffer.

7. *4-Methylumbelliferone Working Standards*: Combine the following volumes of stock standard and glycine buffer:

Concentration (Nanomoles/3.1 ml)	Volume Stock Standard (ml)	Volume Buffer (ml)
0	0	5
0.1	0.05	4.95
0.2	0.1	4.9
0.4	0.2	4.8
0.6	0.3	4.7
0.8	0.4	4.6
1.0	0.5	4.5
1.2	0.6	4.4

REFERENCES

Salafsky, I. S., and Nadler, H. L.: A fluorometric assay of alpha glucosidase and its application in the study of Pompe's disease. *J Lab Clin Med, 81*:450, 1973.

Peters, S. P., Lee, R. E., and Glew, R. H.: A microassay for Gaucher's disease. *Clin Chim Acta, 60*:391, 1975.

FLUOROMETRIC METHOD FOR LIVER α-GLUCOSIDASE

Principle

Activity of liver α-glucosidase is measured fluorometrically as the amount of 4-methylumbelliferone released from methylumbelliferyl-conjugated substrate at pH 4.0. The assay is more sensitive than the colorimetric method, in which activity is measured as glucose liberated by glucose oxidase.

Procedure

1. Homogenize 70 to 80 mg fresh or freshly thawed liver in 0.5 ml demineralized water.
2. Centrifuge at 10,000 g at 4°C for twenty minutes.

3. Collect supernatant fluid, dilute tenfold with demineralized water, measure enzyme activity immediately, and store at 4°C when not in actual use.
4. To each of four 10 ml test tubes add 0.05 ml aliquots of substrate, (which correspond to about 60 mg protein per 0.1 ml of diluted supernatant fluid) acetate buffer, homogenate, and water. Add 2.8 ml glycine buffer to one tube (blank).
5. Incubate all tubes at 37°C for one hour; terminate reaction by adding 2.8 ml glycine buffer to remaining three tubes.
6. Measure fluorescence of blank, sample, and standard tubes on Turner model 110 fluorometer, with primary filter #7-60 and secondary filters #48 and 2-A, overlaid with 10% neutral density filter. If sample readings are off scale, insert 1% neutral density filter and remeasure fluorescence of all tubes.
7. Estimate protein concentrations in homogenate and working standards by combining 50λ aliquots with 2.0 ml aliquots of working alkaline copper reagent.
8. Mix, let stand fifteen minutes, add 0.2 ml dilute phenol reagent, mix, and let stand at least thirty minutes.
9. Measure protein in all tubes at 750 nm on Coleman Jr. spectrophotometer.

Calculations

1. Plot absorbance versus concentration of protein on linear scale.
2. Estimate mg protein per 100 ml homogenate directly from graph, multiply by 0.05, and divide by 100 for mg protein in 50λ homogenate or 3.0 ml final solution.
3. Plot fluorescence versus concentration of 4-methyllumbelliferone standards on linear scale.
4. Estimate nanomoles 4-methylumbelliferone per 3.0 ml final solution liberated in sixty minutes from standard curve, subtract blank, and divide by 60 for nanomoles p r 3.0 ml final solution per minute. Express activity as nanomoles 4-methylumbelliferyl-α-D-pyranoside hydrolyzed per minute per mg protein.

Interpretation

α-Glucosidase activity in normal liver ranges from 0.61 to 1.17 units (nanomoles/min/mg protein) and from 0.00 to 0.01 units in liver from patients with Pompe disease.

Reagents

1. *4-Methylumbelliferyl-α-D-Glucopyranoside Substrate, 1.0 mM*: Dissolve 16.9 mg 4-methylumbelliferyl-α-D-glucopyranoside (Koch-Light) in 50 ml demineralized water.
2. *Sodium Acetate Buffer, 0.2 M, pH 4.0*: Dissolve 0.49 g sodium acetate · 3 H_2O in 80 ml demineralized water. Adjust to pH 4.0 with glacial acetic acid and bring to volume in 100 ml volumetric flask.
3. *Glycine · NaOH Buffer, 1.0 M, pH 10.5*: Dissolve 37.4 g glycine in 400 ml demineralized water. Adjust to pH 10.5 with 10 N NaOH and bring to volume in 500 ml volumetric flask.
4. *4-Methylumbelliferone Stock Standard, 1000 nmoles/3.0 ml*: Dissolve 11.7 mg 4-methylumbelliferone in 200 ml glycine · NaOH buffer.
5. *4-Methylumbelliferone Working Standards*: Combine the following volumes of 4-methylumbelliferone stock standard and glycine-NaOH buffer:

Nanomoles/3.0 ml	Volume Stock Standard (ml)	Volume Buffer (ml)
0	0	10
0.5	0.005	10
1	0.010	10
2	0.020	10
2.5	0.025	10
3	0.025	8.3
*5	0.050	10
*7.5	0.075	10

6. *Protein Stock Standard, 600 mg%*: Combine 1 ml 30% bovine albumin with 49 ml demineralized water.
7. *Protein Working Standard*: Combine the following volumes

---

*If 1% neutral density filter is used.

of protein stock standard and demineralized water:

Mg Protein 100 ml	Volume Stock Standard (ml)	Volume Water (ml)
0	0	4
25	0.25	5.75
50	0.5	5.5
75	0.75	5.25
100	1	5
150	1.5	4.5
200	2	4

8. *Dilute Phenol Reagent*: Just before use, dilute phenol reagent (Fisher) 1:1 with demineralized water.
9. *Alkaline Tartrate Reagent*: Combine 2.0 g Na_2CO_3 and 50 mg Na or K tartrate with 100 ml 0.1 N NaOH.
10. *Copper Sulfate, 0.1%*: Dissolve 100 mg $CuSO_4 \cdot 5 H_2O$ in 100 ml demineralized water.
11. *Alkaline Copper Working Reagent*: Just before use, combine alkaline tartrate reagent and 0.1% copper sulfate, 9:1.

REFERENCE

Salafsky, I. S., and Nadler, H. L.: A fluorometric assay of alpha-glucosidase and its application in the study of Pompe's disease. *J Lab Clin Med*, *81*:450, 1973.

TYPE III (DEBRANCHER)

LEUKOCYTE AMYLO-1, 6-GLUCOSIDASE

Principle

"Debranching" enzyme *in vivo* promotes the depolymerization of glycogen by catalyzing the hydrolysis of the glucose molecules which remain condensed at the polymer's branch points after hydrolysis by phosphorylase. The reaction is reversible, i.e. "debrancher" enzyme can be made to promote branching and formation of the polymer.

The reverse reaction is the basis of the *in vitro* assay for the enzyme, in which the amount of branch point, C^{14}-labelled glucose formed during polymerization is estimated.

Procedure

1. Collect 10 ml blood in EDTA tube, transfer to 250 ml Nalgene centrifuge tube with screw cap, and add 175 ml 0.2% NaCl. Mix by inversion. Exactly two minutes later, add 52.5 ml 3.6% NaCl to restore isotonicity. Mix by inversion.

2. Centrifuge at 1500 g ten minutes at 4°C.

3. Decant supernatant fluid slowly, holding tube with white cell pellet on upper surface. Aspirate last ml of supernatant fluid with Pasteur pipette, completely removing red cell ghosts from top of pellet.

4. Suspend leukocyte pellet in 1.0 ml demineralized water, and homogenize in glass homogenizer with Teflon pestle, using Talboys instrument Bodine motor at maximum speed (5000 R.P.M.) two minutes.

5. Centrifuge homogenate at 14,000 g, fifteen minutes, at 4°C. Transfer supernatant fluid with Pasteur pipette and distribute as described below.

6. To 0.1 ml aliquots leukocyte supernatant fluid in six 16 x 100 mm tubes, add (in the order given) 0.2 ml 20% glycogen, 0.05 ml 0.5 M NaF, 0.1 M phosphate buffer, pH 7.4, 0.05 ml D-glucose C^{14} to four of them. Immediately add 6.5 ml stop solution to two (blanks); mix by inversion. Cap the four tubes containing supernatant fluid, substrate with American Can Parafilm and incubate at 37°C for two hours.

7. In the meantime, add 2.0 ml working protein reagent to the two remaining tubes containing 0.1 ml leukocyte supernatant fluid, and to tubes containing 0.1 ml aliquots albumin working standards or 0.1 ml water (blank). Mix contents of tubes and let stand fifteen minutes.

8. Add 0.2 ml phenol reagent, 1 N, mixing each tube immediately. Let stand twenty minutes.

9. Measure optical density at 750 nm; zero instrument with blank.

10. At the end of the two hour incubation period add 6.5 ml stop solution to incubated tubes. Mix. Centrifuge at three-quarters maximum speed in clinical centrifuge ten minutes.

11. Remove supernatant fluid with Pasteur pipette and discard. Dissolve pellet of glycogen in 2 ml demineralized water. Add

    4 ml ethanol, mix, and centrifuge as in previous step.

12. Discard supernatant fluid, dissolve pellet in 2.0 ml 20% KOH and heat in boiling water bath thirty minutes.

13. Reprecipitate three times with 2.4 ml portions of ethanol and redissolve pellet in 2.0 ml demineralized water. Dissolve final pellet in 0.5 ml demineralized water by heating thirty minutes at 37°C. Spot on Whatman #1 filter paper discs of diameter to fit planchet and let dry overnight.

Calculations

1. Average counts per minute for blanks and samples; subtract blank from sample average CPM for CPM/0.1 ml leukocytes (supernatant fluid).

2. Plot standard curve of optical density at 750 nm against concentration of albumin in mg.

3. Obtain mg leukocyte protein/0.1 ml leukocytes from albumin standard curve.

4. Divide CPM/0.1 ml leukocytes by mg protein/0.1 ml leukocytes for CPM/mg protein.

5. Divide CPM/mg protein by 2 (hrs) for CPM/hr/mg protein.

Interpretation

Enzyme activity in blood from normal adults ranged from 300 to 400 c.p.m./hr/mg protein or 3000 to 4000 c.p.m./hr/10^8 cells. Justice et al.'s (1970) counts of 4042 c.p.m./hr/10^8 white blood cells (WBC) are equivalent when the greater specific activity of their ^{14}C-glucose source is considered. Their data suggests that carrier levels are half the normal range and enzyme from the homozygous patient is practically undetectable.

Reagents

1. *Sodium Chloride, 0.2%*: Dissolve 2.0 g NaCl in 100 ml demineralized water.

2. *Sodium Chloride, 3.6%*: Dissolve 3.6 g NaCl in 100 ml demineralized water.

3. *Alkaline Tartrate Reagent*: Dissolve 2.0 g Na_2CO_3, 50 mg sodium tartrate, and 0.4 g NaOH in 90 demineralized water. Dilute to volume in 100 ml volumetric flask.

4. *Copper Sulfate Reagent, 0.1%*: Dissolve 100 mg CuSO₄ · 5 H₂O in 100 ml demineralized water.
5. *Working Protein Reagent (Fresh)*: Combine 18 ml alkaline tartrate reagent with 2 ml copper sulfate reagent and mix.
6. *Phenol Reagent, 1 N*: Dilute 2 ml Fisher phenol reagent 2 N with 2 ml demineralized water.
7. *Albumin Stock Standard Solution (1 mg/ml)*: Dissolve 100 mg albumin in 90 ml demineralized water and dilute to volume in 100 ml volumetric flask.
8. *Albumin Working Standard Solutions*: Combine the following:

Concentration Albumin Standard (mg)	Volume Stock Standard (ml)	Demineralized Water (ml)
0.1	0.1	0.0
0.08	0.8	0.2
0.06	0.6	0.4
0.04	0.4	0.6

9. *Glycogen, 20%*: Dissolve 400 mg glycogen in 2 ml demineralized water.
10. *Glucose-^{14}C Reagent, 7.3 mC/mmole, 100 μCi in 2.46 mg Glucose*: Dissolve 2.46 mg to 1 ml with demineralized water. Use 50λ aliquots for each sample or blank.
11. *Phosphate Buffer, 0.1 M, pH 7.4, and NaF, 0.5M*: Dissolve 1.39 g K_2HPO_4, 0.27 g KH_2PO_4, and 2.1 g NaF in 90 ml demineralized water and dilute to volume in 100 ml volumetric flask.
12. *Trichloroacetic Acid, 20%*: Dissolve 20 g TCA in 100 ml demineralized water.
13. *Stop Solution*: Mix 5 ml 20% TCA, 40 ml 95% ethanol, 20 ml demineralized water.
14. *Potassium Hydroxide, 20%*: Dissolve 20 g KOH in 50 ml demineralized water and dilute to volume in 100 ml volumetric flask.

REFERENCES

Huijing, F.: Amylo-1,6-glucosidase activity in normal leucocytes and in leucocytes of patients with glycogen-storage disease. *Clin Chim Acta,* 9:269, 1964.

Justice, P., Ryan, C., Hsia, D. Y. Y., and Krmpotik, E.: Amyl-1, 6-glucosidase in human fibroblasts: Studies in type III glycogen storage disease. *Biochem Biophys Res Commun, 39*:301, 1970.

Lowry, O., Rosebrough, N., Farr, A., and Randall, R.: Protein measurement with the Folin phenol reagent. *J Biol Chem, 193*:265, 1951.

Peters, S., Lee, R., and Glew, R.: A microassay for Gaucher's disease. *Clin Chim Acta, 60*:391, 1975.

TYPE IV

LEUKOCYTE α-1,4-GLUCAN:α-1,4-GLUCAN 6-GLYCOSYL TRANSFERASE

Principle

Branching enzyme *in vivo* promotes the synthesis of glycogen by catalyzing the addition of branch points of glucose at every sixth glucose molecule on the developing polysaccharide chain, thereby providing additional sites for linear chain building by phosphorylase.

Branching enzyme activity is measured as the difference in quantity of phosphorus released by the combined action of branching enzyme and phosphorylase and that released by phosphorylase activity alone in the following reaction:

$$\text{G-1-P} < \frac{\text{Enzyme(s)}}{5' \text{ AMP}} > \text{Glycogen} + \text{P}$$

Procedure

1. Collect at least 0.5 ml capillary blood in heparinized hematocrit tubes or venous blood in EDTA (not heparinized) tubes. If heparinized, transfer sample to 50 × 75-mm tube.
2. Combine 0.5 ml blood sample with 50 ml 0.2% NaCl in a 250 ml Nalgene centrifuge tube. Exactly two minutes later add 15 ml 3.6% NaCl. Cover with plastic screw cap and mix by inverting.
3. Centrifuge ten minutes at 1500 g at 4°C.
4. Aspirate supernatant fluid containing hemoglobin and red cells ghosts with Pasteur pipette: Hold tube at 30° angle from

vertical and slide pipette tip along side of tube opposite pellet; remove last ml slowly, removing red cell ghosts from top of pellet.

5. Suspend pellet in 2.5 ml Tris buffer and homogenize suspension in 10 ml glass homogenizing tube with Teflon pestle.

6. Centrifuge at 14,000 g ten minutes at 4°C.

7. Remove supernatant fluid with Pasteur pipette and add to clean 16 × 100-mm test tube.

8. Add 0.2 ml aliquots of supernatant fluid to two 16 × 100-mm test tubes for enzyme measurement and 0.1 ml aliquots to two tubes for protein estimation (step 16).

9. Measure remaining volume of supernatant fluid in 12 ml graduated conical centrifuge. Heat in boiling water bath for five minutes to destroy enzyme activity.

10. Remove tube from water bath, dilute to preboiled volume with demineralized water, and add 0.2 ml aliquots to two 16 × 100-mm test tubes as blank.

11. Equilibrate water bath at 30°C.

12. Combine 0.1 ml aliquots of the following reagent solutions in respective tubes for enzyme measurement and blank: glycylglycine, AMP, phosphorylase a, glucose-1-phosphate, and 2-mercaptoethanol.

13. Mix tubes by swirling. Remove 0.1 ml aliquots immediately and add to 16 × 100-mm tubes containing 0.05 ml 5% TCA. Mix by swirling. Warm TCA-containing tubes (two samples and two blanks) in 30°C water bath, removing 0.1 ml aliquots at fifteen minute intervals up to sixty minutes. Add to tubes containing 50 μl 5% TCA. Centrifuge 10 minutes at 1500 R.P.M. and measure inorganic phosphorus as described in following steps.

14. Add 40 μl 5.0 M H_2SO_4, 80 μl 2.5% ammonium molybdate, and 40 μl ANSA to 100 μl TCA precipitation supernatant fluid. Add 0.9 ml demineralized water, mix, and let stand ten minutes.

15. Measure optical density of samples and phosphorus standards at 730 nm.

16. Estimate protein in leukocyte supernatant fluid (step 8), working albumin standards, and blank (0.1 ml demineralized

water) as described in the following steps.

17. Add 2 ml freshly prepared working copper sulfate reagent to respective 0.1 ml aliquots and mix on Vortex.
18. Fifteen minutes later, add 0.2 ml phenol reagent, mixing each tube *immediately.*
19. Measure optical density at 750 nm.

Calculations

1. Plot standard curve of phosphorus concentration against optical density at 730 nm.
2. Plot standard curve of albumin concentration against optical density at 750 nm.
3. Obtain μmoles phosphorus liberated in 0.1 ml TCA supernatant fluid from the phosphate standard curve at zero O.D. (O.D.$_o$) and again at thirty minutes (O.D.$_{30}$). Subtract μmoles O.D.$_o$ from μmoles O.D.$_{30}$.
4. Multiply by 5.26 for μmoles phosphorus liberated in 0.1 ml leukocyte supernatant fluid per thirty minutes.
5. Obtain mg protein in 0.1 ml leukocyte supernatant fluid directly from standard curve.
6. Divide μmoles phosphorus liberated by 30 for μmoles per minute. Divide by mg protein and express activity as μmoles phosphorus liberated per minute per mg leukocyte protein.

Interpretation

Normal leukocytes contain from 0.6 to 1.5 units of brancher enzyme activity (μmoles P/min/mg protein) (published values); cells from patients with the deficiency have little or no activity.

Reagents

1. *NaCl, 0.2%*: Dissolve 0.2 g NaCl in 90 ml demineralized water and dilute to 100 ml volume.
2. *NaCl, 3.6%*: Dissolve 3.6 g NaCl in 90 ml demineralized water and dilute to 100 ml volume.
3. *Alkaline Tartrate Reagent*: Dissolve 2.0 g sodium carbonate,

50 mg sodium tartrate, and 0.4 g sodium hydroxide in 90 ml demineralized water, and dilute to volume in 100 ml volumetric flask.

4. *Copper Sulfate Reagent, 0.1%*: Dissolve 100 mg $CuSO_4 \cdot 5$ H_2O in 90 ml demineralized water and dilute to 100 ml volume.
5. *Working Reagent (Make Fresh)*: Combine 18 ml alkaline tartrate reagent and 2 ml copper sulfate reagent.
6. *Phenol Reagent, 1N*: Dilute 2 ml Fisher phenol reagent 2N with 2 ml demineralized water.
7. *Albumin Stock Solution, 1 mg/ml*: Dissolve 100 mg bovine albumin in 90 ml demineralized water and dilute to 100 ml volume.
8. *Albumin Working Standard Solutions:* Combine the following:

Concentration Albumin (mg)	Stock Standard Solution (ml)	Water (ml)
0.10	0.1	0
0.08	0.8	0.2
0.06	0.6	0.4
0.04	0.4	0.6
0.02	0.2	0.8

9. *Glycylglycine, 20 mM*: Dissolve 0.0430 g in 1 ml demineralized water.
10. *Adenosine Monophosphate, 4mM*: Dissolve 0.0103 g (mol wt 369) in 1 ml demineralized water.
11. *2-Mercaptoethanol, 20 mM*: Dissolve 0.0098 ml in 1 ml demineralized water.
12. *Phosphorylase a*: Dissolve 50 U Sigma phosphorylase a (rabbit muscle) in 1 ml demineralized water.
13. *Glucose-1-Phosphate (G-1-P), 80 mM*: Dissolve 0.0188 g in 1 ml demineralized water.
14. *TRIS Buffer, 0.05 M*: Dissolve 0.434 g Trizma base in 9 ml demineralized water. Adjust to pH 6.4 with 4 M HCl. Dilute to final volume of 10 ml.
15. *Trichloroacetic Acid, 5%*: Dissolve 5 g TCA in 90 ml demineralized water and dilute to 100 ml volume.

16. *Ammonium Molybdate, 2.5%*: Dissolve 2.5 g ammonium molybdate in 90 ml demineralized water and dilute to 100 ml volume.

17. *Sulfuric Acid, 5 M*: Add 27.8 ml concentrated H_2SO_4 to 90 ml demineralized water slowly (with mixing) and dilute to volume in 100 ml volumetric flask.

18. *1-Amino-2-Naphthol-Sulfonic Acid*: Prepare fresh. Dissolve in order in 10 ml demineralized water: 25 mg 1-amino-2-naphthol sulfonic acid, 1.5 g $NaHSO_3$, and 50 mg Na_2SO_3. Filter, if necessary.

19. *Phosphate Stock Standard Solution* (KH_2Po_4) *0.2 mmoles/100 ml*: Dissolve 27.2 mg KH_2PO_4 in 90 ml demineralized water and dilute to volume in 100 ml volumetric flask.

20. *Working Phosphate Standard Solutions*: Combine the following:

Concentration (mmoles/100 ml)	Stock Standard Solution (ml)	Water (ml)
0.20	0.1 ml	0.0 ml
0.10	2.0 ml	2.0 ml
0.05	1.0 ml	3.0 ml

REFERENCES

Brown, B., and Brown, D.: Lack of an α-1, 4-glucan: α-1,4-glucan-6-glycosyl transferase in a case of type IV glycogenosis. *Proc Natl Acad Sci, USA, 56*:725, 1966.

Fernandes, J., and Huijing, F.: Branching enzyme deficiency — glycogenosis: Studies in therapy. *Arch Dis Child, 43*:347, 1968.

Hsia, David Y. Y., and Inouye, Tohru: *Inborn Errors of Metabolism.* Chicago, Year Book Medical, 1966, pp. 178-180.

Lowry, O., Rosebrough, N., Farr, A., and Randall, R.: Protein measurement with the Folin phenol reagent. *J Biol Chem, 193*:265, 1951.

Peters, S., Lee, R., and Glew, R.: A microassay for Gaucher's disease. *Clin Chim Acta, 60*:391, 1975.

TYPE V (MCARDLE)

MUSCLE PHOSPHORYLASE

Principle

The muscles of patients with McArdle disease (GSD V) are

deficient in phosphorylase. The assay for the enzyme involves the snythesis of glycogen and the dephosphorylation of glucose-1-phosphate, the reverse of the *in vivo* reaction in muscle, as follows:

$$\text{G-1-P} <\frac{\text{Phosphorylase}}{5' \text{ AMP}}> \text{Glycogen} + \text{P}$$

Activity is measured as the increase in concentration of inorganic phosphorus.

Procedure

1. Mince approximately 100 mg muscle tissue with scissors.
2. Incubate in 10 ml glass homogenizing tube with 1.0 ml 0.1 M NaF containing epinephrine ten minutes in a 37°C water bath.
3. Grind tissue three minutes at maximum homogenizer speed (5000 R.P.M. with Talboys instrument Bodine motor). Remove 0.1 ml aliquot and add to 0.9 ml demineralized water (mix) for protein estimation (step 9).
4. Combine 0.3 ml homogenate, 0.1 ml AMP solution, and 0.1 ml demineralized water in two 16 × 100-mm test tubes, the second of which is blank A. In a third tube, blank B, combine 0.3 ml 0.1 M NaF solution containing epinephrine, 0.1 ml AMP, and 0.1 ml demineralized water. Chill tubes in ice water bath ten minutes.
5. Add 1.0 ml of the G-1-P, glycogen, and NaF substrate to sample and blank B tubes and 1.0 ml of the glycogen and NaF solution to blank A. Mix and immediately remove 0.5 ml aliquots from each tube and add to 2.0 ml 0.6 M TCA (zero time samples). Mix and chill five minutes in ice water bath. Centrifuge ten minutes at three-quarters maximum speed in clinical centrifuge.
6. Incubate remainder in 37°C water bath for thirty minutes. Remove similar aliquots, add to TCA, and treat as described above (thirty minute samples).
7. To 100 μl aliquots of TCA precipitate supernatant fluids of zero time and thirty-minute samples and blanks and to 100 μl aliquots of phosphate working standard solutions add 40 μ 5.0 M H_2SO_4, 80 μl 2.5% ammonium molybdate, 40 μl ANSA, and 0.9 ml demineralized water. Mix, let stand at room temperature ten minutes, and measure optical density

at 730 mμ.

8. Add 0.1 ml aliquots of diluted homogenate in triplicate (from step 3), demineralized water as blank, and albumin working standards solutions to respective 16 $\times$ 100-mm test tubes.
9. Add 2.0 ml working protein reagent, mix, and let stand fifteen minutes.
10. Add 0.2 ml Fisher phenol reagent, mix tubes immediately, and let stand twenty minutes.
11. Measure optical density at 750 nm.

Calculations

1 - 3. As in "Calculation" for leukocyte phosphorylase, p. 245.
4. Multiply mmoles P/released by 25 for mmoles P/30 min/0.1 ml muscle homogenate.
5. Plot standard curve of albumin concentration versus optical density at 750 nm.
6. Measure protein (mg) in 0.1 ml muscle homogenate from albumin standard curve.
7. Divide mmoles P per 0.1 ml muscle homogenate per thirty minutes by mg protein for mmoles P/30 min/mg protein.
8. Multiply by 1000 and express activity as mmoles P/30 min/g protein.

Interpretation

Phosphorylase levels in normal muscle range from approximately 4 to 28 units (mmoles P/30 min/g protein). Enzyme activity is minimal (up to about 0.4 unit) or absent in patients with McArdle disease.

Reagents

1. *Adenosine Monophosphate (5'-AMP), 0.02 M*: Dissolve 7.4 mg AMP in 1.0 ml demineralized water.
2. *NaF, 0.1 M*: Dissolve 0.042 g NaF in 10 ml demineralized water containing 20 μg epinephrine.
3. Remaining reagents are the same as those in reagent section on

leukocyte phosphorylase (p. 246), items 5 through 18.

REFERENCES

Fiske, C. H., and Subbarow, Y.: The colorimetric determination of phosphorus. *J Biol Chem,* 2:375, 1925.

Lowry, O., Rosebrough, N., Farr, A. L., and Randall, R.: Protein measurement with the Folin phenol reagent. *J Biol Chem, 193*:265, 1951.

Lubran, M. M.: McArdle's disease: A review. *Ann Clin Lab Sci,* 5:115, 1975.

Schmid, R., and Mahler, R.: Chronic progressive myopathy with myoglobinuria: Demonstration of a glycogenolytic defect in the muscle. *J Clin Invest, 38*:2044, 1959.

Steinitz, Kurt: Laboratory diagnosis of glycogen diseases. In Sobotka, Harry, and Stewart, Corbet P. (Eds.): *Advances in Clinical Chemistry.* New York, Acad Pr, 1967, vol. IX, pp. 299-301.

TYPE VI

LEUKOCYTE PHOSPHORYLASE

Principle

Some patients with deficiency of liver phosphorylase (GSD VI or Hers' disease) also reflect the defect in leukocytes. Assay for the enzyme defect involves the synthesis of glycogen and the dephosphorylation of glucose-1-phosphate, the reverse of the *in vivo* reaction, as follows:

$$\text{G-1-P} < \frac{\text{Phosphorylase}}{5'\ \text{AMP}} > \text{Glycogen} + \text{P.}$$

Activity is measured as the increase in concentration of inorganic phosphate.

Procedure

1. Add 175 ml 0.2% NaCl to 10 ml EDTA blood sample in 250 ml Nalgene centrifuge tube with screw cap. Mix by inversion. Exactly two minutes later add 52.5 ml 3.6% NaCl and mix.
2. Centrifuge at 1500 g ten minutes at 4°C.
3. Decant supernatant fluid carefully, with pellet on upper side of tube. Aspirate last few drops with Pasteur pipette.
4. Suspend pellet in 1.5 ml 0.1 M sodium fluoride solution and transfer to 16 × 100-mm test tube. Cap with American Can

parafilm.

5. Freeze pellet ten minutes at -70°C and thaw. Homogenize 2 minutes in glass homogenizer.

6. Combine 0.3 ml homogenate, 0.1 ml AMP solution, and 0.1 ml demineralized water in a 16 × 100 mm test tube. In a second tube combine 0.3 ml NaF, 0.1 ml AMP, 0.1 ml water (blank A), and in a third tube combine 0.3 ml homogenate, 0.1 ml AMP and 0.1 ml water (blank B).

7. Cool tubes in ice water bath. Add 1.0 ml of the G-1-P, glycogen and NaF substrate to sample and blank A. Add 1.0 ml of the glycogen and NaF solution to blank B. Mix and immediately remove 0.5 ml aliquots from each tube and add to 2.0 ml TCA solution in respective 16 × 100-mm test tubes (zero time samples and blanks). Mix.

8. Incubate remainder thirty minutes at 37°C.

9. Centrifuge the zero time samples and blanks for ten minutes at three-quarters speed in clinical centrifuge. Remove 0.1 ml aliquots and place in 16 × 100-mm test tubes for phosphorus measurement (step 15).

10. Remove and add similar aliquots to TCA at end of thirty minute incubation (thirty-minute samples and blanks). Centrifuge as above and save portions for phosphorus measurement (step 15).

11. Dilute 0.1 ml leukocyte homogenate with 0.9 ml demineralized water and mix. Disperse 0.1 ml aliquots into two 16 × 100-mm test tubes for protein measurement.

12. Add 2.0 ml working protein reagent to diluted homogenate, working albumin standards, and blank (0.1 ml water). Mix.

13. Add 0.2 ml Fisher phenol reagent fifteen minutes later, mixing each tube immediately. Leave at room temperature twenty minutes.

14. Measure optical density at 750 nm.

15. Combine 100 μl supernatant fluid from TCA precipitate and 100 μ demineralized water as blank, in respective tubes, with 40 μl 5.0 M sulfuric acid, 80 μl 2.5% ammonium molybdate, 40 μl ANSA, and 0.9 ml demineralized water. Mix and let stand at room temperature ten minutes.

16. Measure optical density of samples at zero time (O.D.$_o$) and

at thirty minutes (O.D.$_{30}$), standard solutions and blank at 730 nm.

Calculations

1. Obtain difference in O.D. between zero time and thirty minutes incubation in sample and blanks A and B. Subtract O.D. differences of blanks A and B from sample for O.D. change of sample.
2. Plot standard curve of phosphorus concentration versus optical density at 730 nm.
3. Convert O.D. change of sample to mmoles phosphorus/0.1 ml TCA supernatant fluid (P released) directly from standard curve.
4. Multiply mmole P/released by 25×10^6 for mμmole P in 0.1 ml leukocyte homogenate per thirty minutes.
5. Plot standard curve of albumin concentration versus optical density at 750 nm.
6. Measure protein (mg) in 0.1 ml leukocyte homogenate from albumin standard curve.
7. Divide mμmole P in 0.1 ml leukocyte homogenate by 30 for mμmole in 0.1 ml/min. Divide by mg protein in 0.1 ml leukocyte homogenate to obtain activity as mμmole/min/mg protein.

Interpretation

Patients with GSD VI are deficient in liver phosphorylase, some of whom also express the defect in leukocytes. Normal leukocyte phosphorylase levels range from 13 to 55 mμmoles/min/mg protein (published values). Patients with the leukocyte deficiency may have little or no activity; others have up to one-fourth the normal activity (4 mμmoles/min/mg protein).

Reagents

1. *NaCl, 0.2%*: Dissolve 0.2 g in 90 ml demineralized water and dilute to 100 ml volume.
2. *NaCl, 3.6%*: Dissolve 3.6 g in 100 ml demineralized water.

3. *Adenosine Monophosphate (5'-AMP), 0.02M*: Dissolve 7.4 mg in 1.0 ml demineralized water.
4. *NaF, 0.1 M*: Dissolve 0.042 g NaF in 10 ml demineralized water.
5. *Glucose-1-Phosphate (G-1-P), 0.05 M; Glycogen, NaF, 0.05 M Substrate*: Dissolve 0.168 g G-1-P, 5.7 mg glycogen, and 0.021 g NaF in 9 ml demineralized water. Adjust to pH 6.1 with 0.1 M HCl; dilute to 10 ml volume.
6. *Glycogen and NaF, 0.05 M Solution*: Dissolve 5.7 mg glycogen and 0.021 g NaF in 9.0 ml demineralized water. Adjust to pH 6.1 with 0.1 M HCl. Dilute to 10 ml volume.
7. *Trichloroacetic Acid, 0.6 M*: Dissolve 9.8 g TCA in 90 ml demineralized water and dilute to volume in 100 ml volumetric flask.
8. *Alkaline Tartrate Reagent*: Dissolve 2.0 g Na_2CO_3, 50 mg sodium tartrate, and 0.4 g NaOH in 90 ml demineralized water. Dilute to 100 ml volume.
9. *Copper Sulfate, 0.1%*: Dissolve 100 mg $CuSO_3 \cdot 5 H_2O$ in 90 ml demineralized water and dilute to 100 ml volume.
10. *Working Protein Reagent*: Prepare fresh. Combine 18 ml alkaline tartrate reagent and 2 ml copper sulfate.
11. *Albumin Stock Standard Solution, 1 mg/ml.*: Dissolve 100 mg bovine albumin in 90 ml demineralized water and dilute to volume in 100 ml volumetric flask.
12. *Working Albumin Standard Solutions:* Combine the following:

Albumin (mg)	Stock Solution (ml)	Water (ml)
0.1	0.1	0.0
0.08	0.8	0.2
0.06	0.6	0.4
0.04	0.04	0.6

13. *Phenol Reagent, 1 N*: Dilute 2 ml Fisher phenol reagent 2 N with 2 ml demineralized water.
14. *Ammonium Molybdate, 2.5%*: Dissolve 2.5 g in 90 ml demineralized water and dilute to 100 ml volume.
15. *Sulfuric Acid, 5 M*: Add 27.8 ml concentrated H_2SO_4 to 90

ml demineralized water slowly and dilute to volume in 100 ml volumetric flask.

16. *1-Amino-2-Naphthol-Sulfonic Acid:* Prepare fresh. Dissolve (in order): 25 mg 1-amino-2-naphthol sulfonic acid, 1.50 g $NaHSO_3$, and 50 mg Na_2SO_3 in 10 ml demineralized water. Filter, if necessary.

17. *Phosphate Stock Standard Solution (KH$_2$PO$_4$): 0.2 moles in 100 ml:* Dissolve 27.2 mg in 90 ml demineralized water and dilute to volume in 100 ml volumetric flask.

18. *Working Phosphate Standard Solutions:* Combine the following:

Concentration Phosphate (mmoles/100 ml)	Stock Solution (ml)	Water (ml)
0.20	0.1	0.0
0.10	2.0	2.0
0.05	1.0	3.0

REFERENCES

Howell, R. R., Kaback, M. M. and Brown, B. I.: Type IV glycogen storage disease: Branching enzyme deficiency in skin fibroblasts and possible heterozygote detection. *J Pediatrics,78*:638, 1971.

Hsia, David Y. Y., and Inouye, Tohru: *Inborn Errors of Metabolism.* Chicago, Year Book Medical, 1966, p. 178-180.

Huijing, F.: Phosphorylase kinase in leucocytes of normal subjects and of patients with glycogen-storage disease. *Biochem Biophys Acta, 148*:601, 1967.

Hülsmann, W. C., Oei, T. L., and van Creveld, S.: Phosphorylase activity in leucocytes from patients with glycogen-storage disease. *Lancet, 2*:581, 1961.

Williams, H. E., and Field, J. B.: Low leukocyte phosphorylase in hepatic phosphorylase-deficient glycogen storage disease. *J Clin Invest, 40*:1841, 1961.

LESCH-NYHAN SYNDROME

L̲ESCH-NYHAN syndrome is a progressive, neurologic disease of boys, a bizarre feature of which is lip biting to the extent of mutilation. Other neurologic manifestations are choreoathetosis and spasticity. Some patients have seizures; some may be retarded. All are hyperuricemic, the clinical effects of which are gouty arthritis and uric acid stones.

The biochemical error is deficiency of hypoxanthine-guanine phosphoribosyl transferase (HGPRT), an enzyme catalyzing the incorporation of purines into nucleoproteins. The block interrupts the catabolic pathway; as a consequence, purines continue to form, uninhibited by the normal "feed back" mechanism provided by nucleotide precursors. The excessive purines are degraded by an alternative pathway to uric acid.

The disease has X-linked inheritance. Mothers are carriers, if the son's disease is not due to a mutation, and sisters may be. Partial enzyme deficiencies can be demonstrated, in some instances.

Partial HGPRT defects have also been found in adults with gouty arthritis not associated with neurologic signs.

HGPRT defects, complete or partial, are demonstrable in dried blood spots by an isotopic method (p. 248).

LANTHANUM SALT PRECIPITATE METHOD
FOR HYPOXANTHINE-GUANINE PHOSPHORIBOSYL
TRANSFERASE IN DRIED BLOOD SPOTS

Principle

Red cell hypoxanthine-guanine phosphoribosyl transferase is measured as the ^{14}C-labelled lanthanum salt precipitate of inosinic-monophosphate on chromatography paper.

Procedure

1. Place duplicate three-sixteenth-inch Schleicher and Schuell 903 filter paper discs saturated with blood sample into 8 × 100 mm test tubes. Place blank disc in a third tube (blank). Place a fourth disc saturated with the sample in a 10 ml screw-cap tube for hemoglobin estimation later. (step 9)
2. Add 50 μl 0.01 M TRIS buffer, pH 7.4, to all tubes, shake, and incubate in 25°C shaking water bath for thirty minutes.
3. Prepare reaction mixture in 10 × 70-mm cork-stoppered tube in hood.
4. Remove tubes (in rack) from water bath. At thirty-second intervals, add 50 μl reaction mixture to all tubes in hood using Schwarz-Mann Biopipette, mix, and return to 25°C shaking water bath.
5. Exactly thirty minutes later, remove tubes from water bath, one at a time, and, in hood, apply 20 μl reaction mixture to numbered Whatman No. 1 chromatography paper discs (4 cm diameter), impregnated with 0.1 M lanthanum nitrate-0.01 M sodium acetate buffer, pH 5.0.
6. Air-dry discs in hood and rinse quickly with 20 ml aliquots of lanthanum nitrate-sodium acetate buffer in a 150 ml beaker.
7. Immediately place rinsed discs in 150 ml beakers containing 10 ml demineralized water, one for each disc, and let soak five minutes. Repeat five-minute rinse with clean water. Wash discs in sintered glass funnel with 10 ml ethanol and dry with 10 ml acetone.
8. Air-dry discs and attach to planchets with rubber cement. Count ^{14}C in planchet counter.
9. Add 2.5 ml 0.116% ammonium hydroxide (0.5 ml concentrated NH$_4$OH in 125 ml demineralized water) to 10 ml screw-capped tube containing dried blood spot disc for estimation of hemoglobin. Mix (Vortex) and let stand fifteen minutes at room temperature. Mix, decant eluate into cuvettes, and read optical density at 540 nm against blank (0.116% ammonium hydroxide). Multiply O.D.$_{540}$ by the following factors in order to obtain mg Hgb/spot:

$$\frac{O.D._{540} \times 1}{14,800} \times 16,700 \times 2.5$$

or

$$O.D._{540} \times 2.82$$

when 14,800 is molecular extinction coefficient of hemoglobin at 540 nm, 16,700 is the molecular weight of hemoglobin, and 2.5 (ml) is the volume of the hemoglobin eluate measured.

Calculations

1. Calculate average counts per minute for blank and sample discs; subtract blank from sample c.p.m. for net c.p.m./20λ reaction mixture.
2. Multiply by 5 for c.p.m. in 100λ reaction mixture or per dried blood spot.
3. Divide c.p.m./spot by mg Hgb/spot for c.p.m./mg Hgb.

Interpretation

Normal blood contains enzyme activity of from 5000 to 12000 c.p.m./mg Hgb, that from a hemizygous boy contains 228 c.p.m./mg Hgb, and from his mother, 2700 c.p.m./mg Hgb.

Reagents

1. *TRIS Buffer, 0.5 M, pH 7.4*: Dissolve 6.1 g Trizma base in 80 ml demineralized water. Adjust to pH 7.4 with 4 N HCl (34.5 ml concentrated HCl (11.6 N) per 100 ml) and bring to volume in 100 ml volumetric flask.
2. *TRIS Buffer, 0.01 M, pH 7.4*: Combine and mix 0.2 ml TRIS buffer, pH 7.4, and 9.8 ml demineralized water.
3. *Sodium Acetate Buffer, 0.01 M, pH 5.0*: Dissolve 136 mg sodium acetate in 80 ml demineralized water. Adjust to pH 5.0 with 0.1 N acetic acid (0.57 ml glacial acetic acid (17.4 N) per 100 ml) and bring to volume in 100 ml volumetric flask.
4. *Lanthanum Nitrate, 0.1 M,-Sodium Acetate Buffer, 0.01 M Solution, pH 5.0*: Dissolve 4.33 gm lanthanum nitrate in 100

ml 0.01 M sodium acetate buffer, pH 5.0. Adjust to pH 5.0 with solid sodium acetate ($CH_3COONa \cdot 3 H_2O$). Saturate disc of Whatman No. 1 chromatography paper (4 cm diameter) by soaking in lanthanum nitrate-acetate solution for five minutes and air-dry.

5. *Magnesium Chloride, 0.1 M*: Dissolve 203 mg $MgCl_2 \cdot 6 H_2O$ in 10 ml demineralized water.

6. *5-Phosphoribosyl-1-Pyrophosphate (PRPP), 9 mM*: Dissolve 3.9 mg PRPP $\cdot$ 2 H_2O in 1 ml demineralized water or 4.4 mg PRPP $\cdot$ 6 H_2O in 1 ml water.

7. *Hypoxanthine-8-^{14}C, 3.8 mC/mmole, 4.56 mM*: Dilute Schwarz isotope with demineralized water and/or "cold" hypoxanthine according to specific activity, as stated on vial.

REFERENCE

Bakhru-Kishore, Rani, and Kelly, Sally: A rapid method for hypoxanthine-guanine phosphoribosyl transferase in blood. *Clin Chim Acta, 70*:149, 1976.

CHAPTER 10

MUSCULAR DYSTROPHY

DUCHENNE-TYPE muscular dystrophy is a progressive, muscle-wasting disease of boys. Stumbling, awkwardness, and wide stance gait are early clinical signs, usually appearing by the age of seven to eight years. As muscle involvement deepens, the child becomes immobilized and invariably dies by late adolescence.

The basic biochemical defect is unknown. Enzymes normally confined to the muscle cell appear in the serum early in disease, reflecting, perhaps, changes in the permeability of the muscle cell membranes. Of the several enzymes found, lactic dehydrogenase, aldolase, creatine kinase, and pyruvic kinase among them, the kinases are of special value for diagnosis because their presence specifies an enzyme originating chiefly in skeletal muscle, whereas the other enzymes found in serum have various origins. Extremely high levels of creatine kinase, for example, can be found at an early age, even before the clinical signs appear. Concomitantly, the distribution of muscle lactic dehydrogenase isozymes forms a characteristic pattern.

The disease is X-linked. Mothers are carriers, when the son's disease is not caused by a mutation. Sisters, when the mother is an obligate carrier, may or may not be carriers. Carriers sometimes have subclinical disease (muscular fatigue, enlarged calves). In girlhood and adolescence especially, slight excesses of the muscle cell enzymes appear in serum, and the distribution of muscle lactic dehydrogenase isozymes is also slightly abnormal.

Serum creatine kinase and pyruvic kinase activities are measured as described on p. 253 and 255, respectively.

Lactic dehydrogenase isozyme patterns of excised muscle tissue are prepared as described on p. 258.

SERUM CREATINE KINASE

Principle

Creatine kinase in serum is estimated by a spectrophotometric method in which the oxidation of reduced NADH, measured by observing a decrease in optical density at 340 nm, is coupled to the phosphorylation of creatine by a reaction converting pyruvate to lactate.

Procedure

1. Prepare reaction mixture in an 11×75-mm test tube by combining the following: 0.2 ml serum or plasma sample, 1.8 ml saline, (0.85% NaCl), 1.4 ml coenzyme mixture, and 0.1 ml Sigma pyruvate kinase/lactic dehydrogenase suspension. Mix well with a flattened plastic rod and let stand at room temperature fifteen minutes.
2. To 1.0 ml aliquots of reaction mixture in respective cuvettes of 1 cm light path, add 1.0 ml aliquots 0.1 M glycine buffer (blank) or buffer substrate (test cuvette). Mix well with plastic rod.
3. Set blank O.D.$_{340}$ at 0.300. Record O.D.$_{340}$ of test cuvette at zero time as E_1.
4. Exactly ten minutes later, again set blank O.D.$_{340}$ at 0.300 and record O.D.$_{340}$ of test cuvette as E_2.

Calculations

1. Subtract E_2 from E_1 for ΔE_{10}.
2. Simplify the Sigma technical bulletin formula for calculation of activity in Sigma units from

$$\frac{\Delta E_{10} \times \text{Vol liquid} \times 1000 \times \text{Temp Correction Factor (T.C.)}}{\text{Extinction Coefficient}_{340nm} \times \text{Vol sample} \times \text{minutes}}$$

to

$$\frac{\Delta E_{10} \times 2 \times 1000 \times \text{T.C.}}{6.2 \times 0.057 \times 10}$$

or

$$\text{Sigma Units} = \Delta E_{10} \times \text{T.C.} \times 565$$

3. Substitute T.C. from the following table:

Temperature Correction Factors for the Tanzer and Gilvarg Test as Modified in Sigma Bulletin No. 40-UV

Cuv Temperature (°C)	Correction Factor	Cuv Temperature (°C)	Correction Factor
20	1.55	29	0.81
21	1.41	30	0.77
22	1.28	31	0.74
23	1.17	32	0.71
24	1.07	33	0.68
25	1.00	34	0.66
26	0.94	35	0.64
27	0.89	36	0.62
28	0.85	37	0.61

Interpretation

Serum from healthy persons usually contains from 0 to 12 Sigma units. Levels in early or preclinical Duchenne type muscular dystrophy sometimes reach 600 Sigma units or more. Carrier levels are only slightly higher than normal.

Levels in less severe forms of primary muscle disease may be elevated but less so than in the early stages of Duchenne muscular dystrophy. Levels in polymyositis are initially high but fall in response to treatment.

Reagents

1. *Glycine Buffer Stock Solution, 2M, pH 9.0*: Dissolve 37.5 g glycine and 13.05 g $Na_2CO_3 \cdot H_2O$ in demineralized water, adjust to pH 9.0 with 0.1 N NaOH or 0.1 N HCl, and bring to volume in 250 ml volumetric flask. Distribute in large screw-cap tubes (20 ml) in 10 ml amounts. Autoclave twenty minutes at 15 lbs and store at 4°C.
2. *Glycine Buffer, 0.1 M, pH 9.0*: Dilute 2.5 ml 2 M glycine buffer stock solution and bring to volume in 50 ml volumetric flask.

3. *Standard Enzyme, 45 to 60 Sigma Units*: Combine 3.3 mg rabbit muscle creatine phosphokinase (CPK) and 1.0 ml pooled human serum. Shake well to disperse. Add 0.1 ml suspension to 99.9 ml pooled human serum and mix well. Dispense as 0.2 ml aliquots in 11 × 75-mm tubes with rubber stoppers. Freeze in CO_2-ethanol bath and store at -20°C.
4. *Coenzyme Mixture*: To separate aliquots of cold 2 M glycine buffer stock solution, pH 9, add the following reagents and bring to 10 ml volumes with buffer: 11.4 mg Sigma DPNH-Na_2 (one vial dry Sigma reagent reconstituted with 3.3 ml demineralized water and stored at -20°C); 0.91 ml Sigma ATP-glutathione reagent, reconstituted; 10.0 mg phospno(enol)pyruvate; and 26.6 mg $MgSO_4 \cdot 7 H_2O$.
5. *Buffer/Substrate Solution*: Dissolve 43.8 mg anhydrous creatine in 5 ml 0.1 M glycine buffer, pH 9.0: Heat in 40 to 50°C water bath until dissolved. Use larger proportions if necessary.

REFERENCES

The Ultraviolet Determination of Creatine Phosphokinase (CPK) in Serum, or Other Fluids at 340 mμ. Sigma Tentative Technical Bulletin No. 40-UV. St. Louis, Mo., Sigma Chemical Co., 1965.

Tanzer, M. L., and Gilvarg, C.: Creatine and creatine kinase measurement. *J Biol Chem, 234*:3201, 1959.

SERUM PYRUVATE KINASE

Principle

Pyruvate kinase activity in serum is estimated by a spectrophotometric method in which NADH oxidation, measured by decreasing optical density at 340 nm, is coupled to dephosphorylation of phosphoenolpyruvate (PEP) through the conversion of pyruvate to lactate.

Procedure

1. Warm fresh or thawed serum samples and control serum at 25°C for thirty minutes. Samples should not be hemolyzed, to

avoid contamination by red cell pyruvate kinase.
2. Add 2.6 ml reaction mixture to three cuvettes per sample or control; add 0.3 ml sample to cuvette No. 2, 0.1 ml to cuvette No. 3. Bring to equal volumes by adding 0.3 ml demineralized water to cuvette 1 (blank) and 0.2 ml to cuvette No. 3.
3. Start reaction by adding 0.1 ml of 0.06 M phosphoenolpyruvic acid to each cuvette, mix by inversion, and let stand at 23°C for three minutes.
4. Set blank $O.D._{340}$ at 0.500. Record $O.D._{340}$ of cuvettes No. 2 and No. 3 at zero time. Record O.D. of all cuvettes exactly ten minutes later.
5. If ten-minute reading is off scale, repeat incubation with 0.05 ml serum and adjust final volume with water.

Calculations

1. Subtract ten-minute reading of blank from O.D. 0.500 for $\Delta O.D._{10}$ of blank.
2. Subtract the ten-minute readings of cuvettes 2 and 3 from respective zero time O.D. for $\Delta O.D._{10}$ of test cuvettes.
3. Subtract $\Delta O.D._{blank}$ from $\Delta O.D._{test}$ for $\Delta O.D._{10}$ of pyruvate kinase activity (PK).
4. Express PK activity in $\mu moles/ml/hr$ at 23°C from the following formula:

$$\frac{\Delta O.D._{10}\ PK \times 60 \times 0.1 \times 0.3}{10 \times 0.622 \times ml\ serum}$$

or

$$\Delta O.D._{10}PK \times 9.65 \text{ for cuvette 2}$$

or

$$\Delta O.D._{10}PK \times 28.95 \text{ for cuvette 3}$$

Interpretation

Serum PK levels in boys with Duchenne type muscular dystrophy are about twenty times those of normal children. Levels in adult carriers are about twice normal.

Levels of questionable significance should be related to controls of the same age, as there is a slight decline in activity during childhood, from a high of 6 μM/ml/hr in children four-years-old and younger to adult levels, after age fourteen, of no more than 3 μM/ml/hr.

All levels are slightly higher when the volume of serum is 0.1 ml.

Reagents

1. *Triethanolamine-HCl Buffer, 0.05 M, pH 7.5:* At the time of test, dissolve 0.93 g triethanolamine hydrochloride in 80 ml demineralized water. Adjust to pH 7.5 with NaOH and bring to volume in 100 ml volumetric flask.
2. *Potassium Chloride, 2.25 M:* Dissolve 8.4 g KCl in 50 ml demineralized water. Store frozen in 5 ml aliquots.
3. *Magnesium Sulfate, 0.24 M:* Dissolve 2.95 g MgSO$_4$ · 7 H$_2$O in 50 ml demineralized water. Store frozen in 5 ml aliquots.
4. *Adenosine Diphosphate (ADP), 0.024 M:* At the time of test, disperse 120 mg ADP · 2 Na · 1.5 H$_2$O in 10 ml demineralized water.
5. *Lactic Dehydrogenase (LDH) (18 U/0.1 ml:* At the time of test, dilute commercial LDH suspension to give 0.5 ml (Sigma Lot 48B-4090; 400 U/0.1 ml).
6. *NADH, reduced, (1.4 μmoles/ml):* At the time of test, dissolve 19.8 mg NADH in 18 ml demineralized water.
7. *Reaction Mixture (Fifteen samples):* Combine the following:

Reagent	Volume (ml)
0.05 M Triethanolamine-HCl Buffer	22.5
2.25 M KCl	4.5
0.24 M Mg SO$_4$·7 H$_2$O	4.5
0.024 M ADP	9.0
LDH (18 U/0.1 ml	4.5
1.4 mM NADH	18
Demineralized water	54
Total:	117

8. *Phosphoenolpyruvic Acid, 0.06 M:* On the day of test, dissolve 118.2 mg phospho (enol) pyruvate · 3 Na · 5 H$_2$O in 6 ml de-

mineralized water.

REFERENCES

Alberto, M. C., and Samaha, F. J.: Serum pyruvate kinase in muscle disease and carrier states. *Neurology, 24*:462, 1974.

Valentine, W. N., and Tanaka, K. R.: Pyruvate kinase: Clinical aspects. *Methods Enzymol, 9*:468, 1966.

LACTIC DEHYDROGENASE ISOZYMES IN GASTROCNEMIUS

Principle

The lactic dehydrogenase isozymes in muscle from boys with Duchenne-type muscular dystrophy are different from those of normal muscle, as demonstrated by electrophoresis. The enzyme proteins in homogenates move at different rates, according to their structure and electric charge, and appear as multiple bands after incubation with substrate and staining with indicator dye.

Procedure

1. On the day of test, homogenize 300 mg wet weight fresh or frozen gastrocnemius muscle in 1 ml demineralized water in a tissue grinder, and centrifuge at 3000 R.P.M. for twenty minutes. Draw off supernatant fluid for electrophoresis.
2. Apply supernatant fluid of homogenate to cellulose acetate membrane according to method for electrophoretic instrument, and, if using Beckman microzone chamber, apply 150 V for forty minutes through TRIS-HCl-barbit..i buffer.
3. Cut off both ends of the membrane, eliminating holes; lay membrane over reagent gel, rolling it on gently from left to right, forcing air bubbles out ahead. Do not move membrane once laid on gel. Incubate thirty minutes at 37° C or until color development is complete.
4. Rinse membrane under cold water to remove fragments of adhering gel and dip in 10% acetic acid three or four times over a five-minute period.
5. Examine and scan on densitometer. If microzone is used, set

slit width and length at 0.4 cal.
6. Calculate amount of each band and express in percent of total.

Interpretation

The lactic dehydrogenase protein normally separates into five bands. The most anodal are isozymes 1, 2, and 3, in decreasing order. Isozymes 4 and 5 remain close to the origin and are present in greatest amounts. The pattern of isozymes from affected muscles in Duchenne-type muscular dystrophy, especially gastrocnemius, differs in the proportions of the components: Isozymes 4 and 5 are reduced, particularly LDH_5, and isozymes 1, 2, and 3 are relatively increased, as indicated in Table XIII.

Table XIII

DISTRIBUTION OF LACTIC DEHYDROGENASE ISOZYMES
IN NORMAL AND DYSTROPHIC GASTROCNEMIUS*

Muscle	Percent of LDH Isozymes				
	1	*2*	*3*	*4*	*5*
Normal	4.6	7.1	11.7	18.7	58.0
Muscular Dystrophy	9.3	25.5	45.0	16.6	3.6

*Adapted from Lauryssens and Lauryssens (1964)

The pattern in affected muscle from carriers is only slightly different from the normal: The LDH_5 fraction is slightly less and the anodal forms, slightly greater.

Reagents

1. *TRIS-HCl Buffer, 0.2 M, pH 8.3*: When using Beckman Microzone®, dissolve 24.2 g Trizma base in 700 ml demineralized water. Adjust to pH 8.3 with concentrated HCl and bring to volume in 1-liter volumetric flask.
2. *TRIS-HCl-Barbital Buffer, pH 8.4*: Dissolve one package

Beckman B-2 barbital buffer in 1 liter demineralized water. Mix with equal parts of TRIS-HCl buffer. Refrigerate.

3. *Reaction Gel*: For 100 ml gel or 3 150 × 25-mm plastic petri dishes, dissolve 1 g DIFCO Noble agar by heating in 70 ml TRIS-HCl buffer, pH 8.3, cool to 75°C. Add the following, in the order given: 2 ml lactic acid solution (60 mg% syrup), 20 ml nitrobluetetrazolium (NBT) solution (1 mg/ml), 2 ml phenazine methosulfate (1 mg/ml), and 100 mg NAD in 6 ml water. Swirl to mix and dissolve. Pour plates and store in the dark for up to four hours.

REFERENCES

Beckman ® *Methods Manual* RM-TB-010, Spinco Division of Beckman Instruments, Inc., Stanford Industrial Park, Palo Alto, California, August, 1967.

Emery, A. E., Sherbourne, D. H., and Pusch, A.: Electrophoretic pattern of muscle LDH in various diseases. *Arch Neurol, 12*:251, 1965.

Emery, A. E.: Electrophoretic pattern of LDH in carriers and patients with Duchenne muscular dystrophy. *Nature, 201*:1044, 1964.

Lauryssens, M. G., and Lauryssens, M. J.: Electrophoretic distribution pattern of LDH in mouse and human muscular dystrophy. *Clin Chim Acta, 9*:276, 1964.

CHAPTER 11

WILSON'S DISEASE

THE triad of ataxia, liver disease, and psychotic episodes is indicative of Wilson's disease, and any one of the findings is suggestive. Choreoathetoid movements are common. A Kayser-Fleischer ring around the iris is pathognomonic but may be difficult to see without examining with a slit lamp.

The exact biochemical defect is not known. Most but not all patients are deficient in the copper-carrying serum oxidase, ceruloplasmin. The deficiency, furthermore, may not be apparent until after six months of age because the ceruloplasmin level in early infancy is normally low. Copper accumulates in tissues like liver, kidney, iris, and basal ganglia, and interferes with their normal functions. The use of chelating agents, e.g. penicillamine, is prophylactic in preclinical cases and therapeutic in those of long standing.

The disease follows an autosomal recessive pattern of inheritance. In some families the carriers can be identified by partial deficiencies in serum ceruloplasmin.

Ceruloplasmin levels in serum are measured by colorimetric methods for enzyme activity (p. 261 & 264) or an immunologic method for antigenic activity (radial diffusion).

SERUM CERULOPLASMIN

Principle

The copper oxidase, ceruloplasmin, is the chief oxidase of serum which oxidizes p-phenylenediamine (PPD) from the colorless, reduced form to the lavender, semiquinone form. The amount of semiquinone formed is measured by absorption at 525 nm.

Procedure

1. Warm acetate buffer and 0.5% PPD stock solution in 25°C

    water bath fifteen minutes.
2. To respective 1.2 × 12.5-cm cuvettes, add 0.1 ml aliquots sample, control, and standard serum in triplicate. Combine with 2 ml aliquots 0.1 M acetate buffer. Add (by bulb pipette) 1 ml 0.1% sodium azide to one of each triplicate set (sample, control, and standard blanks). Remaining tubes are sample, control, and standard test sera (in duplicate).
3. Mix blanks by swirling and add 1.0 ml 0.5% PPD stock solution to all tubes.
4. Mix by swirling and immerse tubes in 37°C water bath in the dark for one hour.
5. Remove from bath and immediately add 1.0 ml sodium azide (by bulb pipette) to sample, standard, and control test sera to stop reactions. Mix by swirling.
6. Add 6.0 ml 3.0% sodium chloride solution to all tubes. Mix.
7. Record optical density at 530 nm or Klett filter No. 54 (520 to 580 nm), setting zero O.D. with respective blanks.

Calculations

1. Estimate ceruloplasmin concentrations in sample and control test sera in mg per 100 ml as

$$\text{mg}/100 \text{ ml} = \text{O.D.}_{530} \times \frac{\text{concentrated standard serum (mg\%)}}{\text{O.D.}_{530} \text{ standard serum}}$$

Interpretation

    Normal serum contains from 18 to 40 mg ceruloplasmin per ml; serum from homozygous persons has little or none, and that from carriers contains half normal or normal amounts.

Reagents

1. *Acetic Acid, 0.1 N*: Add 0.57 ml glacial acetic acid to 90 ml demineralized water in 100 ml volumetric flask. Mix and dilute to mark with demineralized water.

2. *Acetate Buffer, 0.1 M, pH 6.0*: Dissolve 2.72 g sodium acetate · 3 H$_2$O in 150 ml demineralized water in 300-ml flask or beaker. Add 10 ml 0.1 N acetic acid and mix. Adjust to pH 6, adding in drops 0.1 N acetic acid or 0.1 N NaOH (0.4 g/100 ml), with mixing. Transfer solution and rinses to 200 ml volumetric flask and dilute to mark with demineralized water. Store at 4°C.

3. *p-Phenylenediamine, Recrystallized: CAUTION: AVOID CONTACT.* Recrystallize p-phenylenediamine dye, if the crystals are brown or purple, as follows: In a hood, dissolve 10 g PPD in 10 ml acetone in 50 ml Erlenmeyer flask. Add concentrated hydrochloric acid until no further precipitate forms. Collect precipitate on Whatman No. 40 filter paper and wash with dry acetone. Dry for a week and store in tightly capped brown bottle over anhydrous CaCl$_2$.

4. *PPD Stock Solution, 0.5%*: Dissolve 50 mg recrystallized p-phenylenediamine in 9 ml 0.1 N acetate buffer in screw-capped tube. Adjust to pH 6.0 with 1 N NaOH (approximately 0.4 ml), using narrow range pH paper. Can be stored at 4°C and used within a week.

5. *Sodium Azide Solution, 0.1%*: Dissolve 0.1 gm sodium azide in approximately 50 ml demineralized water in 250 ml Erlenmeyer flask and mix by swirling gently. Transfer solution and rinse carefully (do not pipette by mouth) to 100 ml volumetric flask, and dilute to mark with demineralized water.

6. *Sodium Chloride Solution, 3.0%*: Dissolve 3.0 gm sodium chloride in 100 ml demineralized water.

7. *Standard Serum*: Pool human serum and determine ceruloplasmin concentration by Boehringer radial diffusion assay with commercial antigen. Distribute in 0.5 ml amounts in 10 × 75-mm tubes and store at -20°C. Concentration in new batch of standard serum can be determined by secondary standardization against previous standard serum.

8. *Control Serum*: Pooled rabbit serum, distributed in 1 ml aliquots and frozen at -20°C.

REFERENCES

Ravin, H. A.: Rapid test for hepatolenticular degeneration. *Lancet*, 1:726, 1956.

Henry, R. J., Chiamori, N., Jacobs, S. L., and Segalove, M.: Determination of ceruloplasmin oxidase in serum. *Proc Soc Exp Biol Med, 104*:620, 1960.

CERULOPLASMIN SPOT TEST

Principle

Ceruloplasmin deficiency can be detected in serum or plasma samples when spotted on filter paper discs saturated with PPD.

Procedure

1. Overlay respective PPD filter paper discs in the depressions of Linbro Disposo Tray FB48 with 2 drop aliquots of the sample and control sera. Add 1 drop acetate buffer, pH 6.0.
2. Cover and float tray in 37°C water bath for exactly fifteen minutes.
3. Place tray on white background, remove cover, and observe color of discs.

Interpretation

Normal serum, which contains ceruloplasmin, oxidizes PPD, turning the discs blue. Ceruloplasmin-deficient serum usually fails to oxidize the dye, and disc color remains unchanged.

Reagents

1. *Sample and Control Sera*: Collect capillary or venous blood from patient (sample) and healthy person (control) in heparinized microcapillary tubes. Centrifuge. Break tubes at plasma-red cell interface and discard red cell layers.
2. *Sodium Acetate Buffer, 0.5 M, pH 6.0*: As described in "Serum Ceruloplasmin Assay" (p. 261), using 13.60 g sodium acetate · 3 H_2O and 5 ml 1.0 N acetic acid.
3. *PPD stock solution, 0.5%*: As described in "Serum Ceruloplasmin Assay," (p. 261).
4. *PPD filter paper discs: AVOID CONTACT.* Immerse

Whatman No. 3 filter paper strips, 2 × 6-inches, briefly in PPD solution in shallow glass dish. Blot excess. Dry in dessicator in dark at 4°C in nitrogen. Punch approximately 300 discs with 3/16-inch punch from strip and store in dessicant-containing tubes in dark at room temperature in nitrogen. Use discs only while they remain white or pale pink.

REFERENCE

Aisen, P., Schorr, J. B., Morell, A. G., Gold, R. Z., and Scheinberg, I. H.: A rapid screening test for deficiency of plasma ceruloplasmin and its value in the diagnosis of Wilson's disease. *Am J Med, 28*:550, 1960.

DRUG-INDUCED APNEA
(SUXAMETHONIUM-SENSITIVITY)

CERTAIN patients receiving the muscle re-
laxant, suxamethonium, during anesthesia or shock therapy become apneic from prolonged paralysis of respiratory muscles.

The potential for apnea exists in persons with a defect in choline ester-splitting enzyme. Pseudocholinesterase, the serum enzyme comparable to cholinesterase, the motor end-plate enzyme,
may be deficient or replaced by an atypical, less efficient variant.

The condition has an autosomal recessive pattern of inheritance. Carriers may be heterozygous for the pseudocholinesterase
gene or the gene for variant enzyme. They have half-normal levels
of their respective enzymes, or mixtures of them, and may display
some sensitivity to the drug. Close relatives of affected persons
should be screened for the defect in order to be identified as
suxamethonium-sensitive, in the event they may be given muscle-
relaxing agents in the future.

The enzyme defect is detected by measuring the amount of
pseudocholinesterase present or the activity in relation to that of
atypical variants, as described on p. 266.

PSEUDOCHOLINESTERASE AND VARIANTS

Principle

Pseudocholinesterase, the serum enzyme with the choline ester-
splitting properties of the motor end-plate enzyme, cholinesterase,
can be distinguished from variant, less efficient forms by greater
inhibition by a specific inhibitor, dimethyl carbamate of (2-
hydroxy-5-phenylbenzyl)-trimethyl-ammonium bromide.

The specific inhibitor prevents the hydrolysis of α-naphthyl
acetate by pseudocholinesterase but does not prevent the hydrolysis by variants. Partial hydrolysis proceeds when both nor-

mal and atypical enzymes are present, as in persons heterozygous for either form.

The extent of hydrolysis by either or both forms of enzyme is indicated by the intensity of purple color formed, as freed α-naphthol couples with the diazonium salt, 5-chloro-o-toluidine.

Procedure

1. Dilute serum or plasma (fresh or frozen) one hundred fold with phosphate buffer. (Serum or plasma enzyme is stable several months at -20°C).
2. To 0.5 ml aliquots diluted sample in two tubes, add 0.5 ml aliquot buffer to one (T) and specific inhibitor to the other (T_{In}). Add buffer and inhibitor to a third tube (blank).
3. Add 3.5 ml α-naphthyl acetate substrate to the three tubes, mix and incubate one hour at 37°C.
4. Add 0.5 ml Fast Red TR-Duponal solution, mix, and let stand fifteen minutes. If no color forms in Tube T, repeat procedure with fifty fold dilution of plasma. If blank forms as much color as tube T_{In}, prepare fresh stock substrate and repeat test.
5. Measure optical density at 555 mμ, using blank to zero instrument.
6. Estimate percent inhibition as

$$\frac{\text{O.D. (T) - O.D. (}T_{In}) \times 100}{\text{O.D. (T)}}$$

Interpretation

Hydrolysis by pseudocholinesterase is inhibited 82 to 96% in the presence of specific inhibitor and 43 to 65%, if the sample contains a mixture of normal and atypical enzyme, as in heterozygous persons. Hydrolysis is inhibited slightly, from 9 to 30%, if the sample lacks pseudocholinesterase or contains only variant enzyme, as in persons homozygous for the variant gene. (See Color Illustration 12.)

Avoid hemolysis, as red cell esterases are not inhibited by the specific inhibitor, and hemolyzed samples will give a reaction similar to that for atypical enzyme.

Reagents

1. *Sodium Phosphate Buffer, 0.2 M, pH 7.1*: Dissolve 5.68 g Na_2HPO_4 in demineralized water and bring to volume in 200 ml volumetric flask; dissolve 2.76 g $NaHPO_4$ in demineralized water and bring to volume in 100 ml volumetric flask. Combine 134 ml and 66 ml of the respective solutions and adjust to pH 7.1 with 1 N HCl or 1 N NaOH, if necessary.
2. *Inhibitor: Dimethylcarbamate of (2-hydroxy-5-phenylbenzyl) Trimethylammonium Bromide, 10^{-6}M)*: On the day of test dissolve 4 mg inhibitor (Hoffman-LaRoche) in sodium phosphate buffer, pH 7.1, and bring to volume with buffer in 100 ml volumetric flask (10^{-4}M); dilute one hundred fold with buffer.
3. *α-Naphthyl Acetate Stock Substrate, 0.03 M, in 50% Acetone*: Dissolve 0.2793 g substrate in solution of 50% acetone and bring to volume with 50% acetone in 50 ml volumetric flask. Stable one month at 4°C.
4. *α-Naphthyl Acetate Working Substrate, 0.0003 M*: Immediately before use, dilute 1 ml stock substrate with 20 ml sodium phosphate buffer, 0.2 M, pH 7.1, and bring to volume with demineralized water in 100 ml volumetric flask.
5. *Duponal (Sodium Lauryl Sulfate), 3%*: Dissolve 3 g Duponal in 100 ml of demineralized water.
6. *Fast Red TR Color Reagent*: On the day of test, dissolve 50 mg Fast Red TR salt in 15 ml demineralized water and 10 ml 3% Duponal.

REFERENCE

Morrow, A. C., and Motulsky, A. G.: Screening for atypical pseudo-cholinesterase. *J Lab Clin Med, 71*:350, 1968.

CHAPTER 13

CHILDHOOD CIRRHOSIS AND
EARLY-ONSET FAMILIAL EMPHYSEMA

INFANTS with cirrhosis and adults with early-onset emphysema may have the same biochemical abnormality — familial deficiency of serum alpha-1-antitrypsin. In a few instances, the two diseases have appeared in the same family and, in a rare patient, the emphysema is accompanied by liver damage.

The relationship of the serum defect to the clinical signs is not clear. The deficiency apparently reflects a change in the molecular form or function of the enzyme, confining it to the parent organ (liver), unused. In consequence, the proteases, which alpha-1-antitrypsin normally inhibits, act unchecked, destroying parenchymatous tissue and, indirectly, aging the affected organs prematurely.

The diseases are autosomal recessive. Homozygous persons have abnormally low levels of alpha-1-antitrypsin; carriers may be detected by demonstrating half-normal levels. Screening both healthy and affected families is helpful in locating carriers; even they may be at risk for developing obstructive lung disease from various factors, including smoking, exposure to air pollution or frequent untreated respiratory infections.

Alpha-1-antitrypsin deficiency in serum is detected by noting the absence of the alpha-1-globulin fraction in serum protein electrophoretograms or can be measured by radial diffusion (p. 269). Allelic forms are distinguishable by a combination of acid starch gel electrophoresis and agarose gel immunoelectrophoresis.

ALPHA-1-ANTITRYPSIN DEFICIENCY BY RADIAL DIFFUSION

Principle

Alpha-1-antitrypsin, a serum enzyme with antigenic properties, forms precipitin zones by radial diffusion through gels containing specific antiserum. The precipitin zone is directly proportional to the antigen concentration.

Procedure

1. As indicated in instructions with the Miles Laboratory's kit for α trypsin inhibitor (KATI), measure 5λ aliquots of serum samples onto plate in rows A and C and 5λ aliquots of standards in row B, using a Hamilton microliter syringe.
2. With Pasteur pipette, add a few drops of water to moisture trough.
3. Incubate plate eighteen hours at room temperature.
4. Measure diameter of precipitin rings, using Miles' viewer/ magnifier or hand lens.
5. Plot curve of diameters versus concentration of standards on semilogarithmic paper supplied with Miles kit.
6. Obtain concentration of alpha-1-antitrypsin in serum sample from standard curve.
7. If concentration in sample is higher than that of highest standard, dilute serum 1:2 with saline and repeat test.

Interpretation

The serum of normal persons contains from 180 to 340 mg per 100 ml alpha-1-antitrypsin, serum from heterozygotes contains 100 to 180 mg per 100 ml, and serum from homozygotes has less than 100 mg per 100 ml. Acute inflammation or necrosis, estrogen therapy, and pregnancy raise normal levels; severe chronic liver disease lowers them.

REFERENCE

Lieberman, J.: A new "double ring" screening test for α_1-antitrypsin variants. *Am Rev Respir Dis, 108*:248, 1973.

IMMUNODEFICIENCY DISEASES

HUMORAL IMMUNITY DEFECTS

R ECURRING severe, pyogenic infections are the clue to complete deficiencies of the immunoglobulins. One form of the deficiency is X-linked, affecting only the boys in a family (Bruton's agammaglobulinemia). Survivors may develop mesenchymal diseases (arthritis, vasculitis, dermatomyositis), lymphomas, or chronic respiratory disease, ending in respiratory failure despite regular treatment with high doses of gamma globulin to prevent infections.

Another form affects both sexes, is transient, and corrects itself by the age of two years (transient hypogammaglobulinemia of infancy).

Isolated deficiencies of the immunoglobulins may occur in healthy persons (immunoglobulin A) or in association with gastrointestinal infections or mesenchymal diseases (immunoglobulin A) or sino-pulmonary infections (immunoglobulin E or E and A combined).

These serum defects reflect overall impairment of the humoral immune response. The progenitor organs and tissues, e.g. Peyer's patches, tonsils, plasma cells, and other lymphoid tissue are absent or, at best, structurally abnormal, and hence fail to produce antibody in response to normal antigenic stimuli.

Immunoglobulin defects are detected by radial diffusion assays of serum antigen through commerically prepared immunodiffusion gels, as indicated on p. 271.

IMMUNOGLOBULIN A DEFICIENCY
BY RADIAL DIFFUSION

Principle

Deficiency of immunoglobulin A in the serum is detected by

271

measuring precipitin zones formed by radial diffusion of antigen in the sample through gels containing specific antiserum. The precipitin zone is directly proportional to the antigen concentration.

Procedure

1. As indicated in instructions accompanying Meloy immunodiffusion plate, fill wells in gel with serum samples in duplicate and three standards, using capillary pipettes supplied with kit.
2. Incubate plates eighteen to twenty-two hours at room temperature.
3. Measure diameter of precipitin rings against a dark background, using a Bausch and Lomb measuring magnifier.
4. Plot curve of diameters versus concentration of standards on semilogarithmic paper.
5. Obtain IgA concentrations of samples from standard curve in mg/100 ml.
6. If concentrations in samples are below those of standards, repeat assay with plates containing less antibody (Meloy low-level IgA radial immunodiffusion plates), using standards accompanying the low level plates.

Interpretation

Normal IgA levels are age-related, rising gradually from lows of 100 mg/100 ml or less at six months, to over 300 mg/100 ml as adults. Within the age groups there is a considerable range between lowest and highest concentrations expected, and test sample values should always be compared with the laboratory's own or published (Stiehm and Fudenberg, 1966) data.

IgA levels in the patient with ataxia telangiectasia and agammaglobulinemia will be well below the lowest value in the normal range for the age. The serum of some healthy persons may also contain little or no IgA.

REFERENCE

Stiehm, E. R., and Fudenberg, H. H.: Serum levels of immune globulins in health and disease: A survey. *Pediatrics, 37*:715, 1966.

CELLULAR AND COMBINED IMMUNITY DEFECTS

Repeated viral and mycotic infections, impaired delayed hypersensitivity reactions (negative tuberculin and other skin test responses in infected persons, for example, and progressive vaccinia, miliary T.B., or giant cell pneumonia after exposure to the respective infectious agents), and impaired allograft rejection are some of the clinical signs associated with deficiencies in cellular, i.e. thymus-mediated, immunity mechanisms. The deficiencies may be total or partial and may be isolated or combined with defects in humoral immune mechanisms.

The kind and intensity of the immune defect affect the severity of clinical signs. Infants with a total deficiency of cellular immunity mechanisms, for example, as in agenesis of the III and IVth pharyngeal pouches (from which the thymus, parathyroid, and part of the thyroid gland develop), do not survive. Newborns are hypocalcemic, develop tetany, and succumb to repeated bouts of mycotic, viral, or chronic bacterial infections (DiGeorge's syndrome), despite the intactness of the humoral immune system.

Most of the defects in cellular immunity, however, occur in combination with defects in humoral immunity. In lymphopenic (Swiss-type) agammaglobulinemia, for example, an extreme form of a combined immunodeficiency disease, neither cellular nor humoral immune mechanisms develop normally. The respective progenitor organs are absent or hypoplastic, and infants homozygous for the recessively inherited disease usually die from infections during the first year.

Thymic alymphoplasia, an X-linked recessive condition, is similar but less severe. Affected boys have severe, recurring infections as infants and usually die from viral or mycotic infections by seven years of age. Bone marrow transplants from sibling donors, however, have recently improved the prognosis.

Infants with Wiskott-Aldrich syndrome, another X-linked recessive condition of combined deficits, have severe, recurring infections, thrombocytopenic purpura, and eczema. Later they become lymphopenic and express greater deficits in cellular immunity. They respond normally to some antigens, variably to protein, and poorly or not at all to polysaccharide antigens. The affected boys die as children or in early adolescence, usually from infections, hemorrhagic events, or neoplastic disease (reticulum cell sarcoma and lymphosarcoma). Their prognosis has improved recently, however, by the partial replacement of the deficits by bone marrow transplants.

Late-occurring dysgammaglobulinemias consist of immunoglobulin and cellular immunity deficiencies of varying degrees and present from infancy through adulthood. The clinical signs reflect both kinds of defects, e.g. recurrent severe pyogenic infections and impaired development of delayed hypersensitivity, respectively. Lymphomas and mesenchymal diseases develop later. Infections or malignancies are the usual cause of death.

Ataxia telangiectasia, an autosomal recessive disease appearing in young children, consists of progressive ataxia, telangiectasia on sclera, earlobes, and skin, and impaired immunologic responses. Survivors beyond childhood may be sexually immature and at high risk for lymphoreticular neoplasms. Both cellular and humoral immunity mechanisms are impaired, e.g. abnormal delayed hypersensitivity reactions and prolonged survival of skin homografts, decreased serum, and salivary immunoglobulin A, and serum immunoglobulin E, accompanied by recurring infections. The thymus is usually hypoplastic, the lymphocyte complement of thymus-dependent lymph organs is low and lymphopenia is common. The relationships among the immunologic defects, vascular proliferation, and neurologic signs, however, are not clear.

The deficits in cellular immunity described above are identified in the laboratory by discovering profound lymphopenia and observing absence or depletion of thymus-dependent lymphoid tissue. The deficits in humoral immunity are detected by demonstrating immunoglobulin deficiencies (p. 271). The combined deficits are found by uncovering defective components of both systems.

Hereditary Angioneurotic Edema

Hereditary angioneurotic edema, a dominantly inherited trait, presents with clinical signs reflecting yet another type of immuno-logic defect. Patients have spontaneous, recurring attacks of lo-calized edema or abdominal pain which are self-limiting. Some crises, however, are life-threatening, e.g. edema of the larynx, and must be terminated quickly with adrenalin. The defect lies in the absence of the complement system inactivator, C^1 esterase in-hibitor. The episodes are thought to be responses to the activated complement system.

The major diagnostic laboratory criterion is demonstration of a deficiency of C^1 esterase inhibitor in serum.

THE FAMILIAL
HYPERLIPOPROTEINEMIAS

$\mathbf{X}$ANTHOMAS, abdominal distress, and ather-osclerotic manifestations early in life are common presenting signs of the hereditary hyperlipoproteinemias. Infants are affected by Type I, children and adolescents by Type II, and young adults by Types III, IV, and V. While age of onset is important in the clinical diagnosis, data pertaining to kinds and amounts of plasma lipids in excess are necessary for the final diagnosis.

Plasma lipids are for the most part bound to proteins, forming a series of lipoproteins, the properties of which relate to the proportions of the component lipids, e.g. cholesterol, triglyceride, and phospholipids. The particular kinds of hyperlipidemia, therefore, can be identified by the particular lipoprotein in excess. In Type I disease, for example, chylomicrons appear, the chief lipid of which is dietary triglyceride. The triglycerides remain in the circulation of Type I patients longer than in the healthy person since they lack the triglyceride-splitting enzyme, lipoprotein lipase, normally released from the blood vessel walls by heparin. In Types II, III, and IV hyperlipoproteinemia, the excesses appear in the β- and pre β- fractions. These lipoproteins are synthesized in the liver and stored in adipose tissue, the defective metabolism of which pertains chiefly to endogenous mechanisms. In Type V disease, on the other hand, both chylomicrons and β- fractions are excessive, indicating both exogenous and endogenous sites of metabolic error.

The primary hyperlipoproteinemias are familial. Some have clear-cut patterns of inheritance. Type I and the other hyperlipoproteinemias have autosomal recessive patterns of inheritance. Some (II, III, and IV) also have autosomal dominant forms.

Certain dietary factors and drugs, e.g. alcohol, estrogens, and steroids, may precipitate hyperlipoproteinemia in the genetically disposed patient.

276

The plasma lipoprotein fractions are separated and the characteristic patterns identified by agarose gel electrophoresis (p. 277). Triglyceride and cholesterol levels are needed for accurate interpretation.

SERUM LIPOPROTEIN ELECTROPHORESIS ON BIO-GRAM ® PRECAST AGAROSE SLIDES

Principle

The serum lipoproteins separate into chylomicron, beta, prebeta, and alpha fractions during electrophoresis on precast agarose gel slides. The patterns, in conjunction with the concentrations of serum cholesterol and triglyceride, form the basis of the Frederickson and Lees (1965) method for the classification of the familial hyperlipoproteinemias.

Procedure

1. Remove Bio-Gram precast agarose slide (three samples/slide) carefully from sealed slide package; do not touch agarose surface.
2. Stand slide on paper toweling (with letters at top of slide) and let dry fifteen minutes. (DO NOT OVERDRY.)
3. Place Beckman ® paper wicks in Durrum cell and fill with electrophoresis buffer. Complete contact from wicks to slides with smaller wicks.
4. Add fresh serum samples from fasting patients to respective Bio-Gram A sample cups with Pasteur pipette (DO NOT BLOW OUT), keeping slides, applicator, and sample cup in respective lettered order. Serum sample may be kept at 4°C overnight before testing. Do not freeze. Use Bio Gram tracking dye in one cup.
5. Fill sample applicator from sample cups using the white Bio-Gram A applicator guide. Push sample cups to back of applicator guide with dry slide, thus lining up slide with applicator tips.
6. Apply samples to slide by depressing applicator gently into gels and holding there three seconds.

7. Place slides *face down* on wicks in Durrum cell so that letters on slide are at the cathode (-) end of the cell. Place wicks on outside in slot.
8. Apply 150 volts (10 ma) for twenty minutes at room temperature or when tracking dye has moved 4 cm from origin.
9. Remove slides from Durrum cell and *immediately* immerse in 220 ml fixing solution fifteen minutes. Shake gently occasionally.
10. Repeat immersion in second portion of fixing solution.
11. Dry slides in vented oven at 60°C until gel becomes a thin film. Store slides overnight at room temperature if necessary.
12. Place in developing stain two hours and dry at room temperature at least two hours.
13. Remove black background by quickly dipping slide in 95% ethanol. Rinse in tap water until water runs smoothly, but do not overrinse.
14. Inspect pattern and compare with that of normal serum, or scan with Beckman Microzone using red filter slit width of 0.2 mm and slit length of 1.4 mm.

Interpretation

The normal lipoprotein pattern and those of five familial lipoproteinemias, abeta lipoproteinemia and Tangier disease can be discerned and, when related to cholesterol and triglyceride levels, are diagnostic (Figure 9). An abnormal band of chylomicrons appears at the origin in Type I, a second, or β-band, is elevated in Type II; β- and pre β-, or "broad β-", bands are increased in Type III, the pre β-band in Type IV, and chylomicron and pre β-bands in Type V.

In abetalipoproteinemia and Tangier disease, on the other hand, the β- and α-lipoproteins, respectively, are absent or greatly decreased.

Triglycerides are elevated in four of the five familial lipoproteinemias (I, III, IV, V); cholesterol is the excessive serum lipid in Type II.

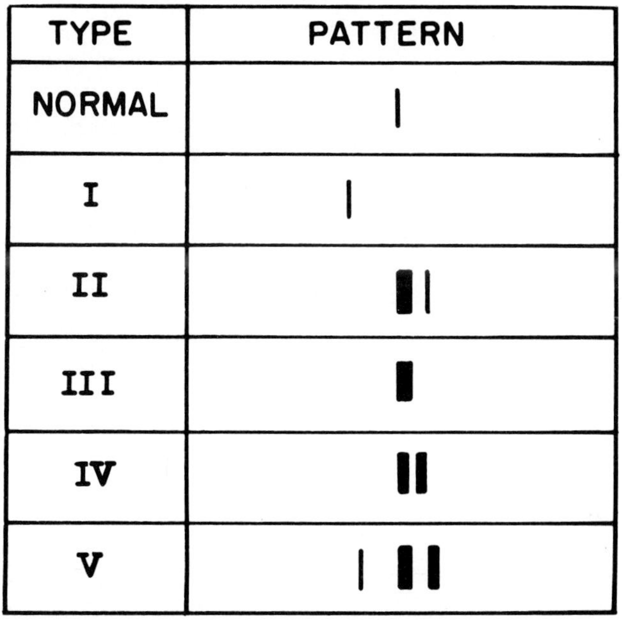

TYPE	PATTERN
NORMAL	I
I	I
II	▮I
III	▮
IV	II
V	I ▮▮

Figure 9. Electrophoretic patterns of serum lipoproteins on agarose in the hereditary hyperlipoproteinemias. From left to right are chylomicron, beta and prebeta fractions, respectively. In the lipoprotein deficiency diseases the beta or alpha bands may be missing. (The alpha fraction, not shown here, appears as a diffuse band beyond the prebeta fraction).

Reagents

1. *Barbital Electrophoresis Buffer, 0.05 M, pH 8.6*: Dissolve one package Beckman B-2 Buffer in 1900 ml demineralized water.
2. *Fixing Solution*: On the day of test, combine and mix: 300 ml 95% ethanol, 25 ml glacial acetic acid, and 175 ml demineralized water.
3. *Developing Stain (Sudan Black B)*: On the day of test, combine, mix with stirring bar, and filter: 110 ml Bio-Gram A stain concentrate, 66 ml 95% ethanol, and 44 ml demineralized water.

REFERENCES

Bio-Gram A Lipoprotein Profile Instruction Manual. BioRad Laboratories, Richmond, California, 1970.

Sanbar, Shafeek S.: *Hyperlipidemia and Hyperlipoproteinemia.* Boston, Little, 1969.

Frederickson, D. S., and Lees, R. S.: System for phenotyping hyperlipoproteinemia. *Circulation, 31*:321, 1965.

CHAPTER 16

FAMILIAL LIPOPROTEIN
DEFICIENCY DISEASES

CONGENITAL ABETALIPOPROTEINEMIA

THE diagnosis of abetalipoproteinemia in infants is difficult, as the early clinical signs are nonspecific, e.g. failure to thrive, gastrointestinal symptoms (diarrhea, steatorrhea), and abdominal distension. The discovery of acanthocytes in the peripheral smear, however, should suggest the diagnosis of abetalipoproteinemia and the need for obtaining the serum lipoprotein pattern. Neurologic signs (ataxia, tremors, and athetosis) appear later, and muscle weakness with its skeletal sequelae (kyphosis, lordosis, and pes cavus) is a progressive event. Retinitis pigmentosum is an even later manifestation.

The array of symptoms suggests a widespread or fundamental defect in, for example, the competency of cell membranes, the structure and function of which depend on adequate lipid-carrying protein, e.g. β-lipoprotein.

The disease is autosomal recessive, with the homozygous person expressing the mutant gene biochemically as hypolipidemia and absence of the serum β-lipoprotein fraction. Obligate carriers, however, have not consistently displayed abnormal lipid or β-lipoprotein levels.

The absence of the β-lipoprotein fraction in serum from homozygous persons is detected by lipoprotein electrophoresis (p. 277).

TANGIER DISEASE

Patients with deficiency of serum α-lipoproteins may appear healthy; others experience paresthesias, muscle wasting, and weakness (Tangier disease). The tonsils in either patient are grey-reddish orange and enlarged. The spleen may be enlarged and, in time, hypersplenism ensues. The disease was named "Tangier" after the Chesapeake Bay island on which the first patients lived.

The defect is congenital absence of α-lipoprotein. The molecular error may be a disproportional synthesis of the two major apoproteins involved. Derived abnormalities are storage of cholesterol esters in lymph organs (reflected in the size and color of the tonsils and in the splenomegaly), fat-staining foam cells in the marrow, orange spots on rectal mucosa, and corneal deposits. The depositions suggest that α-lipoproteins are necessary for the mobilization and/or transport of cholesterol.

Inheritance of the defect is autosomal recessive. Homozygous persons have subnormal levels of serum cholesterol and no discernible normal α-lipoprotein fraction The serum of carriers contains low levels of the fraction.

Alpha-lipoprotein deficiency is detected by electrophoresis of serum lipoproteins (p. 277).

PHYTANIC ACID STORAGE
DISEASE (REFSUM)

RETINAL degeneration is associated with peripheral neuropathy and ataxia in phytanic acid storage disease (Refsum). The degeneration causes night blindness, pigment mottling, and narrowing of the visual fields. In addition, cataracts, skeletal defects, cardiac changes, and renal disease are sometimes part of the clinical picture. The disease progresses slowly and intermittently; some patients, however, die suddenly from cardiac arrythmias or respiratory arrest.

The defect involves the initial oxidation of phytanic acid, i.e. the conversion of phytanic acid to α-hydroxyphytanic acid. The clinical signs may derive from phytanic acid storage; indeed, interference with vitamin A metabolism is a possible cause of the retinal degeneration, and some improvement follows when patients consume less of the phytol-rich foods.

The disease is transmitted as an autosomal recessive trait; homozygous persons have excessive phytanic acid in serum; carrier levels, for the most part, are normal.

The serum phytanic acid excess of homozygous persons is demonstrable by thin-layer chromatography (p. 283). A defect of phytanic acid oxidation is found in cultured fibroblasts. A partial defect can be detected in fibroblasts from carriers.

SERUM PHYTANIC ACID

Principle

Serum phytanic acid associated with the triglycerides is extracted with chloroform, developed by thin-layer chromatography, and stained with iodine vapor.

283

Procedure

1. Combine 0.5 ml aliquots of sample and control sera in respective 16 × 125-mm screw-cap test tubes in duplicate with 10 ml chloroform:methanol solution and shake by hand two minutes.
2. Centrifuge tubes ten minutes at 1500 R.P.M.
3. Remove liquid layer from *under* precipitated protein film with Pasteur pipette and place in 16 × 125-mm screw-cap tube.
4. Add a boiling chip (not a glass bead) to each tube. Heat tubes in 55 °C water bath in hood five minutes. (Solutions will boil immediately).
5. Repeat centrifugation and removal of fluid below precipitated protein film.
6. Measure volumes and, in 16 × 125-mm screw-cap tubes, combine with demineralized water in amounts estimated to change the relationship of chloroform:methanol:water from 2:1:0 to 8:4:3 (V:V:V).
7. Centrifuge tubes ten minutes at 1500 R.P.M.
8. Prepare iodine vapor chamber, seal, and let equilibrate three hours.
9. Remove bottom layer in tubes with Pasteur pipette and evaporate to dryness in hood under N_2.
10. Mark channels for five samples on 20 × 20 cm Eastman Chromagram sheet of 13179 silica gel, 100 μ thickness, as lines 1.5 cm long, spaced 1.5 cm apart, beginning 3 cm from edges and 2 cm from bottom of sheet.
11. Dry sheet thirty minutes at 100°C.
12. Dissolve dried extracts in 0.1 cm chloroform and apply to sheet in 15λ aliquots.
13. Develop sheet with hexane:ethyl ether:acetic acid solvent until front is 4 cm from the top (about one and one-half hours).
14. Dry sheet in hood thirty minutes.
15. Stain in iodine chamber.

Interpretation

    The serum lipids normally separate into five bands. Phytanic acid combines with three, chiefly the triglycerides, causing them to separate as double bands (Figure 10).

Reagents

1. *Chloroform-Methanol Solvent, 2:1, (V:V)*: Combine 20 ml chloroform and 20 ml methanol.
2. *Hexane-Diethyl Ether-Acetic Acid Developing Solvent 90:10:1, (V:V:V)*: Combine 90 ml hexane, 10 ml diethyl ether, and 1 ml glacial acetic acid.

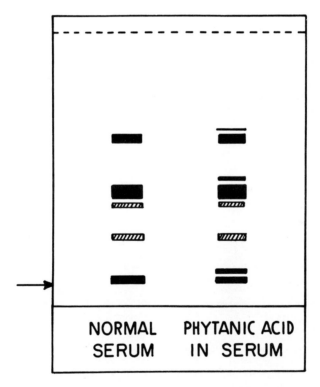

Figure 10. Paper chromatographic separation of serum lipids, iodine-stained. Arrow indicates origin. Phytanic acid combines chiefly with the triglyceride (prominent, second from top) fraction.

REFERENCES

Karlsson, K. G. Norrby, A., and Samuelsson, B.: Use of thin-layer chromatography for preliminary diagnosis of Refsum's disease. *Biochem Biophys Acta, 144*:162, 1967.

Karlsson, K. A., Nilsson, K., and Pascher, I.: Separation of lipids containing phytanic acid by thin-layer chromatography. *Lipids, 3*:389, 1968.

ACID PHOSPHATASE DEFICIENCY

VOMITING, fever, and lethargy, followed by bleeding and death, are clinical signs in infants which Dr. Henry Nadler associates with familial deficiency of acid phosphatase. Two infants improved temporarily with prednisolone treatment but did not survive.

Doctor Nadler discovered a deficiency of acid phosphatase in cell homogenates, especially in the lysosomal fraction. In one family, the defect was reflected in other fractions, and in some families it was even evident in serum.

Clinical and biochemical pedigrees of families affected suggest an autosomal recessive mode of inheritance.

The deficiency can be tested for initially by measuring serum acid phosphatase levels (p. 287).

SERUM ACID PHOSPHATASE

Principle

A deficiency of lysosomal acid phosphatase in cells is reflected in the serum by a decrease in the normal activity of the enzyme. The level of serum enzyme is measured with p-nitrophenyl phosphate as substrate.

Procedure

1. Prewarm 0.5 ml aliquots acid buffer substrate in two 16 × 100-mm tubes in 37°C water bath five minutes. Leaving tubes in bath, add 0.1 ml serum sample to one tube and 0.1 ml demineralized water to the other (water blank).
2. Continue heating for thirty minutes. Add 2 ml 0.1 N NaOH to both tubes, remove from bath, and mix. To a third tube containing 0.1 ml aliquot serum sample, add 2.5 ml 0.1 N NaOH

and mix (serum blank).
3. Read absorbance of samples, standards, and blanks at 410 nm, zeroing instrument with 0.2 N sodium hydroxide.

Calculations

1. Plot standard curve of optical density at 410 nm versus enzyme equivalents in standard solutions (IU/1).
2. Subtract $O.D._{410}$ values of blanks from O.D. value of sample.
3. Obtain enzyme equivalents in sample from standard curve and express activity of serum acid phosphatase in IU/1.

Interpretation

Normal levels in the newborn (13.4±3.0 IU/1) are slightly higher than in children and adults (10.8±2.2 IU/1). The activity of enzyme in the serum of Doctor Nadler's patients was less than 10% of normal (1973).

Reagents

1. *Acid Buffer*: Dissolve 1.89 g citric acid in 18 ml 1 N NaOH. Add 10 ml 0.1 N HCl and dilute to 90 ml with demineralized water. Add 3 drops chloroform and bring to pH 4.8 with 1 N NaOH or 0.1 N HCl. Dilute to volume with demineralized water in 100 ml volumetric flask.
2. *NaOH, 1.0 N*: Dissolve 4 g NaOH in 90 ml demineralized water and bring to volume in 100 ml volumetric flask.
3. *NaOH, 0.2 N*: Dilute 20 ml 1.0 N NaOH to 100 ml with demineralized water in a volumetric flask.
4. *NaOH, 0.1 N*: Dilute 10 ml 0.2 N NaOH with 10 ml demineralized water.
5. HCl, *0.1 N*: Dilute 0.85 ml concentrated HCl with 90 ml demineralized water and dilute to volume in 100 ml volumetric flask.
6. *Buffer Substrate*: Dissolve 0.1 g Sigma p-nitrophenyl phosphate disodium, in about 20 ml demineralized water. Add 25 ml acid buffer and dilute to volume in 50 ml volumetric flask

with demineralized water.
7. *Nitrophenol Standard Stock Solution*: Dilute exactly 0.5 ml 10 μmoles/ml Sigma p-nitrophenol stock solution with demineralized water and bring to volume in 100 ml volumetric flask. Mix.
8. *Nitrophenol working standard solutions (enzyme equivalent solutions)*: Combine the following volumes of nitrophenol standard stock solution and demineralized water:

Stock Standard (ml)	Water (ml)	0.2 N NaOH (ml)	Enzyme Equivalent (IU/liter)
0	0	10	0.0
1	9	1.1	3.8
2	8	1.1	7.8
4	6	1.1	15.7
6	4	1.1	23.3
8	2	1.1	31.2
10	0	1.1	39.0

REFERENCES

Nadler, Henry L.: Treatment of acid phosphatase deficiency disorders. In Bergsma, Daniel (Ed.): *Enzyme Therapy in Genetic Diseases.* Birth Defects: Original Articles Series, vol. IX. Baltimore, Williams & Wilkins, 1973, pp. 195-197.
Nadler, H. L.: Personal communication, 1976.
O'Brien, Donough, Ibbott, Frank A., and Rodgerson, Denis O.: *Laboratory Manual of Pediatric Micro-Biochemical Techniques,* Fourth Ed. New York, Har-Row, 1968.

CHAPTER 19

THE ENZYME-DEFICIENT
HEREDITARY HEMOLYTIC ANEMIAS

GLUCOSE-6-PHOSPHATE DEHYDROGENASE DEFICIENCY

THE clinical signs of the hereditary hemolytic anemias due to red cell enzyme deficiencies vary with the particular defect, the commonest of which are caused by defects and variants of glucose-6-phosphate dehydrogenase (G-6-PD). Patients of Mediterranean, Chinese, or African descent who have defective G-6-PD undergo hemolytic crises (back and abdominal pain, jaundice, and darkening of the urine) when exposed to certain drugs and agents, or may be jaundiced as infants. The quinoline antimalarials, e.g. primaquine, are the chief offenders, and, for the Mediterranean, ingestion of fava beans. Antibiotics (sulfonamides, furadantin), other medicinals (acetylsalicylic acid), and naphthalene have been among the common chemicals and pharmaceuticals cited.

Although well-studied, the pathogenesis is not complete. The hemolytic reaction to drugs may be related to G-6-PD's role as a catalyst in the red cells' "pentose shunt." The red cells' oxidative pathway is interrupted, in particular, the steps regulating the supply of sulfhydryl groups through reduction of NADP to NADPH and the maintenance of glutathione in the reduced state.

The disease has an X-linked pattern of inheritance, i.e. more men than women have hemolytic crises, sons inherit the mutant gene from mothers only, and daughters inherit from either or both parents. Sons will be affected if they inherit the gene (hemizygous); daughters, on the other hand, are seldom affected or only mildly so, unless they inherit the gene from both parents (homozygous).

Many variants of the enzyme are known. Some are recognized by locality of origin, others by red cell activity, electrophoretic mobility, kinetic characteristics, and heat stability. About twenty have been sufficiently characterized to establish their distinctness with certainty, in addition to the normal Caucasian, or "B," form of the enzyme. The properties of others have been less thoroughly examined and have yet to be accepted as distinct. Most of the variants are less active in the red cell than the "B" form and, aside from the normal Negro or "A" variant, occur chiefly in localized populations. Some variants of normal activity and a few of low activity are not associated with clinical signs. The variant in Mediterranean and oriental groups tends to cause more severe disease than that in African populations.

The defect can be detected in affected males by measuring the activity of red cell enzyme, preferably after the patient is no longer exposed to the drug. The blood of carrier females may or may not reflect a partial deficiency, depending upon the proportion of red cells derived from stem cells containing the mutant gene on the "active" X-chromosome.

Red cell G-6-PD activity is measured and a defect discernible by several methods, most of which are based on colorimetric or fluorometric indicators of change in the assay system's redox potential (p. 291). Characterization of variants requires further study, usually with purified preparations of the enzyme.

GLUCOSE-6-PHOSPHATE DEHYDROGENASE FLUORESCENT SPOT TEST

Principle

Glucose-6-phosphate dehydrogenase in red cells dried on filter paper retains the capacity to oxidize G-6-PD to 6-phosphogluconate, with concomitant reduction of the coenzyme NADP to NADPH. NADPH is fluorescent, and the development of fluorescence in aliquots of reaction mixture spotted, dried on filter paper, and observed in long wave ultraviolet is an indication of G-6-PD activity.

Procedure

1. Spot Schleicher and Schuell 903 filter paper card (PKU card)

with heparinized blood until circle is saturated through. Air dry.

2. Place 3/16-inch discs of test and control blood samples in depressions of Linbro Disposo Tray and overlay with 0.2 ml reaction mixture.

3. Mix with nonheparinized microhematocrit tube (with finger over one end) and immediately drop aliquot onto prelined and prenumbered Whatman No. 1 filter paper sheet (dried in dessicator before use in damp weather).

4. Cover and incubate tray in 37°C water bath for fifteen minutes.

5. Remix, respot, and dry sheet at room temperature for at least ten minutes.

6. Observe fluorescence in long wave ultraviolet.

Interpretation

Reaction mixtures containing normal blood fluoresce in fifteen minutes. If deficient in G-6-PD, mixtures remain nonfluorescent. (See Color Illustration 13.)

Reagents

1. *Saturated Digitonin*: Dissolve 0.1 g digitonin in 50 ml demineralized water, allow excess to settle, remove, and save supernatant fluid.

2. *Potassium Phosphate Buffer, 0.25M, pH 7.4*: Dissolve 3.49 g K_2HPO_4 and 0.68 g KH_2PO_4 in 50 ml demineralized water. Adjust to pH 7.4 with 0.1 N solutions of NaOH or HCl and bring to volume in 100 ml volumetric flask.

3. *Reaction mixture for 500 tests*: Dissolve 57.4 mg NADP (M.W. 765) and 28.2 mg glucose-6-phosphate, sodium salt (M.W. 282), in 30 ml demineralized water, both corrected for water of hydration (See vials) by the formula:

$$mg = 57.4 \times \frac{\text{hydrated mol. wt.}}{\text{mol. wt.}}$$
$$\text{or}$$
$$28.2$$

Transfer to 100 ml volumetric flask, add 20 ml saturated digitonin, 30 ml 0.25 M potassium phosphate buffer, and bring to volume with demineralized water. Store as 10 ml aliquots in 20 ml screw cap tubes at -20°C.

REFERENCE

Beutler, E.: A series of new screening procedures for pyruvate kinase deficiency, glucose-6-phosphate dehydrogenase deficiency, and glutathione reductase deficiency. *Blood, 28*:553, 1966.

QUANTITATIVE GLUCOSE-6-PHOSPHATE DEHYDROGENASE ASSAY (ERYTHROZYME®)

Principle

Levels of G-6-PD activity in lysed red cells are estimated by measuring the increase in absorption at O.D.$_{340\ nm}$ by the reduction of NADP to NADPH, the coenzyme form with specific absorption at wavelength 340_{nm}.

Procedure (Erythrozyme® assay from Princeton Biomedix)

1. Warm substrate tube, reconstituted with 2.5 ml demineralized water, in 30°C water bath.
2. Add 10λ fresh whole blood (capillary or collected in EDTA) to lysing tube, reconstituted with 0.5 ml demineralized water, and incubate seven minutes in 30°C water bath.
3. Add warmed substrate to the lysing tube and pour back and forth to mix. Transfer to microcuvette.
4. Measure optical density changes at 340 nm at one-minute intervals, between two and five minutes, in Beckman DU spectrophotometer. Record temperature during the reaction time and correct for deviation from standard temperature of reaction at 30°C (T_f) from temperature correction factor table. No correction is needed if O.D. changes are measured at 30°C.

Calculation

1. Calculate change in O.D./min. as the average of the 3 one-

minute $\triangle$ O.D. readings between two and five minutes.

2. Express activity as:

$$\text{IU/ml erythrocytes} = \frac{0.484 \times \triangle \text{ O.D.}/\min \times 10^2 \times T_f}{\text{Hematocrit} \times \text{ml sample}}$$

where T_f is one of the following correction factors for a standard temperature of 30°C:

°C	
27	1.21
28	1.12
29	1.07
30	1.00
31	0.94
32	0.88
33	0.83

Interpretation

Fresh normal blood contains approximately $2.38 \text{ IU} \pm 0.26$/ml erythrocytes (by hematocrit). Blood from hemizygous males will be markedly deficient. Levels in heterozygous carriers may or may not be partially deficient. Since the reaction mixture contains an excess of substrate, kinetic variants may not be detected by this method.

Reagents

1. *NADP lysing tube:* Erythrozyme glucose-6-phosphate dehydrogenase UV Set.
2. *Buffered glucose-6-phosphate substrate tube (pH 7.5):* Erythrozyme glucose-6-phosphate dehydrogenase UV Set.

CYTOCHEMICAL ASSAY OF GLUCOSE-6-PHOSPHATE DEHYDROGENASE ACTIVITY

Principle

Granules of formazan precipitate within red cells when hemoglobin is exposed to and reduces a tetrazolium dye in a histochemical reaction indicating the presence or absence of "pentoseshunt" enzymes. Methemoglobin, formed by oxidation with nitrite before incubation, is reduced to hemoglobin during incubation of enzyme-containing red cells with glucose, NADP, and indicator dye.

The amount of activity can be estimated from the number of formazan granules formed.

Procedure

1. Collect 2 ml heparinized blood and test on the day of collection. If blood must be stored before testing, collect 2 ml blood in 1 ml Alsever's solution and store at 4°C for no more than a week.
2. Centrifuge sample for ten minutes at approximately 2000 R.P.M. and remove supernatant fluid.
3. Transfer exactly 0.5 ml packed red cells to a 12 ml Sorvall tube containing 9.0 ml isotonic saline and 0.5 ml 0.18 M sodium nitrite. Mix by inverting gently; incubate undisturbed at 37°C for twenty minutes.
4. Centrifuge at 2300 R.P.M. for fifteen minutes at 4°C. Discard supernatant fluid without disturbing buffy coat or red cells.
5. Wash pellet three times with 9.0 ml volumes isotonic saline; remove buffy coat after last wash, leaving only red cells.
6. Mix packed red cells with swab stick; transfer 50λ to screw-capped tube containing 1.0 ml incubation mixture. Incubate undisturbed at 37°C for thirty minutes.
7. Gently resuspend red cells in 0.2 ml MTT tetrazolium after thirty minutes incubation. Incubate at 37°C for another sixty minutes.
8. Resuspend red cells thoroughly after incubation. Place a drop of suspension adjacent to a drop of 0.6% saline on glass slide. Mix drops thoroughly, add cover slip, and examine under oil immersion lens (Figure 11).
9. Score granularity in 100 cells as follows:

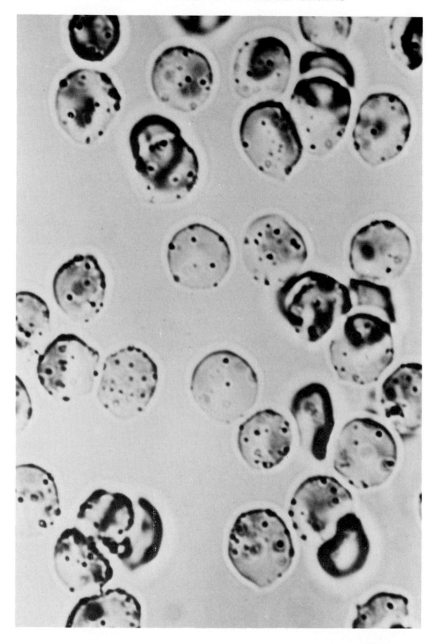

Figure 11. Photomicrograph of normal red cells after incubation and staining with MTT tetrazolium. Cells deficient in glucose-6-phosphate dehydrogenase contain few or no formazan granules. 1562 X.

Cells with no granules:	0
Cells with 1-3 granules:	1+
Cells with 4-6 granules:	2+
Cells with 7+ granules:	3+

10. Multiply scores by number of cells per score. The sum of multiplied scores is total granule score (TGS) of 100 cells.

Interpretation

Total granule scores of 100 cells from normal persons range from 265 to 300, from 200 to 225 in carriers, and are less than 50 in hemizygotes. Published values are slightly lower.

Reagents

1. *Sodium Nitrite Solution, 0.18 M*: Dissolve 6.2 g $NaNO_2$ in 500 ml demineralized water.
2. *Incubation Mixture*: Combine 4 ml 0.85% sodium chloride, 1.0 ml 5.0% glucose (5 g/100 ml), 2.0 ml 0.3 M phosphate buffer, pH 7.0 (dissolve 4.08 g KH_2PO_4 in 40 ml demineralized water; adjust to pH 7.0 with 0.5 N NaOH and bring to volume in 100 ml volumetric flask), 1.0 ml 11 mg% Nile blue sulfate (or Nile blue A) (11 mg/100 ml), and 2.0 ml demineralized water.
3. *Saline Solution, 0.85%*: Dissolve 0.85 g NaCl in 100 ml demineralized water.
4. *MTT Tetrazolium* [3-(4,5-Dimethyl thiazolyl-2-)-2,5-diphenyl tetrazolium bromide]: Dissolve 5 mg MTT tetrazolium in 1.0 ml 0.85% saline solution.
5. *Saline Solution, 0.6%*: Add 7.1 ml 0.85% saline to 2.9 ml demineralized water.

REFERENCE

Fairbanks, V. F., and Lamps, L. T.: A tetrazolium-linked cytochemical method for estimation of glucose-6-phosphate dehydrogenase activity in individual erythrocytes: Applications in the study of heterozygotes for glucose-6-phosphate dehydrogenase deficiency. *Blood, 31*:589, 1968.

GLUCOSE-6-PHOSPHATE DEHYDROGENASE ISOZYMES BY ELECTROPHORESIS ON CELLULOSE ACETATE

Principle

The commonest electrophoretic forms of human red cell G-6-PD, types A+ and B+ separate on cellulose acetate.

Procedure

1. Centrifuge 2 to 3 ml whole blood at maximum speed in clinical centrifuge for fifteen minutes. Heparinized blood should be processed within twenty-four hours of collection. ACD or EDTA blood can be stored for up to two weeks at 4°C before processing.
2. Discard plasma and buffycoat.
3. Wash packed red cells twice with 10 ml 0.9% NaCl. Add 0.5 ml aliquot of the packed cells to 0.5 ml cold distilled water after last wash. Freeze and thaw twice in alcohol · CO_2 bath.
4. Add 0.4 ml toluene, shake, and centrifuge at maximum speed in clinical centrifuge for twenty minutes.
5. Remove and filter clear middle solution (hemolysate) through Whatman No. 1 filter paper.
6. If only smaller volumes of blood are available, the preceding steps are modified for 0.5 ml whole blood. Add 10 ml cold 0.9% NaCl, mix by inversion, and separate cells as above. Lyse by freezing and thawing three times with 0.2 ml lysing solution. Use two applications of sample for electrophoresis when prepared by this method.
7. Refrigerate Beckman Microzone electrophoresis cell one hour before use. Soak Gelman Sepraphore III cellulose polyacetate membrane for ten minutes in cold soaking buffer.
8. Blot, position membrane in chamber, deposit samples at the cathodal end (-) of strip (first groove), and apply 450 V for sixty minutes.
9. Stain a blank cellulose acetate membrane in staining solution for three to five minutes, blot gently, and keep moist in Petri

dish lined with wet tissue paper (staining strip). Remove test strip from electrophoresis chamber and immediately place it on top of staining strip. Do not let strips slip once they have made contact. Cover dish, seal with tape, and incubate in the dark fifteen to thirty minutes at room temperature.

Interpretation

The A+ and B+ isozymes of G-6-PD are more anodal than hemoglobin A, the A+ form migrating faster than B+. Protein with 10% or more enzyme activity will stain as isozyme.

Reagents

1. *TRIS-EDTA-Borate (TEB) Buffer, 0.14 M, pH 9.1*: Dissolve 16.5 g Sigma Trizma base, 1.48 g EDTA (disodium salt), and 0.93 g boric acid in 800 ml demineralized water. Adjust to pH 9.1, if necessary, and bring to volume in 1000 ml volumetric flask. Store at 4°C.
2. *Soaking Buffer*: Dissolve 5 mg NADP in 100 ml 0.14 M TEB, pH 9.1.
3. *Saturated Digitonin for Alternate Sample Preparation*: Dissolve 10 mg digitonin in 10 ml demineralized water for ten to fifteen minutes on magnetic stirrer and filter.
4. *TEB Buffer, 0.014 M, pH 9.1, for Alternate Sample Preparation*: Combine 10 ml 0.14 M TEB buffer, pH 9.1, and 90 ml demineralized water.
5. *Lysing Solution for Alternate Sample Preparation*: Combine 5 ml saturated digitonin and 10 ml 0.014 M TEB.
6. *TRIS · HCl Stain Buffer, 0.1 M, pH 8.0*: Dissolve 12.1 g Sigma Trizma base and 80 ml demineralized water. Adjust to pH 8.0 with 4 N HCl and bring to volume in 100 ml volumetric flask.
7. *Phenazine Methosulfate Solution*: *Just before use,* dissolve 5 mg phenazine methosulfate in 5 ml demineralized water. Cover tube with aluminum foil to prevent reaction to light.
8. *Staining Solution*: Dissolve 4.0 mg NADP, 10 mg glucose-6-phosphate (sodium salt), and 2 mg Sigma MTT tetrazolium in 9.4 ml 0.1 M TRIS · HCl Buffer. Add 0.6 ml phenazine

methosulfate solution just before use.

REFERENCE

Sparks, R. S., Baluda, M. A., and Townsend, D. E.: Cellulose acetate electrophoresis of human glucose-6-phosphate dehydrogenase, *J Lab Clin Med*, 73:531, 1969.

RED CELL PYRUVATE KINASE DEFICIENCY

Variable degrees of jaundice, splenomegaly, and gall stones are the common presenting signs of a chronic hemolytic process in persons with deficiency of red cell pyruvate kinase. The disease usually begins in childhood; length of survival often depends upon severity of the particular form and prevention of secondary effects.

The relation of hemolysis to the enzyme defect is not entirely clear. The red cells require an intracellular supply of the coenzymes, ATP and NAD, the former generated by normal pyruvate kinase activity. The reticulocytes, which form a disproportionately high fraction of the red cells in hemolytic reactions, are particularly susceptible to the limited supply of coenzymes. Some reticulocytes are destroyed when formed; others are "caught" in the spleen as shrunken, rigid cells which eventually are lysed. Splenectomy relieves the severe anemia of the disase, chiefly because it removes the "trap."

The disease follows an autosomal recessive pattern of inheritance.

Affected persons have little or no red cell pyruvate kinase; carriers have partial enzyme defects or molecular variants of varying efficiency.

Red cell pyruvate kinase is measured by fluorescent or colorimetric methods in which the indicator system is linked to the specific enzyme reaction, (pp. 301, 302) as in assays for G-6-PD. The assays are practically pathognomonic, since other conditions have not been associated with a deficiency of the kinase. The severity of the disease, however, is not necessarily correlated with the degree of the defect.

PYRUVATE KINASE FLUORESCENT SPOT TEST

Principle

Pyruvate kinase in dried blood spots catalyzes the splitting of phosphate from phosphoenolpyruvate to form pyruvic acid and, with adenosine diphosphate, a new molecule of adenosine triphosphate. Pyruvic acid is reduced to lactic acid by lactic dehydrogenase in the hemolysate. The indicator in the reaction mixture, the fluorescent, reduced form of NADH, is oxidized to nonfluorescent NAD. The disappearance of fluorescence in aliquots of reaction mixture indicates activity.

Procedure

1 - 3. As in the fluorescent screening test for G-6-PD, p. 291.
4. Cover and incubate tray in 37°C water bath for thirty minutes.
5. Remix, respot, and dry sheet at room temperature for at least ten minutes.
6. Observe fluorescence in long-wave ultraviolet.

Interpretation

Reaction mixtures containing normal blood become nonfluorescent in about thirty minutes; those from blood deficient in pyruvate kinase remain fluorescent.

Reagents

1. *Phosphoenol pyruvate, 0.15 M*: Dissolve 304.7 mg PEP (M.W. 465.6) in 4.2 ml demineralized water, corrected for water of hydration by the ratio:

$$mg = 304.7 \times \frac{\text{hydrated mol. wt.}}{\text{mol. wt.}}$$

Store in 0.6 ml aliquots at -20°C.
2. *Adenosine Diphosphate, 0.03 M*: Dissolve 133.1 mg ADP (M.W. 449.2) in 9.1 ml demineralized water, corrected for

hydration, as above. Store in 1.3 ml aliquots at -20°C.

3. *Nicotinamide Adenine Dinucleotide, Reduced, 0.015 M*: Dissolve 101.7 mg NADH in 9.1 ml demineralized water, corrected for hydration, as above. Store in 1.3 ml aliquots at -20°C.

4. *Magnesium Sulfate, 0.08 M*: Dissolve 179.5 mg MgSO₄ in 9.1 ml demineralized water. Store in 1.3 ml aliquots at -20°C.

5. *Potassium Phosphate Buffer, 0.25 M, pH 7.4*: Dissolve 3.49 g K_2HPO_4 and 0.68 g KH_2PO_4 in 75 ml demineralized water. Adjust to pH 7.4 with 0.1 N HCl or NaOH, and bring to volume in 100 ml volumetric flask with demineralized water.

6. *Reaction Mixture (For Fifty Tests)*: On the day of test, combine the following:

> 0.3 ml PEP
> 1.0 ml ADP
> 1.0 ml NADH
> 1.0 ml MgSO₄
> 0.5 ml phosphate buffer
> 6.2 ml demineralized water

REFERENCE

Beutler, E.: A series of new screening procedures for pyruvate kinase deficiency, glucose-6-phosphate dehydrogenase deficiency and glutathione reductase deficiency. *Blood* 28:253, 1966.

QUANTITATIVE PYRUVATE KINASE ASSAY (ERYTHROZYME)

Principle

Levels of pyruvate kinase activity in lysed red cells are estimated by measuring the decrease in absorption at O.D.$_{340\ nm}$ by the oxidation of NADH, reduced to the oxidized form, NAD, when the specific reaction, dephosphorylation of phosphoenol pyruvate by the kinase, is coupled with pyruvate conversion by lactic dehydrogenase and its fluorescent coenzyme, NADH.

Procedure (Erythrozyme assay from Princeton Biomedix)

1. Warm substrate tube, reconstituted with 2.5 ml demineralized

water, in 30°C bath.

2. Remove plasma and leukocytes from 0.5 ml sample of fresh whole blood, or blood stored at 4°C for up to as long as twenty days, as follows: Draw up phthalate oil mixture (sp. gr. 1.062) to 5 mm in a hematocrit tube and fill to 90% volume with the blood sample. Seal the oil end with Seal-Ease® or Critoseal®; centrifuge in hematocrit centrifuge. Score and break tube at sealant end of packed red cell layer. Transfer red cells to 5λ pipette.

3. Add 5λ packed red cells to the NADH lysing tube, reconstituted with 0.5 ml demineralized water, and incubate for five minutes in 30°C water bath.

4. Add warmed substrate to the lysing tube and pour back and forth to mix. Transfer immediately to microcuvette.

5. Measure optical density changes at 340 nm at one minute intervals, between two and five minutes, in Beckman DU spectrophotometer. Record temperature of solution and correct for deviation from standard temperature of reaction at 30°C (T_f) from temperature correction factor table. No correction is needed if O.D. changes are measured at 30°C.

Calculations

1. Calculate change in O.D./min as the average of the 3 one-minute Δ O.D. readings between two and five minutes.

2. Express activity as

$$\text{IU/ml erythrocytes} = \frac{\Delta \text{ OD/min} \times 1000 \times T_f \times 3}{6.2 \times 10^3 \times \text{ml of sample}}$$

where 6.2×10^3 is the extinction coefficient, 3 is the volume of test solution in ml, and T_f is one of following correction factors for a standard temperature of 30°C:

°C	
27	1.16
28	1.10
29	1.05
30	1.00
31	0.95

32	0.91
33	0.86

3. To express as $IU/10^{10}$ erythrocytes, multiply IU/ml erythrocytes $\times$ 1.15, where 1.15 is the normal value for $100/$mean corpuscular volume (μ^3)

Interpretation

Pyruvate kinase activities range from 1.77 to 2.25 IU/ml erythrocytes in normal blood, when measured at 30°C, and from 0.85 to 1.99 IU/ml erythrocytes in blood from heterozygous persons. Blood from homozygous persons displays little or no activity.

Reagents

1. *NADH Lysing Tube*: Erythrozyme Pyruvate kinase UV set.
2. *Buffered Adenosine Diphosphate-Phosphoenol Pyruvate Substrate Tube, pH 7.5*: Erythrozyme Pyruvate kinase UV set.
3. *Phthalate Oil Mixture,sp.g.1.062*: Erythrozyme pyruvate kinase UV set.

TRIOSEPHOSPHATE ISOMERASE DEFICIENCY

Only a few patients with deficiency of red cell triosephosphate isomerase have been described. Most have been severely anemic infants and, if older than a year, developed neuromuscular signs of spasticity, muscular atrophy, and weakness. Respiratory and other recurrent infections were common, the course of which ended in sudden and unexpected death.

The enzyme defect interrupts the red cells' glycolytic pathway at the interconversion of the 3-carbon isomers, 3-phosphoglyceraldehyde (G-3-P) and dihydroxyacetone (DHAP), formed by the cleavage of fructose-1,6-diphosphate. Since only G-3-P is metabolized further, a defect in isomerase greatly reduces the cleavage product available for energy production and leads to the intracellular accumulation of DHAP.

The disease follows an autosomal recessive mode of inheritance.

The red cells of homozygous persons have little or no isomerase activity; white cell, skeletal muscle, and cerebral spinal fluid isomerase activities are low also. The activity of the carrier's red cell isomerase is about half normal.

The enzyme defect is discernible by a fluorescent screening test of dried blood spots (p. 305) and by quantitative assay of enzyme in whole blood.

TRIOSEPHOSPHATE ISOMERASE
FLUORESCENT SPOT TEST

Principle

Isomerase activity in dried blood spots is indicated by the disappearance of fluorescence as the reduced form of NADH is oxidized to NAD in a linked reaction between the isomerization of glyceraldehyde-3-phosphate and DHAP and the conversion of DHAP to α-glycerol phosphate by added α-glycerol phosphate dehydrogenase.

Procedure

1 - 3. As in procedure for glucose-6-phosphate dehydrogenase screening, p. 291.
4. Cover and incubate tray at room temperature for twenty minutes.
5. Remix, respot, and dry sheet at room temperature for at least ten minutes.
6. Observe fluorescence in longwave ultraviolet.

Interpretation

Reaction mixtures containing normal levels of enzyme become nonfluorescent within twenty minutes; those deficient in enzyme remain fluorescent during the test period.

Reagents

1. *Triethanolamine Buffer, 0.1 M, pH 8.0*: Dissolve 1.856 g triethanolamine in 50 ml demineralized water, add 3 ml 2 N NaOH (8 g/100 ml), and bring to volume in 100 ml volumetric flask with demineralized water. Store at 5 to 10°C.
2. *Disodium Ethylenediaminetetraacetic Acid (EDTA), 0.05 M*: Dissolve 1.861 g EDTA in demineralized water and bring to volume in 100 ml volumetric flask. Store at 5 to 10°C.
3. *Reaction mixture, 10 ml (for fifty tests)*: On the day of test, combine the following reagents in a 20 ml test tube, in the order given, and mix:

	(ml)
Triethanolamine buffer, 0.1 M, pH 8.0	5.0
Demineralized water	3.0
EDTA, 0.05 M	1.0
NADH, reduced, 0.5 mg/ml	1.0
DL-Glyceraldehyde-3-phosphoric acid, 50 mg/ml	0.100
α-glycerolphosphate dehydrogenase, 4.0 mg/ml	0.001

REFERENCE

Kaplan, J. C., Shore, N., and Beutler, E.: The rapid detection of triose phosphate isomerase deficiency. *Am J Clin Pathol, 50*:656, 1968.

GLUTATHIONE REDUCTASE DEFICIENCY

Patients with partial deficiencies of glutathione reductase (GR) present with a variety of clinical signs, including severe hemolytic anemia, drug-induced pancytopenia, and hemolytic anemia accompanied by mental retardation or other neurologic manifestation.

Recent data suggest that GR deficiency is not the primary defect. The reductase is a flavin enzyme, which provides the cell with a steady supply of reduced glutathione (GSH) by catalyzing the transfer of hydrogen ions from the nicotinamide adenine dinucleotide phosphate system (NADPH $\leftrightarrow$ NADP) to oxidized glutathione (GSSG). The enzyme in normal hemolyzates can be activated by the addition of the prosthetic group, flavin-adenine dinucleotide (FAD), or by the ingestion of the precursor vitamin, riboflavin. GR deficiency, therefore, may be a secondary expression of abnormality, reflecting a more basic defect, as, for example, decreased affinity of apoenzyme for FAD, dietary deficiencies of riboflavin, or defects in the enzymatic conversion of riboflavin to FAD.

The various clinical signs, however, may relate directly to the GR defect, as the target tissues, bone marrow, and brain are comprised of rapidly metabolizing cells, in constant demand for reduced glutathione. Thus, the cell partially deficient in GR has a limited supply of the tripeptide, which protects against oxidative damage, stabilizes glycolytic enzymes and promotes the conversion of disulfides to sulfhydryl groups.

The mode of inheritance of GR deficiency is unclear. The disease has a dominant pattern in at least one family; in others, the pattern is autosomal recessive.

Patients are screened for GR deficiency by a fluorescent spot test (p. 307). If apparently deficient, they should be retested after increasing the dietary riboflavin. Quantitative tests of enzyme activity are based on fluorescence or ultraviolet absorption.

GLUTATHIONE REDUCTASE FLUORESCENT SPOT TEST

Principle

Glutathione reductase maintains reduced glutathione in red cells at a level which protects them from oxidative damage. The enzyme retains its activity in dried blood spots and is measured by the defluorescence of reaction mixtures, containing fluorescent TPNH, during the reduction of glutathione.

Procedure

1 - 3. Steps as described for G-6-PD on p. 291.
4. Cover and incubate tray in 37°C water bath for forty-five minutes.
5. Remove aliquot, spot, and dry sheet at room temperature for

at least ten minutes.
6. Observe fluorescence in longwave ultraviolet.

Interpretation

Reaction mixtures containing normal blood become nonfluorescent in from thirty to forty-five minutes; those from blood containing little or no reductase remain fluorescent.

Reagents

1. *Saturated Digitonin*: Dissolve 0.1 g digitonin in 50 ml demineralized water, let excess settle, remove, and save supernatant fluid.
2. *Potassium Phosphate Buffer, 0.25 M, pH 7.4*: Dissolve 3.4 g K_2HPO_4 and 0.68 g KH_2PO_4 in 50 ml demineralized water and bring to volume in 100 ml volumetric flask.
3. *Reaction Mixture, 5 ml (for fifty tests)*: On the day of test dissolve 3.1 mg nicotinamide adenine dinucleotide phosphate, reduced form (NADPH), corrected for water of hydration by the formula

$$mg = 3.1 \times \frac{\text{hydrated mol. wt.}}{833.4}$$

and 5.0 mg oxidized glutathione (GSSG) in 3 ml phosphate buffer. Add 1 ml saturated digitonin and 1 ml demineralized water. Mix.

REFERENCE

Beutler, E.: A series of new screening procedures for pyruvate kinase deficiency, glucose-6-phosphate dehydrogenase deficiency, and glutathione reductase deficiency. *Blood, 28*:553, 1966.

CHAPTER 20

HEMOGLOBINOPATHIES

HEMOLYTIC crises are the hallmark of sickle cell disease. The anemia caused by spontaneous exacerbations of red cell sickling is severe and occurs chiefly in persons of African or Mediterranean descent. The defect is one of hemoglobin structure, in which normal hemoglobin A is replaced by a less soluble variant, hemoglobin S. Carriers of hemoglobin S (hemoglobin AS) are usually free of crises and other clinical signs, although their red cells contain only half the normal quantity of hemoglobin A. The disease is recessively inherited, i.e. both parents must carry the trait to produce children with sickle cell anemia. The sickling trait and the mutant hemoglobin itself, however, are dominantly inherited, so that all children of a homozygous parent will, at the least, be carriers. Since extreme anoxia may precipitate episodes of sickling in the carrier, it is important to detect and alert carriers of their heterozygosity.

Hemoglobin S is readily demonstrable by electrophoretic pattern. The sickling phenomenon is seen in blood smears of patients with sickle cell anemia and may be induced in the carrier's red cells by lowering the oxygen tension.

Other hereditary hemolytic anemias due to structural defects in hemoglobins are recognizable by their electrophoretic mobilities, as, for example, hemoglobin C disease, hemoglobin E disease, and combinations with hemoglobin S or thalassemia. Methemoglobinemia from Hb M is also the result of a structural error.

The anemias of the thalassemias are the result of an imbalance in the proportions of the α and β peptide chains comprising the hemoglobin molecule. The defect in individuals with β thalassemia, for example, is underproduction of the β chains of hemoglobin A, resulting in a severe anemia. Carriers have relatively normal levels of hemoglobin A; their red cells, however, contain variable amounts of fetal hemoglobin and an excess of hemoglobin A_2.

SEPARATION OF STRUCTURAL
VARIANTS BY ELECTROPHORESIS

ELECTROPHORESIS OF HEMOGLOBINS
S, C, AND A ON CELLULOSE ACETATE

Principle

Structural variants of hemoglobin can be detected in both dried blood spots and whole blood by electrophoresis on cellulose acetate, according to changes in the molecule's electric charge.

Procedure

1. Prepare whole blood samples as follows: Centrifuge approximately 3 ml whole blood at maximum speed in clinical centrifuge for ten to fifteen minutes. Wash three times with saline (2 × vols), centrifuging after each wash.
2. Remove supernatant fluid after last wash, and add 1.75 ml demineralized water and 0.4 ml toluene per 1.0 ml volume packed red cells. Shake vigorously for five minutes and centrifuge at maximum speed for twenty minutes. Remove hemolysate (clear red layer) with syringe, filter, and store at 4°C.
3. Prepare dried blood spot samples, as follows: Elute approximately ten 1/4 inch discs of dried blood on 3 MM filter paper (PKU) cards in an 11 × 75-mm test tube for one-half hour with 0.2 ml Helena Laboratories hemolysate reagent.
4. Wet and blot cellulose acetate membrane, as described in Beckman "Instruction Manual," position on frame, and place in Beckman Microzone electrophoresis cell.
5. Apply samples and standards with Beckman applicator.
6. Apply 400 V for thirty minutes at room temperature. Disconnect from power source, remove membrane, and stain immediately with Gelman Ponceau S for five to ten minutes.
7. Wash in 5% acetic acid three to four times with one-minute washes until red background fades.

8. Dry membrane at room temperature, interpret, and store in plastic envelope, unless the level of Hgb A_2 by densitometry is to be measured, in which instance the membrane wet from the last acetic acid wash is covered with 95% ethanol for exactly 1.0 minute, rinsed in clearing solution 1.0 minute, and dried in 60°C vented oven on a glass drying frame.

Interpretation

Compare electrophoretic patterns of whole blood hemolysate and blood spot eluate samples with hemolysates and eluates, respectively, of control hemoglobin samples.

Reagents

1. *TRIS-Glycine Buffer, pH 9.3*: Dissolve 69.1 g Sigma Trizma base and 10.5 g glycine in 1700 ml demineralized water, and adjust to pH 9.3 with 1 N NaOH or 1 N HCl, if necessary. Bring to volume in 2000 ml volumetric flask.
2. *Whole Blood Hemolysate Standards*: Use Gelman Instrument complete hemoglobin control set (A, AA_2 AS, AC, SC, F, AFSC).
3. *Dried Blood Spot Standards:* Saturate PKU card (Schleicher and Schuell filter paper #903) with whole blood from patients with known hemoglobinopathies. Air-dry for at least one hour. Stable at -20°C for at least six months.
4. *Acetic Acid, 5%:* Dilute 100 ml glacial acetic acid to 1900 ml with demineralized water.
5. *Clearing Solution: Just before use,* mix 79 ml 95% ethanol with 10 ml glacial acetic acid.

REFERENCES

Beckman Methods Manual, *Model R-100 Microzone Electrophoresis System,* Spinco Div. Beckman Instrument, Palo Alto, Calif., 1967.

Beckman Instruction Manual, *Model R-100 Microzone Densitometer,* Spinco Div. Beckman Instrument, Palo Alto, Calif., (RM-TB-005, Oct. 1967).

Kohn, J.: Separation of haemoglobins on cellulose acetate. *J Clin Pathol,*

22:109, 1969.

Breen, M., and Weinstein, H. G.: An improved method for the mass screening of hemoglobin diseases. *Biochem Med, 2*:35, 1968.

ELECTROPHORESIS OF HEMOGLOBIN S AND D ON CITRATE AGAR

Principle

Hemoglobin D, which migrates at the same rate as hemoglobin S during electrophoresis on cellulose acetate at alkaline pH, separates from S on agar gel at acid pH.

Procedure

1. Centrifuge whole blood at maximum speed in clinical centrifuge; wash packed red cells three times with two volumes of saline (0.85% sodium chloride); add 1.0 volume demineralized water and 0.2 volume toluene after the last wash, shake vigorously, and let stand overnight in refrigerator. Centrifuge at 3000 R.P.M., remove clear hemolysate, and filter through Whatman #1 paper.
2. Apply hemolysates to cooled gel, as follows: Make a series of slits with spatula tip, one inch from anodal end, 3/4 inches long at 1/2 inch intervals along the width (10 inches) of the gel. Insert strips of Whatman #3 filter paper, 5/8 × 1/8-inch, saturated with sample and control hemolysates.
3. Lay Whatman #3 MM paper wicks, 8 1/2 × 3-inch, along cathodal and anodal ends of gel and coat entire plate twice with Bordon Krylon® plastic spray 1301.
4. Apply current of 20 ma for sixteen hours at 4°C.
5. Strip plastic coating from gel; stain twenty minutes in Amido Schwarz 10B. Pour off stain and rinse gel carefully in 2% acetic acid until rinse is clear (three or four times).

Interpretation

The common hemoglobins migrate cathodally in this system.

Hemoglobin D moves faster than hemoglobin S, at a rate similar to hemoglobin A, and slower than hemoglobin F. Hemoglobin C remains at or near the origin.

Reagents

1. *Citric Acid-Sodium Citrate Stock Buffer, pH 6.0:* Dissolve 147 g sodium citrate · 2 H_2O in 600 ml demineralized water. Adjust to pH 6.0 with concentrated citric acid (60%) and dilute to 1 liter.
2. *Citric Acid-Sodium Citrate Working Buffer, 0.5 M, pH 6.2:* Dilute stock buffer with demineralized water 1:9 and adjust to pH 6.2 with concentrated (60%) citric acid solution.
3. *Agar Gel:* Dissolve 1 g Difco Bacto-agar in 100 ml citrate working buffer in 300 ml Erlenmeyer flask; heat in boiling water bath until clear. Cool to 55°C and pour approximately 25 ml of solution onto a 4 × 10-inch thin glass plate. Cool at room temperature until set (fifteen to thirty minutes).
4. *Amido Schwarz 10B Stain:* Dissolve 0.5 g Amido Schwarz 10B stain in 100 ml solution of methyl alcohol:water:acetic acid, 50:50:5, and filter before use.

REFERENCE

Robinson, A. R., Robson, M., Harrison, A. P., and Zuelzer, W. W.: A new technique for differentiation of hemoglobin. *J Lab Clin Med, 50*:745, 1957.

ELECTROPHORESIS OF HEMOGLOBIN M
ON STARCH GEL

Principle

The oxidation product of hemoglobin M, methemoglobin M, migrates at a slower rate than methemoglobin A during electrophoresis in starch at neutral pH.

Procedure

1. Prepare starch gel, as described in method for hemoglobin H

electrophoresis on starch gel, p. 315.

2. Prepare 10% hemolysate, as described in the section on electrophoresis on cellulose acetate, p. 310.

3. Oxidize hemolysate to methemoglobin, as follows: Combine 120λ untreated hemolysate with 30λ 5% potassium ferricyanide (500 mg per 10 ml) in 1/15 M phosphate buffer, pH 6.6.

4. Apply samples of untreated and oxidized hemolysates from patient and healthy control, as described in method for hemoglobin H electrophoresis on starch gel, p. 315.

5. Apply constant current of 35 ma at 4°C overnight with origins toward anode (+).

6. Slice gel horizontally, as described in method for separation of galactose-1-phosphate uridyl transferase isozymes on p. 116. Examine.

Interpretation

Untreated hemolysate from normal persons forms a single cathodal band of hemoglobin A during electrophoresis in starch at neutral pH; untreated hemoglobin M forms a diffuse band of three zones. The methemoglobins of both form single bands, methemoglobin M migrating slower than methemoglobin A.

Reagents

1. *Sodium Phosphate Electrophoresis Buffer, 0.04 M, pH 6.8:* Dissolve 28.4 g $Na_2HPO_4 \cdot 12\ H_4O$ in 1800 ml demineralized water. Adjust to pH 6.8 with phosphoric acid and bring to volume in 200 ml volumetric flask.

2. *Sodium Phosphate Gel Buffer, pH 6.8:* Dilute 27 ml electrophoresis buffer to 200 ml with demineralized water.

3. *Starch Gel:* Dissolve 23 g Connaught starch in 200 ml gel buffer.

4. *Phosphate Buffer, 1/15 M, pH 6.6:* Combine 9.0 g $Na_2HPO_4 \cdot 12\ H_2O$ and 5.7 g KH_2PO_4 in 1000 ml demineralized water.

REFERENCES

Gerald, P. S.: The electrophoretic and spectroscopic characterization of Hgb M. *Blood, 13*:936, 1958.

Huehns, Ernst, R.: Haemoglobins. In Smith, Ivor (Ed.): *Chromatographic and Electrophoretic Techniques. Volume II Zone Electrophoresis,* 2nd ed. New York, Interscience, 1968, pp. 291-324.

ELECTROPHORESIS OF HEMOGLOBIN H ON STARCH GEL

Principle

Hemoglobin H (β_4^A) and its fetal counterpart, hemoglobin Bart's (γ_4^F), migrate anodally during electrophoresis on starch gel at pH 8.6.

Procedure

1. On the day of use, prepare gel early, as follows: Add gradually 200 ml freshly prepared gel buffer to 23 g Connaught starch in a 500 ml suction flask, apply low heat, and stir at slow speed. When boiling begins, i.e. bubbles of approximately 2 to 3 mm diameter form at the flask bottom, remove immediately from heat and boil under vacuum for exactly one minute. (Protect face with shield; insert flask in 2000 ml Nalgene beaker during evacuation.)

2. Fill electrophoresis tray (glass plate framed with plexiglass) with starch solution and cool for one hour at room temperature.

3. Cover tray with plastic film and store at 5 to 10°C until used (within 12 hours).

4. Remove gel tray from storage; add 1-liter portions of buffer to both compartments of electrophoresis chamber at 4°C; attach leads to power supply; insert 5 1/2 × 5-inch wicks (Whatman #3MM) in buffer compartments.

5. Insert 8 × 4-mm sections of 3 MM paper saturated with sample or control hemoglobin solutions in a series of 8 mm-wide slots, made in gel with tip of spatula, about 1 1/2-inch

from cathode.
6. Place gel tray across buffer compartments at 4°C, with application slots near cathode.
7. Connect wicks to gel and apply a potential of 250 V. One-half hour later blot gel at application points, cover with plastic film, and continue electrophoresis overnight at 4°C.

Interpretation

Except for hemoglobin I, hemoglobin H migrates anodally at pH 8.6 to a greater degree than other hemoglobins (Figure 12). It separates anodally from hemoglobin I during electrophoresis at pH 6.5.

Reagents

1. *TRIS-EDTA-Borate Stock Buffer:* Dissolve 109 g TRIS, 5.84 g ethylenediaminetetraacetic acid and 30.9 g boric acid in 800 ml demineralized water. Adjust to pH 8.6 and bring to volume in 1000 ml volumetric flask.
2. *Gel Buffer:* Dilute 10 ml of stock buffer to volume in a 200 ml volumetric flask with demineralized water.
3. *Electrophoresis Buffer:* Dilute 286 ml stock buffer to volume in a 2000 ml volumetric flask with demineralized water.

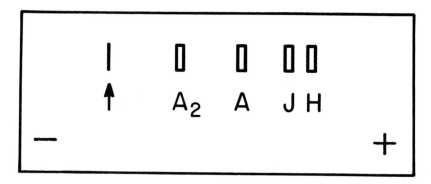

Figure 12. Electrophoretic mobility of hemoglobin H on starch gel at pH 8.6.

4. Hemolysates: As prepared in the method for unstable hemoglobin screening by precipitation, on p. 322.

REFERENCES

Huehns, E. R., and Shooter, E. M.: Human hemoglobins. *J Med Genet, 2*:48, 1965.
Porter, I. H., Boyer, S. H., Watson-Williams, E. J., et al.: Variation of glucose-6-phosphate dehydrogenase in different populations. *Lancet, 1*:895, 1964.

OTHER TESTS FOR HEMOGLOBIN S

ORTHO DIAGNOSTICS SICKLEDEX® TUBE TEST

Principle

The insolubility of reduced hemoglobin S in Sickledex test solution is the basis of the test. Turbidity produced by hemoglobin S and other sickling hemoglobins is easily distinguishable from clear solutions of the soluble hemoglobins. The test is a quick, easy, proprietary method for screening for sickle cell anemia and the carrier state.

Procedure

1. Add 0.02 ml sample of whole blood to 2.0 ml Sickledex test solution in a 12 × 75-mm tube, equilibrated to room temperature. Repeat with a control sample (hemoglobin A).
2. Mix by inversion and let stand at least five minutes.
3. Observe turbidity or transparency in tubes by holding against ruled lines or printed copy.

Interpretation

Solutions of hemoglobin A and other soluble hemoglobins remain transparent (ruled lines or printed copy are visible through solution). Hemoglobin SS, AS, and other sickling hemoglobins form turbid suspensions (ruled lines or copy are not visible through suspension).

Reagents

1. *Sickledex Test Solution (Ortho Kit):* Reconstitute vial of Sickledex reagent powder by adding to bottle of Sickledex diluent buffer, equilibrated to room temperature. Shake vigorously. The test solution is stable for one month at 4°C.

FERROHEMOGLOBIN SOLUBILITY

Principle

Hemoglobin S can easily be distinguished from hemoglobin D, a hemoglobin with similar electrophoretic mobility on cellulose acetate at alkaline pH, by its lower solubility in phosphate solutions. Reduced hemoglobin S precipitates while hemoglobin D remains soluble in concentrated phosphate solutions. The percent solubility is calculated from relative optical densities of reduced hemoglobin in phosphate and water solutions and is characteristic of the hemoglobin (Itano's test).

Procedure

1. Prepare test and normal (A) hemolysates, as described in method for screening for unstable hemoglobins by precipitation, on p. 322. Add 0.20 ml aliquots to 1.8 ml phosphate buffer, 2.48 M, containing 20 mg sodium hydrosulfite, $Na_2S_2O_4$. Mix well, let stand fifteen minutes, and filter through Whatman #5 filter paper.
2. Dilute 0.1 ml aliquots of filtrates with 3.9 ml buffer containing 20 mg sodium hydrosulfite, $Na_2S_2O_4$, and measure optical density at 422 mμ against reagent blank (3.9 ml buffer containing 20 mg sodium hydrosulfite).
3. Dilute 0.020 ml aliquots of test and normal (A) hemolysates in 8.0 ml demineralized water, and measure $O.D._{422}$ against water blank.

Calculations

Compare solubilities in phosphate and water as:

$$\frac{O.D._{.p} \times 100}{O.D._{.w}}$$

and express as percent solubility.

Interpretation

Hemoglobin SS is only slightly soluble in phosphate (6 to 23%), while hemoglobins A, AD, and DD are from 88 to 102% soluble. Hemoglobins from persons heterozygous for the sickle gene, i.e. hemoglobins AS, SC, and SD, are of intermediate solubility (from 35 to 44 or 68%).

Reagents

1. *Phosphate Buffer, 2.48 M:* Dissolve 43.4 g K_2HPO_4 (anhydrous) and 33.8 g KH_2PO_4 (anhydrous) in 180 ml CO_2-free distilled water (boiled). Bring to volume in 200 ml volmetric flask with CO_2-free water.

REFERENCES

Goldberg, C. A. J.: Hemoglobins. In Seligson, David (Ed.): *Standard Methods of Clinical Chemistry.* New York Academic Press, 1961, vol. III, pp. 138-149.

Jonxis, Jean H. P., and Huisman, Titus, H. J. (Eds.): *A Laboratory Manual on Abnormal Hemoglobins,* 2nd ed. Oxford, Blackwell, 1968, p. 37.

SOLUBILITY SPOT TEST

Principle

The spot-plate method is based on the greater solubility of hemoglobin S in phosphate-urea solution than in phosphate alone. The test is sufficiently sensitive to distinguish hemoglobins AS and SC from SS in samples of dried blood on filter paper.

Procedure

1. Punch pairs of filter paper discs (1/4-inch) from PKU cards saturated with sample blood and hemoglobin standards (A-A, A-S, S-S, A-C) and dried for at least one hour. Place in adjacent cups of a clean plastic Linbro Disposo tray.
2. Add 0.2 ml Sickledex reagent to the first members of the pairs and 0.2 ml Sickledex reagent with 3 M urea to the other discs of the pairs, stir with plugged capillary tubes, and leave at room temperature for one hour.
3. Stir again, remove discs, and observe color of solutions in cups against a white background.

Interpretation

The pair of solutions from each hemoglobin type is colored, as follows:

Hemoglobin Type	Sickledex	Sickledex + Urea
A-A	Orange or pink	Red
A-S	Yellow	Orange or red
S-S	Colorless	Yellow
S-C	Yellow	Orange or red
A-C	Orange or pink	Red

(See Color Illustration 14.)

Reagents

1. *Ortho Diagnostics Sickledex Reagent:* Reconstitute according to Ortho directions.
2. *Sickledex Reagent with 3 M Urea:* Add 1.8 g urea to 10 ml reconstituted Sickledex reagent and stir to dissolve. The reconstituted Sickledex solutions are stable three weeks at 4°C.

REFERENCE

Kelly, S., and Desjardins, L.: Spot test for detection of sickling hemoglobin.

Clin Chem, 18:934, 1972.

INDUCTION OF SICKLING IN VITRO

Principle

Hemoglobin S's property of relative insolubility under anoxic conditions is taken advantage of in the *in vitro* sickling test. Hemoglobin AS becomes less soluble when the red cell's oxygen potential is reduced chemically, precipitating and distorting cell structure into sickle forms.

Procedure

1. Mix single drops of heparinized blood and bisulfite reagent on a glass slide with a wooden applicator, cover, and seal coverslip with air-tight lubricant.
2. Examine for sickling with four hundred-fold magnification immediately and hourly for three hours.

Interpretation

Cells containing hemoglobin S may be sickle-shaped upon initial observation. Cells containing hemoglobin AS will sickle within a few hours.

Reagents

1. *Bisulfite Reagent, 2%:* On the day of test, dissolve 0.5 g sodium metabisulfite ($Na_2S_2O_5$) in 25 ml demineralized water.

REFERENCE

Wintrobe, Maxwell M. (Ed.): *Clinical Hematology,* 7th ed. Philadelphia, Lea and Febiger, 1974, p. 838.

UNSTABLE HEMOGLOBINS

SCREENING BY PRECIPITATION FROM NONPOLAR SOLUTION

Principle

One method of detecting unstable hemoglobins is by denaturing the protein with nonpolar solvents. As the solution's polarity decreases, the molecule's bonding weakens; hemoglobin becomes less soluble and begins to precipitate. Normal hemoglobin remains soluble in 17% isopropanol for a longer period than the unstable hemoglobins.

Procedure

1. Prepare hemolysates of test and control samples of whole blood, as follows:
   Centrifuge samples at 2000 R.P.M. ten to fifteen minutes, discard plasma and wash red cells three times with 0.85% NaCl (2 volumes). Add 1.2 volume of water and 0.4 volume toluene to the packed red blood cells after the last wash. Shake vigorously for five minutes, centrifuge at 2000 R.P.M. for twenty minutes, remove clear red layer with a syringe, and filter through coarse, fluted filter paper. Store at 4°C if not used immediately.
2. Equilibrate 2 ml aliquots of 17% isopropanol/buffer solution in 10 × 75-mm cork-stoppered tubes in a shaking water bath at 37°C for five minutes. Stopper tubes to prevent evaporation.
3. Add 0.2 ml freshly prepared hemolysates to equilibrated tubes.
4. Restopper tubes, mix by inversion, incubate in 37°C water bath, and examine for cloudiness and/or precipitate after five, ten, twenty, and forty minutes of incubation.

Interpretation

Seventeen percent isopropanol/buffer solutions of normal hemoglobin remain clear when incubated at 37°C for up to forty minutes. Solutions of unstable hemoglobins become cloudy in about five minutes and form flocculent precipitates within twenty minutes.

Reagents

1. *Seventeen percent isopropanol/buffer solution:* Mix 17 ml isopropanol and 83 ml 0.1 ml TRIS · HCl, pH 7.4 buffer (1.58 g TRIS-HCl/100 ml demineralized water).

REFERENCE

Carrell, R., and Kay, R.: A simple method for the detection of unstable hemoglobins. *Br J Haematol, 23*:615, 1972.

RED CELL INCLUSION BODIES

Principle

Intracellular precipitates of labile hemoglobin (Heintz bodies) form in the red cells or erythroid precursors of patients with unstable hemoglobin disease or the homozygous thalassemias. They are spontaneously present (preformed) in the blood of splenectomized patients (in whom the filtering action of the spleen has been eliminated), but must be induced by incubation or redox dyes in blood from patients with intact spleens.

Procedure

1. Mix equal amounts of whole (EDTA) blood sample and brilliant cresyl-blue stain. Repeat with control sample. Make thin film on glass slides, let dry, and examine.
2. Incubate blood-and-stain mixture at 37°C for one hour; make films, dry, and examine.
3. Incubate mixture overnight at 37°C, make films, dry, and examine.

Interpretation

Brilliant cresyl-blue-stained red cells, containing unstable hemoglobin, e.g. hemoglobin H (hemoglobin Seattle) form green-blue, reticular-filamentous inclusions of reticulocytes. The preformed inclusions of splenectomized patients are larger than the induced inclusions. Hemoglobin H inclusions also form in occasional cells of patients heterozygous for α-thalassemia-1.

Reagents

1. *Brilliant Cresyl-Blue Stain:* Dissolve 1.3 gm sodium oxalate and 1.0 gm brilliant cresyl-blue in 100 ml demineralized water. Let stand a few days at room temperature. Filter and store in dark bottle at 4°C.

REFERENCES

Folayan Esan, G. J.: Hgb Bart's in newborn Nigerians, *British J Hematology,* 22:73, 1972.

Jonxis, Jean H. D. and Huisman, Titus H. J. (Ed.): *A Laboratory Manual on Abnormal Hemoglobins,* 2nd ed. Oxford, Blackwell, 1968, p. 116.

Wintrobe, Maxwell, M. (Ed.): *Clinical Hematology,* 7th ed. Philadelphia, Lea and Febiger, 1974, pp. 879-880.

FETAL HEMOGLOBIN

PERIPHERAL BLOOD FILMS

Principle

Hemoglobin F is not eluted by acid from ethanol-fixed red cells in peripheral blood films and can be stained by hematoxylin-erythrosin B.

Procedure

1. Fix thin films of peripheral blood on glass slides in 80% ethanol in a coplin jar for five minutes. Slides may be stored at 5 to 10°C for at least one week before fixing.
2. Rinse thoroughly with demineralized water (until water runs

off the slide freely).

3. Incubate slides for five minutes in prewarmed buffer containing 26.6 ml of 0.2 M disodium phosphate solution and 73.4 ml of 0.1 M citric acid solution, adjusted to pH 3.2, in a 37°C water bath. Agitate slides occasionally.

4. Rinse slides in demineralized water in coplin jars. Air-dry *thoroughly* (an hour or longer) to avoid artifacts when stained.

5. Stain in coplin jar with hematoxylin for three minutes.

6. Rinse thoroughly with demineralized water, three to each coplin jar, and stain with 0.1% erythrosin B for four minutes.

7. Rinse slides with demineralized water, three to each coplin jar, air-dry, and mount in 50% glycerol.

8. Count number of stained cells per 100 red cells at 400X magnification.

Interpretation

At birth, from 90 to 100% of red cells contain fetal hemoglobin, by six months of age only 5% of cells, and at a year, less than 1%. The relative proportions of hemoglobins A and F in individual cells determine the depth of color.

Reagents

1. *Citric Acid Solution, 0.1 M:* Dissolve 2.1 g of citric acid ($C_6H_8O_7 \cdot H_2O$) in demineralized water and dilute to volume in a 100 ml volumetric flask. Store at 5 to 10°C.

2. *Disodium Phosphate Solution, 0.2M:* Dissolve 2.8 g of anhydrous disodium phosphate (Na_2HPO_4) in demineralized water and dilute to volume in a 100 ml volumetric flask. Store at 5 to 10°C.

3. *Hematoxylin Stain:* Dissolve 5.0 g hematoxylin crystals in 50 ml absolute ethanol, and combine with a prewarmed liter of 10% aluminum ammonium sulfate (alum). Stir and bring to a rapid boil. Remove immediately from heat and gradually add 2.5 g mercuric oxide (red). Reheat at a simmer until solution becomes dark purple, remove from heat immediately, and cool flask in cold water. Add 2 to 4 ml glacial acetic acid and store

at room temperature.
4. *Erythrosin B, 0.1%:* Dissolve 0.1 g erythrosin B in 100 ml demineralized water.
5. *Hemoglobin F Standard:* Prepare thin films of umbilical cord blood and store at room temperature.
6. *Hemoglobin A Standard:* Prepare thin films of peripheral blood from healthy adults and store at room temperature.

REFERENCES

Shepard, M. K., Weatherall, D. J., and Conley, C. L.: Semi-quantative estimation of the distribution of fetal hemoglobin in red cell populations. *Bull Johns Hopkins Hosp, 110-111:*293, 1962.

Wadsworth, Augustus B.: Histologic Procedure. In *Standard Methods of the Division of Laboratories and Research of the New York State Department of Health,* 3rd ed. Baltimore, Williams and Wilkins Company, 1947, p. 548.

CHARACTERIZATION OF HEMOGLOBIN VARIANT

VERTICAL ACRYLAMIDE GEL SEPARATION OF HEMOGLOBINS

Principle

The E. C. Apparatus Corporation vertical gel electrophoresis system enables one to separate the hemoglobins in approximately 1 ml blood and recover individual types in from 10 to 20 mg amounts.

Procedure

1. Melt 5 ml aliquot of 1% Oxo ionagar in boiling water bath.
2. Coat contact plates of electrophoresis chamber with 10% Eastman Kodak Photo-Flo,® using a small brush, and let dry approximately ten minutes.
3. Assemble electrophoresis chamber, inserting yellow sponge in bottom and attaching tubes for water flow. Let cooling water flow five to ten minutes.
4. Rest chamber on its side on two test tube racks, pour ionagar

over the rubber seal, and let dry five minutes. Repeat on other side of chamber.

5. Prepare separating gel and set aside 75 ml.
6. Turn chamber so that gel slot is parallel to counter and slightly canted (<45°). Add 0.17 ml freshly dissolved catalyst ammonium persulfate (AP), to remaining 25 ml separating gel, and quickly pour down canted gel slot. Let polymerize twenty to thirty minutes in the dark (cover with black cloth). Aspirate and discard unpolymerized gel with Pasteur pipette.
7. Add 0.51 ml catalyst (AP) to the 75 ml separating gel and quickly pour down canted gel slot to within 3.5 to 4.0 cm of the top.
8. Slowly return chamber to vertical position and gently overlay top of gel with 5 ml demineralized water. Let polymerize twenty to thirty minutes in the dark (cover with a black cloth). Store gel at this point for use next day, if necessary.
9. Aspirate and discard water and unpolymerized gel with a Pasteur pipette.
10. Prepare stacking gel.
11. Rinse gel slot with 5 ml stacking gel, remove it immediately, and add 8-10 ml stacking gel. Overlay with 5 ml demineralized water.
12. Polymerize in the light by exposing to a light source four inches from the face of the chamber for about ten minutes.
13. Aspirate and discard water layer and add a 3 mm layer of sucrose (5 g/10 ml TEB).
14. Add 800 ml buffer to lower compartment, insert overflow tube, and fill top compartment with buffer to just below gel slot.
15. Connect power supply (connect positive electrode to lower chamber).
16. Overlay sucrose in gel slot with 0.8 to 0.9 ml hemolysate.
17. *Carefully* add buffer to gel slot until slot is filled.
18. Fill buffer compartment *slowly,* until upper compartment and gel slot are in contact.
19. Apply a potential difference of 100 V; a few minutes later add remaining buffer to upper compartment.
20. When the hemoglobins are in the stacking gel (ten to fifteen

minutes), increase voltage to 250 V (110 to 130 ma), and continue electrophoresis at room temperature until the variant band is separated (four to five hours).

21. Cut out variant band, elute from gel with multiple portions of demineralized water, and concentrate to approximately 5 g/100 ml by vacuum dialysis.

Interpretation

The variant band is identified according to its mobility established in previous electrophoretic assays.

Reagents

1. *Photo-Flo 200, 10%:* Dilute 10 ml Eastman Kodak Photo-Flo 200 solution with 90 ml demineralized water.

2. *Ionagar, 1%:* Suspend 1 g Oxo ionagar No. 2 in 100 ml demineralized water and dissolve by heating in a boiling water bath. Dispense in 5 ml aliquots in 10 ml screw-cap tubes. Autoclave and store at 4°C.

3. *Stock Solution A for Separating Gel:* Combine 10 ml conc HCl and 100 ml demineralized water in a 250 ml volumetric flask; add 90.8 g Sigma Trizma base and 0.58 ml N, N, N', N' tetramethylethylenediamine (TMED). Dilute to volume with demineralized water. Adjust to pH 8.8 to 9.0. Filter under vacuum and store in a brown bottle.

4. *Stock Solution C for Separating Gel:* Combine in a 250 ml volumetric flask 70.0 g acrylamide and 1.837 g N, N' methylene-bis-acrylamide (bis). Dilute to volume with demineralized water. Filter under vacuum and store in a brown bottle.

5. *Catalyst (AP) 2: Just before use,* dissolve 0.4 g ammonium persulfate in 2.0 ml demineralized water.

6. *Separating Gel: Just before use,* combine 25 ml solution A, 25 ml solution C, and 50 ml demineralized water.

7. *Stock Solution B for Stacking Gel:* Combine 14.9 g Sigma Trizma base, 100 ml demineralized water, 10 ml conc HCl, and 1.15 ml TMED in a 250 ml volumetric flask. Dilute to

volume with demineralized water. Adjust to pH 6.6 to 6.8.

8. *Stock Solution D for Stacking Gel:* Combine 25 g acrylamide and 6.25 g bis acrylamide in a 250 ml volumetric flask. Dilute to volume with demineralized water.

9. *Stock Solution E for Stacking Gel:* Dissolve 4.0 mg riboflavin in demineralized water. Bring to volume in a 100 ml volumetric flask.

10. *Stock Solution F for Stacking Gel:* Dissolve 40 g sucrose in demineralized water. Bring to volume in a 100 ml volumetric flask.

11. *Stacking Gel:* Combine 2.5 ml aliquots of solutions B and E, 5.0 ml Solution D, and 10 ml solution F.

12. *Stock Electrophoresis Buffer (TEB 10x):* Dissolve 186.0 g Sigma Trizma base, 24.0 g sodium EDTA, and 14.4 g boric acid in 2 liters of demineralized water.

13. *Working Electrophoresis Buffer:* Dilute 100 ml stock electrophoresis buffer to 1000 ml with demineralized water.

REFERENCES

Technical Bulletin No. 130. Procedure for electrophoretic analysis of hemoglobins. E. C. Apparatus Corp., Philadelphia, 1964.

Heideman, M. L. J.: Disc electrophoresis of I[131]-labelled protein hormone preparations and their reaction products with antibodies. *Ann NY Acad Sci, 121*:501, 1964.

IDENTIFICATION OF VARIANT CHAIN BY HYBRIDIZATION

Principle

Human and canine hemoglobins are dissociated in acid conditions and allowed to recombine, forming two hybrid species. One hybrid hemoglobin contains canine hemoglobin β-chain and human hemoglobin α-chain; the other contains canine hemoglobin α-chain and human hemoglobin β-chain. Since the recombination is incomplete, some human and canine hemoglobins remain. The mutation in a variant hemoglobin can be localized to the affected chain by comparing the electrophoretic pattern of its canine hybrids with the canine hybrids of normal hemoglobin (A).

Procedure

1. Prepare solutions of variant, canine, and normal human (A) hemoglobins, as follows: Isolate the three hemoglobins from appropriate sources by acrylamide gel electrophoresis, as described on p. 326. Vacuum dialyze to volumes containing hemoglobin concentrations of from 5 to 10 g/100 ml. (Measure hemoglobin concentration, as described on p. 122.) Reconstitute to give approximately 1 ml of solution containing hemoglobin in concentration of 3 g/100 ml (3%).
2. Combine in respective tubes, in duplicate, the diluted and variant hemoglobin solutions with equal volumes (0.1 ml) of diluted canine hemoglobin solution. Add 0.2 ml aliquots of acetate buffer, pH 4.7, or demineralized water to the duplicates, respectively. Adjust buffer-containing tubes to pH 4.7.
3. Incubate tubes in an ice water bath for four hours, transfer contents to 6-inch lengths of presoaked dialysis tubing, 1/4-inch diameter.
4. Dialyze overnight at 4°C against separate liter volumes of soidum phosphate buffer, pH 6.8.
5. Dialyze solutions again for approximately eight hours against fresh liters of phosphate buffer.
6. Apply to cellulose acetate membranes and apply a potential difference of 400 volts for forty minutes in Beckman Microzone electrophoresis chamber with TEB buffer, pH 9.0.

Interpretation

The electrophoretic positions of the two hybrids of canine-variant hemoglobin are compared to those of canine-normal (A) hemoglobin (Figure 13). If the mutation is in the β chain, there will be no canine-variant hybrid corresponding to the canine-normal hybrid which contains β chains of normal hemoglobin (A). In its place will be a canine-variant hybrid which migrates differently from either canine-normal hybrid. Conversely, if the

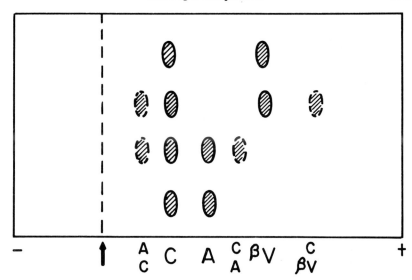

Figure 13. Electrophoretic patterns formed during hybridizations of A and canine hemoglobins (channels 1-4), and β-chain variant and canine hemoglobins (channels 5 and 6).

mutation is in the α chain, there will be no canine-variant hybrid corresponding to the canine-normal hybrid which contains α chains of normal hemoglobin (A), and the hybrid containing the mutant chain will migrate differently from either of the canine-normal hybrids.

Reagents

1. *Acetate Buffer, I=0.1, pH 4.7:* Dissolve 1.23 g Na acetate in 80 ml demineralized water. Adjust to pH 4.7 with glacial acetic acid ($\approx$0.5 ml) and bring to volume in 100 ml volumetric flask with demineralized water.

2. *Sodium Phosphate Buffer, I=0.02, pH 6.8:* Dissolve 6.48 g Na_2HPO_4 and 15.79 g NaH_2PO_4 in 7500 ml demineralized water. Adjust to pH 6.8 and bring volume to 8000 ml in a 9-liter bottle.

3. *TEB Electrophoresis Buffer, 0.13 M, pH 9.0:* Combine and dissolve 32.2 g Trizma base, 3.12 g EDTA, and 1.84 g boric

acid in 2 liters of demineralized water. Adjust to pH 9.0 with 1 N HCl or 1 N NaOH, if necessary.

REFERENCE

Gammack, D. B., Huehns, E. R., and Shooter, E. M.: Identification of the abnormal polypeptide chain of haemoglobin G_{Ib}. *J Mol Biol, 2*:372, 1960.

IDENTIFICATION OF VARIANT CHAIN BY CHAIN ELECTROPHORESIS

Principle

The mutation site in a variant hemoglobin can be localized to the α and β chain locus by comparing the electrophoretic mobility of chains cleaved by p-hydroxymercurybenzoate (HMB) with similarily-cleaved chains of normal human hemoglobin (A).

Procedure

1. Prepare hemolysates of variant and normal human hemoglobin (A); as described on p. 322.
2. Prepare starch gel plate, as described for galactose-1-phosphate uridyl transferase isozymes, on p. 116.
3. Saturate 8×5-mm pieces of Whatman #3 MM filter paper with hemolysates, apply at cathode end of starch gel, and apply a potential difference of 250 volts overnight at 4°C.
4. Prepare a second starch gel plate late in the afternoon on the day before use and store at 4°C.
5. Cut out appropriate band of hemoglobin from first starch gel plate and insert a portion (about one-third) in slot made in second starch gel plate.
6. Soak 8×5-mm piece of Whatman #3 MM filter paper in HMB solution, and insert in slot with, but ahead of, hemoglobin gel segment, so that the variant hemoglobin solution passes through it during migration toward the anode. Apply a potential difference of 225 V (6.5V/cm) for four hours with borate buffer.

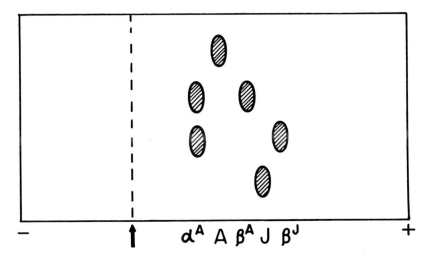

Figure 14. Photograph of electrophoretic separation of α- and β-chains of hemoglobins A and the β-chain variant, J β Baltimore.

Interpretation

The chain containing the mutation has a different electrophoretic mobility from the corresponding α or β chain of normal human hemoglobin (A) (Figure 14).

Reagents

1. *Stock TEB Buffer:* Combine the following: 109 g TRIS base, 5.84 g EDTA and 30.9 g boric acid in 800 ml demineralized water. Adjust to pH 8.6 and bring to volume in a liter volumetric flask; store at 4° C.
2. *TEB Gel Buffer for Hemoglobin Electrophoresis:* Dilute 10 ml stock TEB buffer to 200 ml in a volumetric flask.
3. *TEB Electrophoresis Buffer for Hemoglobin Electrophoresis:* Dilute 286 ml stock TEB buffer to volume in a 2-liter volumetric flask.
4. *TEB Gel Buffer for Chain Electrophoresis:* Dilute 10 ml stock TEB buffer to 250 ml and adjust to pH 8.1.
5. *TEB Electrophoresis Buffer for Chain Electrophoresis:* Dis-

solve 43.2 g boric acid in 1800 ml demineralized water, adjust to pH 9.0, and bring to volume in a 2-liter volumetric flask.

6. *Starch Gels:* Prepare plates from 23.0 g Connaught starch in 200 ml gel buffer, as described in method for galactose-1-phosphate uridyl transferase isozymes, p. 116.

7. *Hemolysates:* Prepare 10% hemolysates as described in method for unstable hemoglobins by precipitation, p. 322.

8. *Sodium p-hydroxymercurybenzoate, 0.5 M:* Dissolve 360 mg HMB in 1 ml 0.1 N NaOH (4 g/1).

REFERENCE

Schwantes, A. R., and Schwantes, M. L. B.: An improved technique for rapid identification of hemoglobin chains by starch gel electrophoresis. *Experientia, 26*(8):928, 1970.

IDENTIFICATION OF VARIANT HEMOGLOBIN BY PEPTIDE MAPPING

Principle

The variant hemoglobin is identified by comparing a map of its peptides with a peptide map or fingerprint of normal hemoglobin (A). The map is derived by procedures which split the molecule into peptide fragments of predictable number and composition, each of which has a characteristic electrophoretic and chromatographic mobility on paper.

The proteolytic enzyme, trypsin, is used for catalyzing hydrolysis, as it cleaves the molecule at predictable intervals – at lysine and arginine linkages only. The fragments are separated by high voltage electrophoresis in one direction and paper chromatography in the other. They appear as spots in characteristic positions when stained with ninhydrin. Specific stains reveal their amino acid composition, in some instances, while elution and amino acid analysis of spots are required for the identification of other peptides.

The mutation is usually apparent by the displacement of a normal peptide, i.e. absence of an expected peptide and appearance of a new peptide.

Procedure

1. Dialyze a 5% solution of purified hemoglobin (2 ml or more) for three days against liter volumes of cold demineralized water containing 1.0 ml of 1.0 M phosphate, pH 7.2, changed once daily. Use dialysis tubing long enough to allow for doubling of the initial volume. Centrifuge dialyzed hemoglobin (now 2 1/2% solution) at 4°C.
2. Adjust an 8 ml aliquot in a Pyrex test tube to pH 8.0 with 1 N NaOH and denature by heating at 90°C (water bath) for four minutes. Cool tube immediately. It should contain a fine brown suspension.
3. Flush suspension in a small plastic beaker with nitrogen gas. Add 0.1 ml trypsin solution per 80 mg hemoglobin and digest ninety minutes at 37°C, continuing the nitrogen flush throughout. Monitor pH, adjusting to between 7.95 and 8.00 with 0.5 N NaOH in 0.001 ml amounts.
4. Adjust to pH 6.5 with 1.0 N HCl. Centrifuge at 5000 R.P.M. and distribute digest (supernatant fluid) as 0.3 ml aliquots in small cork-stoppered tubes. Store at −20°C.
5. Thaw 0.3 ml aliquots of control and variant hemoglobin digests, evaporate to dryness on a spot plate under vacuum, and reconstitute with 0.015 ml demineralized water.
6. Prepare electrophoresis tank.
7. Dip 27 × 60-cm sheet of Whatman #3 MM sheet in electrophoresis solvent, blot, and place in chamber.
8. Spot 0.010 ml concentrated digest at anodal (+) end of sheet. If using Savant chamber, spot 1 1/2 inches from lower edge and 6 inches from anode end. Spot a similar amount of digest from control hemoglobin (A) on separate sheet.
9. Close chamber and apply 2500 V for thirty minutes, followed by 2000 volts for forty minutes.
10. Turn off power, remove sheets from chamber, and air-dry at room temperature in vented oven (no heat) or hood for three to four hours.
11. Bring anodal and cathodal edges of sheets together to form circular drum. Staple.
12. Place drums in chromatography tank saturated with chroma-

tography buffer and develop by ascending chromatography overnight (eighteen hours).

13. Dry sheets in hood about three hours and dry in vented oven at 70°C for approximately thirty minutes.

14. Stain sheets by dipping in ninhydrin solution. Heat at 70°C in vented oven for approximately twenty minutes.

15. Mark ninhydrin-positive spots and overstain with specific amino acid stains for identification of specific peptides, as described in the following steps. Three peptide maps are needed to stain for arginine, tryptophane, histidine, tyrosine, and methionine. Two should be stained with ninhydrin, as described, and the peptides circled in pencil. The third sheet should be unstained.

16. For arginine stain, dip ninhydrin-stained peptide map into Sakaguchi reagent solution A. Dry thoroughly. Dip into Sakaguchi reagent solution B. Arginine-containing peptides are orange spots which fade quickly. Observe and mark immediately.

17. Bleach ninhydrin-stained paper by dipping into 10% HCl in acetone. Air dry.

18. For methionine stain, dip bleached paper into methionine reagent. Methionine-containing peptides appear as white or pale yellow spots on greyish-purple background.

19. For tyrosine stain, dip dry methionine-stained paper into tyrosine solution A. Drain, and rapidly dip into tyrosine solution B. Drain quickly and heat in vented oven at 70°C. Tyrosine-containing peptides appear as red spots against a green background. Tryptophane-containing peptides form faint grey spots.

20. For histidine stain, use map not stained with ninhydrin. Mix together 2 ml aliquots of solutions A, B, and C. Scratch side of test tube and cool at 0°C for five minutes to promote crystallization. Add 6 ml demineralized water and shake. Spray onto both sides of the paper till damp. Avoid inhaling solutions as amyl nitrite is a cardiac stimulant. Two to three minutes later, spray with 5% (w/v) Na_2CO_3 solution. Histidine-containing peptides are reddish-orange against a very pale yellow background; tyrosine-containing peptides are

yellow-orange.

21. For tryptophane stain, dip histidine-stained paper (or fresh or ninhydrin-stained paper) in Ehrlich's reagent. Tryptophane-containing peptides appear as purple spots within a few minutes.

Interpretation

The peptide maps of the control (Hgb A) and variant hemoglobin digests will differ slightly. Since the substituted amino acid in the variant peptide may affect its electric charge and solubility, and hence its electrophoretic and chromatographic mobilities, respectively, its R_f will differ from that of the analogous normal peptide. Therefore, a normal peptide will be missing from the map of the variant hemoglobin, and a new mutant peptide appears, generally in a different position. Staining for specific amino acids is helpful in locating specific peptides and defining the amino acid composition of mutant peptides.

Reagents

1. *Phosphate Buffer for Tryptic Digest, 1.0 M, pH 7.2:* Dissolve 17.9 g Na_2HPO_4 and 7.7 g $NaH_2PO_4 \cdot H_2O$ in 200 ml demineralized water. Adjust to pH 7.2, if necessary.
2. *NaOH, 1 N:* Dissolve 4 g NaOH in 100 ml demineralized water.
3. *Trypsin, 0.5%:* Dissolve 50 mg trypsin in 10 ml 0.001 N HCl (0.1 ml 1 N HCl in 100 ml water).
4. *NaOH, 0.5 N:* Dissolve 4 g NaOH in 200 ml demineralized water.
5. *HCl, 1.0 N:* Dilute 8.6 ml concentrated HCl to 100 ml volume with demineralized water.
6. *Electrophoresis Buffer:* Combine pyridine:acetic acid:demineralized water in proportion of 10:0.4:90. Adjust to pH 6.4.
7. *Chromatography Buffer:* Combine isoamyl alcohol:pyridine:demineralized water in proportion of 35:35:27.
8. *Ninhydrin, 0.2%:* Dissolve 400 mg ninhydrin in 200 ml ace-

tone.

9. *Sakaguchi Reagent Solution A:* Dissolve 0.5 g 8-hydroxy-quinoline in 500 ml acetone. Store at 4°C indefinitely.

10. *Sakaguchi Reagent Solution B: Just before use,* combine 0.3% solution Br_2 (v/v) in 0.5 N NaOH (2 g/100 ml).

11. *Methionine Reagent:* Combine 207.5 mg KI, 12.0 ml demineralized water, 19.4 mg K_2 Pt Cl_6, and 0.4 ml concentrated HCl in a 25 ml graduated cylinder. Bring to volume with demineralized water (23:23 ml). Rinse into reagent bottle with 380 ml acetone. Solution is stable in dark for several weeks at 4°C.

12. *Tyrosine Reagent Solution A:* Dissolve 0.5 g α-nitroso-β-naphthol in ethanol, 95%. Stable at 4°C in the dark.

13. *Tyrosine Reagent Solution B: Just before use* mix 5 ml concentrated nitric acid with 45 ml acetone.

14. *Histidine Solution A:* Dissolve 1 g sodium salt of sulphanilic acid in 100 ml 50% ethanol. Stable at 4°C.

15. *Histidine Solution B:* Combine 10 ml concentrated HCl with 90 ml absolute ethanol.

16. *Histidine Solution C:* Combine 10 ml anyl nitrite with 90 ml absolute ethanol.

17. *Tryptophane Reagent: Just before use,* dissolve 0.5 g p-dimethylaminobenzaldehyde in 5 ml concentrated HCl and 45 ml acetone.

REFERENCES

Lehmann, Hermann, and Huntsman, Richard G.: *Man's Haemoglobins.* Lippincott, Philadelphia, 1966, pp. 303-306.

Ingram, V. M.: Abnormal human haemoglobins: I. The comparison of normal human and sickle-cell haemoglobins by "fingerprinting." *Biochim Biophys Acta, 28:*539, 1958.

Baglioni, C.: An improved method for the fingerprinting of human hemoglobin. *Biochim Biophys Acta, 48:*392, 1961.

Huehns, Ernst R.: Hemoglobins. In Smith, Ivor (Ed.): *Chromatographic and Electrophoretic Techniques, Volume II Zone Electrophoresis,* 2nd ed. New York, Interscience, 1968, pp. 291-324.

INDEX

A

Abetalipoproteinemia, 278, 281-282
Acetoacetic acid, 39
N-Acetyl-α-D-glucosaminidase, 132, 133, 150-152
Acid-albumin turbidity test, 135-136
Acid esterase (lipase), 178-182
Acid phosphatase deficiency disease, 287-289
Alanine, 18
Albinism, 35, 81-83
α-Lipoproteins, 282
Alkaptonuria, 33, 39, 86-91
Alpha-1-antitrypsin, 269-270
Amino acids, 14-34
  general, 14-34
  specific, 15, 18-27
    bacterial-inhibition assays, 14, 28-32, *see also name of amino acid or disease*
    chemical assays, 14, 32, *see also name of amino acid or disease*
    chromatography, 14, 17-27, *see also name of amino acid or disease*
Aminoacidopathies, 14-35, *see also name of disease*
α & γ-Aminobutyric acid, 16
β-Aminoisobutyric acid, 19
Amniocentesis, 11, 213
Amniotic cells, 11, 12, 211-218
  fluid, 12, 210
Amylo-1,6-glucosidase, 232-236
Anthranilic acid, 83-86
Apnea, drug-induced, 266-268
Arginine, 18, 19, 52, 65, 336
Argininosuccinase, 65
Argininosuccinate lyase, 30, 35, 65
Argininosuccinicaciduria, 15, 29, 35, 65
Aspartylglycosamine, 165-166, 182-184
Aspartylglycosaminuria, 164-166, 182-184
Ataxia telangiectasia, 272, 274

B

Bacterial-inhibition assays, 28-32, *see also name of aminoacidopathy*
Bilirubin, 38
Biochemical defects, *see name of disease*
Biotin, 70
Blood samples, dried, 17
  use, *see name of disease*
"Blue-diaper syndrome," 83
Borohydride, in nitroprusside reaction, 55-56
Branched chain keto acid decarboxylases, 35
"Branching" enzyme deficiency disease (GSD IV), 236-240
"Branching" enzyme, leukocyte, 236-240
Brilliant cresyl blue stain, 323-324

C

Calcium oxalate, *see* Hyperoxaluria
Carbon-14 isotopes, use in tests
  cystathionine synthetase, 59-64
  "debrancher" enzyme, 232-236
  galactokinase, 126-130
  hypoxanthine-guanine phosphoribosyl transferase, 248-251
Carrier detection, 10, *see also name of disease*
Cell cultures
  in cystathionine synthetase assay, 57-64
  in hexosaminidase assay, 211-214
Ceruloplasmin, 261-265
C'esterase inhibitor, 275
Cetylpyridinium chloride turbidity, 136-137
Chloramine T, 33, 70, 72
Cholesterol, 278, 282
Chondroitin sulfate, 134, 136, 142, 143
Cirrhosis, childhood, 269-270
Citrate agar, in hemoglobin electro-